Practical Approaches to Patient Teaching

Practical Approaches to Patient Teaching

Edited by
Donald A. Bille, R.N., Ph.D.
Associate Professor
Department of Nursing
De Paul University, Chicago

Foreword by John C. Weaver, Ph.D.
President Emeritus, University of Wisconsin System
Distinguished Professor of Geography, University
of Southern California, Los Angeles

Little, Brown and Company, Boston

To Bertha ("Bert") Clark
colleague, mentor, and best of all, friend

Contents

Part III   Roles and Settings for Patient Teaching

Appendixes

Foreword

It is interesting, if a bit confounding, for a nonprofessional to be asked to write a foreword for a book designed for the health-care professional. It was asked that my comments be made from the standpoint of the receiver in the health-care system, the point of view of the patient.

Certainly, my present personal history has given me abundant opportunities to observe health professionals at work. Having had a myocardial infarction, subsequent heart catheterization, and bypass heart surgery, I am not exactly unacquainted with health-care teams, the health-care environment, or the Intensive Care Unit.

As a patient, I can certainly commend this volume to its readers for its perceptions and insights of many kinds. It brings together a variety of wisdom clearly based on common sense. There is much that is familiar, and certainly much with which both patient and practitioner can agree.

I observe that the word *patient* is an interesting one. It is a well-chosen word used to designate the receiver of health care, for certainly one of the most obvious needs in the realm of sickness calls for a high level of patience, both on the part of the one who treats and the one who is treated.

The book says much about the importance of education in the health-care professional's relationship to the patient. Having given my life to education, I believe most firmly in the importance of effective teaching in any setting or circumstance. The emphasis given throughout the chapters of this book to teaching is well taken and soundly defended.

Certainly, in the care of the ill, teaching must be firmly based on the three C's: compassion, concern, and continuity. One who has been a patient shudders a bit at the statement that "automated teaching devices and learning aids produce better results than conventional teaching." I tend to doubt the validity of such a concept, conscious as I am through long experience, of the real strengths that come from the establishment of warm personal relationships between learner and teacher. I fear that I could, however, at least on occasion, agree with the later comment that "the quality of patient teaching done by health-care professionals often leaves much to be desired." Whenever the rush of time and insensitivity robs the teaching process of humaneness, it is a much-to-be-regretted circumstance. The treatment and the education of a patient desperately need to be tailored to individual needs. Never should the concern be lost for dealing with patients one by one, rather than in generalized categories.

This book gives extensive reference to many people in the health-care field, ranging from the physician to the nurse, the pharmacist, and the librarian. The emphasis, however, is clearly on the nurse and the nurse's role. From a patient's perspective, this is a welcome emphasis that seems fully justified and extremely basic. As one of the authors of this book puts it: "Each time the patient and the nurse interact, the nurse is meaningfully affecting the patient's body-mind-spirit. Each time she identifies and meets a patient's needs her response affects the whole patient."

Unquestionably, the nurse-patient relationship is "a teaching-learning experience." For this reason, if for no other, the nurse, to be an effective teacher, must be given the benefit of all possible facts from all other members of the health-care team. As a teacher, the nurse must carry the encouragement of independence and bring sustaining help through individualized and well-informed action. The sense of reassuring faith that a good nurse is able to establish in the patient is an enormously fundamental achievement and of vital significance. Once the trust of this relationship has been firmly established, *continuity* becomes extremely important. The patient's morale and well-being are certainly best served when the nurse who has gained the patient's confidence can stay with the case, or at the very least, in close touch with it, throughout its duration.

In this book, recognition is given to the contributions of family members. It might be observed that while family members can be expected to give vital support to the patient, the health-care team should not neglect its obligation to aid the attending family in overcoming anxiety, in avoiding inappropriate actions, and in stabilizing morale through a full disclosure of the vital facts in the case.

Illumination is also offered on the environmental stresses affecting a hospital patient, and the need for guarding to the maximum the patient's opportunity for rest and uninterrupted sleep. Anyone who has spent days in an Intensive Care Unit is very conscious of disturbing noise, a hustle and bustle on every hand, and a bright illumination that often extends through the night. Sleep deprivation becomes a serious hindrance to recovery. Surely such sleep as an ICU patient can achieve should not be unnecessarily interrupted by thermometers or even the taking of sleeping pills!

As recognized in this volume, even critically ill patients can be taught, and it is imperative that they be permitted to know enough to participate in the decision-making that surrounds them. Nothing can be more stressful to a patient than the sense that information is being withheld.

It is so true, as Dr. Bille points out, that "the patient needs to recognize that a health problem exists before he or she will engage in learning how to solve that problem." Be it alcoholism or heart damage, the patient cannot cope with his problem unless he has within himself recognized and accepted the reality of the situation. Surely this is a concept at the elemental heart of teaching and learning.

John C. Weaver

Preface

The complexities of the health-care system, as well as the continued changes in the technology of health care, present a challenge, not only to the health-care worker, but also to the patient (client) of the health-care system. When a person enters the health-care system at any point (the physician's office, the hospital, the ambulatory care clinic, in the home through community health service), he may be subjected to life-altering changes in daily routine and body structure. Human beings have not learned to cope with disease and injury before they happen.

During the period of time that the patient is coping with disease or injury, assistance in the form of guidance and information from the health-care professional helps the patient regain and maintain control over body and environment. An uninformed patient is unable to exert any lifestyle control. Loss of control results in fear, anxiety, and emotional and intellectual paralysis. To prevent or remedy this loss of control, health-care professionals have the responsibility to the patient, as a person, to facilitate adaptation to change; facilitation in the form of patient education.

This book is designed as a text for a basic education program preparing the health-care professional, especially the nurse, for patient teaching. It is also designed as a text for continuing education and staff development for health-care professionals who are responsible for implementing patient education programs, either to meet the needs of their own patients or the broader needs of an organization (e.g., in the role of administrator, patient education coordinator, or staff development instructor). A continuing education workshop entitled, "Patient Teaching Workshop: A Multidisciplinary Approach" has provided the impetus for this text. During the workshop, health-care professionals throughout the United States asked questions and described problems that arose when they attempted to teach their patients. These questions form the basis for each chapter in the text.

The book is divided into three major parts, supplemented by appendixes, with materials collected from around the nation. Part I establishes the structural elements necessary to succeed in patient teaching activities. An historical overview of teaching-learning, adult education, and patient education is presented to give the reader a feel for the current state of the art and how it has developed. Guidelines for establishing a comprehensive patient education program are developed and illustrated. The text presents a structured approach to patient teaching. The reader should be cautioned that this means a systematic, structured *process*, not standardized or structured content. Patient teaching, to be optimally effective, must be developed for each patient on an individual basis.

As educators realize that adults learn in a different way than children, a theory of adult education is developing. This text presents a philosophy that encompasses adult education theory, as well as how this theory changes when the adult becomes a patient.

Medicolegal aspects of health care are an increasing concern of health-care professionals, especially as consumers become more aware of their rights. The patient's right to know is a legal "hot potato," an issue that is complicated by arguments concerning the health-care professional's right and responsibility to teach.

The teaching-learning process is often perceived as a complicated task, especially since many health-care professionals have never been taught how to teach. The structured approach presented in this text simplifies the teaching-learning process, rendering it more easily accomplished by any health-care practitioner, even though he or she may not have an advanced academic degree in education. The patient teacher often encounters barriers to teaching and learning; the comment "We taught them, but they didn't learn" sometimes echoes through the halls of the modern medical center.

Information is presented to help the patient teacher break down barriers to teaching-learning, including separate chapters dealing with how to approach teaching of various ethnic minorities, and how to include the patient's family in the teaching program.

Part II describes the tasks involved in carrying out patient teaching activities. Discharge planning, like patient teaching, should begin with admission to the hospital (or entry into others areas of the health-care system). Discharge planning and patient teaching share common ground, and activities in one area satisfy requirements of the other.

Evaluation of patient teaching, especially in the face of cries for cost containment, must be carried out. Evaluation may take the form of program evaluation, evaluation of the individual's learning, or performance appraisal of the teacher. Evaluation efforts interface with the institution's quality assurance program, and may also have an impact on the analysis of cost-benefit and cost-effectiveness. Patient teaching may be an expensive activity, especially in terms of staff salaries. Thus, evaluation activities may become necessary to analyze the cost of teaching an individual patient, and hard data, gained through evaluation, may be used to negotiate with a third party for reimbursment of specific fees for individual patient teaching activities.

Automation and technology are beginning to make an impact on patient teaching. Audiovisual aids to patient teaching are proliferating as manufacturers identify a market for commercially "canned" presentations. This forces each patient educator to analyze the impact of media on patient teaching efforts and outcomes in light of his or her own patient education philosophy. Computers have been available in many hospitals for a long rime. This form of technology, however, has been virtually ignored as a useful aid to patient teaching. Careful planning for patient education programs can make the various media and computers useful allies in achieving successful patient learning outcomes.

Patient teaching is the responsibility of *everyone* who "touches" the patient. Part III describes the role of some of the various health-care professionals, such as the patient education coordinator, the director of nursing service, the physician, the pharmacist, and the librarian, each of whom has a specific responsibility for patient education programs. A glance through this and other sections of the text indicates that many terms are currently being used to describe the roles of those who contribute to patient education (patient teacher, patient education specialist, nurse-educator); no attempt has been made to standardize role titles, even though the different names often designate more or less the same role. Part III also describes how patient education theory may differ in the areas of critical care, pediatrics, and psychiatric-mental health.

It was impossible to include a chapter specifically dealing with every component or professional in the health-care system. Most obviously absent are theories about patient teaching in a community health setting. Specific chapters for the dietitian, physical therapist, and social worker, are also absent. It must be realized, however, that the principles of patient teaching remain the same, regardless of the setting, the disease-specific content, or the title of the teacher's health-care profession.

In summary, this book will be a major resource for any health-care professional who has or will have patient teaching responsibilities, whether inside or outside a health-care institution. Many chapters are written for the nurse (e.g., staff nurse, patient education coordinator, nursing service administrator, or inservice-continuing educator), but other health-care professionals may simply read their own titles into the text whenever it says "nurse." Many questions and concerns of patient teachers are answered, and practical approaches to teaching patients are offered.

Gratitude is expressed to William A. Ledger for his encouragement and help while this manuscript was in progress.

D.A.B.

Contributing Authors

Donald A. Bille, R.N., Ph.D.
Associate Professor
Department of Nursing
De Paul University
Chicago, Illinois

Ann Marie T. Brooks, R.N., D.N.Sc.
Assistant Professor of Psychiatric Nursing
Rush University
Chairperson, Department of Psychiatric Nursing
Rush-Presbyterian St. Luke's Medical Center
Chicago, Illinois

Janice C. Colwell, R.N., E.T.
Enterostomal Therapist
University of Chicago Hospitals and Clinics
Chicago, Illinois

Mary Crabtree, R.N., M.S.N.
Director of Nursing, Passavant Pavilion
Northwestern Memorial Hospital
Chicago, Illinois

Sondra G. Ferguson, R.N., M.S.N.
Clinical Nurse Specialist for Cardiac Surgery
Veterans Administration Hospital
Lexington, Kentucky

Carelyn P. Fylling, R.N., M.S.
Patient Education Consultant
Diabetes Education Center
St. Louis Park Medical Center Research Foundation
Minneapolis, Minnesota

Cathie E. Guzzetta, R.N., C.C.R.N., Ph.D.
Assistant Professor and Chairperson, Cardiovascular Nursing
The Catholic University of America
Washington, D.C.

Katherine M. Hedberg, R.N., B.S.N.
Patient Education Coordinator, Nursing
St. Mark's Hospital
Salt Lake City, Utah

William L. Holzemer, Ph.D.
Coordinator, Program Research and Development
Assistant Professor
Department of Nursing in Biological Dysfunction
Associate Appointment, Nursing Services
Division of Education and Research
University of California, San Francisco
San Francisco, California

David J. Kinsey
Director of Instructional Media
Kettering Medical Center
Kettering, Ohio

Mary Ann Klis, R.N.
Assistant to Vice President of Medical Affairs
Copley Memorial Hospital
Aurora, Illinois

Rebecca R. Martin, M.A.
Chief, Library Service
Veterans Administration Medical Center
San Francisco, California

Claire Gavin Meisenheimer, R.N., M.S.N.
Clinical Assistant Professor, Nursing
University of Wisconsin—Milwaukee
Assistant Vice President, Quality Assurance
Froedtert Memorial Lutheran Hospital
Milwaukee, Wisconsin

Barbara J. Mohr, R.N., M.S.N.
Consultant, Quality Assurance
Spokane, Washington

Penny O'Malley, R.N., B.S.N.
Director of Nursing-Ambulatory Services
Cleveland Metropolitan General Hospital
Cleveland, Ohio

Pamela Kay Owen, B.S., R.N.
Inservice Coordinator, Nursing Service
All Saints Episcopal Hospital
Fort Worth, Texas

Clayton M. Press, Jr., A.B., M.Ed.
Cresap, McCormick and Paget, Inc.
Chicago, Illinois

William H. Roach, Jr., M.S., J.D.
Assistant Professor, Health Systems Management
Rush University
Partner
Gardner, Carton and Douglas
Chicago, Illinois

Michael R. Ryan, R.N.
Clinical Instructor, Nursing Education and Research
Mercy Hospital Medical Center
Chicago, Illinois

Ronald K. Schaffner
Assistant Professor of Education
Kettering College of Medical Arts
Director, Educational Design
Kettering Medical Center
Kettering, Ohio

Karen K. Sedlacek, R.N., M.S.N., C.P.N.P.
School Nurse and Nursing Inservice Coordinator
Anchorage School District
Anchorage, Alaska

Marita McSherry Sension, R.N., B.S.N.
Director of Health Education
Mennonite Hospital
Bloomington, Illinois

David K. Solomon, Phar. D.
Associate Professor and Director
Graduate Studies in Hospital Pharmacy
Wayne State University
Director of Pharmacy Services
Detroit Receiving Hospital
Detroit, Michigan

Barbara J. Stevens, R.N., Ph.D.
Director, Division of Health Services, Sciences and Education
Teachers College
Columbia University
New York, New York

Richard E. Thompson, M.D.
Thompson, Mohr and Associates, Inc.
Oak Brook, Illinois

Edward J. Wygonik
Assistant Director, Hospital Information Services
University of Illinois Hospital
Chicago, Illinois

Sen Yee, M.L.S.
Librarian, Patient Education Resource Center
Veterans Administration Medical Center
San Francisco, California

The Structure for Patient Teaching

I

Donald A. Bille

An Overview of Patient Teaching

Should nurses and other health care workers teach patients?
Do patients want to learn?
What information is important for patients to learn?
What teaching methods are most effective in patient education?
Does patient education make a difference?

Patient education has been identified as an integral component of comprehensive patient care throughout most of this century. Nevertheless, current patient education programs often leave much to be desired. The following chapter examines some of the historic and philosophic background in patient education. An extensive review of the literature is presented to demonstrate that education is often an imprecise science and that research does not always provide solutions to teaching-learning problems.

The information in this chapter should help the reader to

1. *Describe various philosophies that identify teaching as a means toward reaching nursing goals*
2. *List categories of information that patients need to learn*
3. *Compare and contrast the effectiveness of several teaching methods in achieving learning outcomes*
4. *List several factors that may affect patients' compliance with the medical regimen*
5. *Identify areas of personal interest for further study in patient education*

When a person is hospitalized for a disease or injury, a change in lifestyle may become necessary to adapt to new limitations on the body or the personality. Yet, patients are not always given enough of the information they need in order to adequately reorder their lives. Part of the reason for this failure may be that the quality of patient teaching done by various health care workers is often inadequate. Patients may complain of lack of information, and they may be readmitted to hospitals because of lack of compliance with discharge prescriptions. An overview of the field of patient education will describe the state of the art and its evolution. The overview will deal with theory, rationale, and research relevant to patient teaching and teaching formats, the patient's need to learn, and patients' compliance with posthospitalization prescriptions.

HISTORIC AND PHILOSOPHIC BACKGROUND

Teaching has been identified as a function of nursing for many years. As early as 1918 the National League for Nursing Education issued a statement that reflected a concern with preparing nurses for teaching tasks [74]. By 1937 the curriculum guide extended the earlier idea by stating that "The nurse is essentially a teacher and an agent of health in whatever field she may be working . . ." [75]. Further extension of the place of teaching in nursing was evident in 1950, when the components of the curriculum were identified as "teaching, contributing subject matter, psychology (especially principles of learning) . . . knowledge of principles of learning and teaching . . . [and] teaching skills" [76].

Many of the contemporary leaders in nursing theory are increasingly interested in the scientific bases of the teaching-learning process. Kreuter, for instance, believes that nursing operations should include the teaching of self-care, and counseling on health matters [52]. Henderson, whose philosophy of nursing is widely utilized as a basis for nursing curricula, says that nursing assists the individual (sick or well) to perform health activities he would do unaided if only he possessed the strength, will, or knowledge to do so [44]. Nursing assistance, which includes teaching, has a goal of increasing the patient's independence. Lambertsen describes nursing as an "educative process" [53], and Peplau characterizes nursing as a maturing force—an educative instrument [80]. Hall describes the nurse as a facilitator of learning. The nurse reflects the patients' verbal expressions so they will hear what they are saying and thus come to grips with themselves, and learn to be well [39]. Travelbee further describes teaching as an interactive process in which both the nurse and the patient learn [98].

The similarity of teaching and nursing is brought out in the philosophies of many nurses. Each of these nursing leaders views teaching as one means toward the goal of nursing—that is, the development of independence in the client—with both the nurse and the patient assuming responsibility for reaching that goal.

PATIENTS WANT TO LEARN

When an individual is hospitalized, he or she not only wants but also expects to know about his or her condition. This fact is supported by Lineham, who studied more than 400 patients in Cleveland. These patients indicated that they wanted to know about changes in their conditions, as well as about the medications they were taking [56]. Newman studied acutely ill patients who also identified the need for information regarding their diagnosis or their routine care [72].

Skipper found that "patients desired information about their illness, technical procedures, and the general social organization of the hospital" [90]. Alt surveyed the opinions of 450 patients, and found that 49 percent of them were discharged from the hospital with one or more of their questions unanswered. Sixty-five percent of these same patients had been given no specific information about their postdischarge care [2]. The questions of the patients in Alt's study fell into these categories:

1. Activity after discharge
2. The real diagnosis
3. Their own reluctance to ask questions
4. Symptoms they wanted explained
5. Suggestions for obtaining more information
6. Reason for treatment
7. Prognosis
8. Confusion about medications
9. Operation
10. Personal care
11. Diet
12. Personal problems
13. Nursing care and nurses
14. Miscellaneous
15. Finances
16. Marital relations
17. Tests that were done

Abdellah and Levine found many patients who reported unfulfilled needs relating to information about their illness. One classic statement encountered was, "I have confidence in my nurses and doctors, but they just won't take the time to explain my illness or treatment" [1].

Deficiencies of Nursing Practice in Patient Teaching

Although the philosophies of nursing leaders include teaching as a part of nursing, and although patients need and want to know about their illnesses, the quality of patient teaching done by various professionals often leaves much to be desired. Organized teaching plans, aimed at increasing the efficiency and effectiveness of the teaching-learning process, are often inadequate or nonexistent. Brown, an anthropologist whose studies detect the thready pulse of nursing practice in patient care, conducted a study of employed nurses. She found that systematic plans for teaching patients self-care after leaving the hospital are quite rare [12]. Streeter investigated several hospitals' medical/-surgical units in a metropolitan area and found no organized teaching programs. None of the nurses thought that patients learned enough about disease prevention and health promotion. Teaching by nurses about disease was almost completely nonexistent. Rehabilitation was found to be most neglected; in six of the eight hospitals studied, no organized program existed [96].

While other authors have described the inadequate teaching done by nurses [60,73,91], Safford and Schlotfeldt identified five essential categories of nursing care. In their study, they found that patients, physicians, and nurses rate teaching and preparation for home care as being consistently less well accomplished than physical care, emotional care, nurse-physician relationships, and administration [87].

The usefulness of patient teaching as a tool of nursing practice has been approved for years. Yet patient teaching continues to be ineffective, inadequate, or completely absent. Gibson has found that as a result, "our patient's knowledge . . . is a hodge-podge of folklore, handed-down family experience, hearsay, bits of advertising, much misinformation, many misconceptions, a jot from the family doctor, and (if he was lucky) a smattering from a school course in health, hygiene or biology" [35].

Redirection of Nursing Practice

Nursing research, then, shows that patients want to learn. Yet nurses may fail to provide patient teaching as a part of their total nursing care. Current leaders in the nursing profession, however, have begun to challenge the traditional roles of health-care practitioners as they develop a working definition of "quality patient care." The momentum for establishing quality patient care has been accelerated by "voluntary standards of professional associations and accrediting agencies as well as vigorous action by citizens who are demanding that their right to the highest quality health and illness care is assured" [106].

The nursing profession bears accountability for the care that clients (patients) receive [4]. Through self-evaluation and peer review, nursing practitioners are required to establish the degree of excellence of nursing care they provide. Each statement of definition reviewed by this author listed patient teaching as an integral part of quality patient care [4, 5, 42, 99, 106].

Accrediting agencies such as the Joint Commission for Accreditation of Hospitals (JCAH) have also established standards for evaluating care. The commission's standards for accreditation require evidence that patient and family teaching is being done [48], and they also provide guidelines for evaluating this teaching [49].

Other voluntary associations such as the American Hospital Association

(AHA) have taken on roles as patient advocates, as they demand better nursing care. The AHA has drafted A Patient's Bill of Rights, through which it expects to realize more effective patient care. One important right the Association has spelled out is the patient's right to obtain "complete current information concerning his diagnosis, treatment and prognosis in terms the patient can be reasonably expected to understand" [3]. (The complete list of patient's rights formulated by the AHA can be found in Appendix I.)

Patients (or health-care consumers) are coming to realize that knowledge about illness and medical care is not the exclusive property of health professionals [95]. As they have come to realize their right to know, health-care consumers have become more vocal in asserting this right. The growing number of malpractice suits alleging a failure to disclose sufficient information to the patient [30] is evidence that patients seek recompense when they feel their rights have been abused.

The responsibility for health care and thus for patient teaching, "like an Olympic torch, is passed on in a relay from one health worker to another. This is true whether the patient is hospitalized or not. Unlike the Olympic torch, however, much is often lost or changed when the responsibility for patient care changes hands. Continuity of care is frequently only an ideal instead of an acutal fact" [84]. Streeter feels that by standardizing the content and using written materials, we can prevent the confusion that occurs when each nurse teaches a patient differently [96].

The potential for a structured teaching program with hospitalized patients is tremendous. Many chronic diseases impose life-altering conditions on people as they grow older, and old age alone imposes a need for change in some health habits. Providing health education for these patients is expensive and time-consuming. The health professionals, however, must demonstrate that their teaching efforts are effective—that their efforts do produce change in their client, the patient.

Research in Effectiveness of Teaching Formats

Hundreds of research projects comparing the effectiveness of various teaching formats accumulated in the 1970s. The results have been largely inconclusive, in that "if a study can be found denying a position on teaching, another can usually be found which confirms it; if no position can be said to be clearly demonstrated [right], none can be said to be clearly wrong" [93]. As the reader reviews some of the research, a word of caution is advised. Most studies have been done on healthy subjects, whereas the author believes that illness changes one's perspectives and abilities to learn. Thus, research done on healthy subjects may not apply to unhealthy subjects.

"Teaching involves providing conditions under which learning will occur" [85]. Various learning conditions have been researched, using the amount of information acquired as a measure of relative effectiveness. Many studies found that the lecture and discussion methods are equally effective in stimulating learning [6, 13, 34]. Hurst also found that no particular method leads effectively to student change [45]. Longstaff found no significant differences [58] between lecture and lecture-quiz methods.

Studies comparing teacher-centered with group-centered classes also found no significant difference in effectiveness between the two approaches [10, 24, 25, 28, 36, 38, 66, 104]. Haar developed a program with phenylketonuria (PKU) children and their mothers; using a group approach, she obtained change in the behavior of the mothers, pointing to the effectiveness of this group approach to teaching patients [37]. Mezzanotte used a group approach to preoperative teaching. She found that patients also prefer to learn in groups [67]. Both Haar and Mezzanotte demonstrated the effectiveness of group teaching, but only in the terms of the nurses' savings of time and effort were they able to say that group instruction is superior.

Smith found no significant difference between the effectiveness of conventional classroom methods and programmed instruction [92]. Bartz and Darby found that supervised programmed instruction is more efficient than unsupervised programmed instruction [7]. Davis, Denny and Marzocco found no significant difference in learning outcomes with different modes of presenting programmed instruction [23].

Miller found that automated teaching devices and learning aids produce better results than conventional modes [68]. McDaniel and Filiatreau, on the other hand, obtained results that favor conventional over mediated instruction [65].

The amount of structure or standardization of presentation has been studied. Bille found that the teaching format, along with the amount of standardized content presented, is not related to the achievement of knowledge about life after a heart attack [9].

The plethora of research on modes of teaching leaves one with the overall impression that the various methods are about equally effective. Knowles states that each of the principal methods of teaching "has unique characteristics that render it peculiarly useful in certain situations and out of place in others. Usually the methods are most effective when used in combination—as when a lecture includes several demonstrations, is followed by a question and answer period, and then is discussed. Over the span of a whole course the teacher may find an opportunity to use almost *every* method effectively" [51].

PATIENTS NEED TO LEARN

Human beings have certain beliefs and behaviors that affect their health. These beliefs and behaviors also affect the patient's ability to profit from health education. Rosenstock studied the motivation of clients in a public health setting. He found evidence that a person will only be likely to take a health action if [86]:

1. He believes himself susceptible to the disease in question

2. He believes that the disease would have serious effects on his life if he should contract it
3. He is aware of certain actions that can be taken and believes that these actions may reduce his likelihood of contracting the disease or reduce the severity of it
4. He believes that the threat of taking the action is not as great as the threat of the disease itself

Couture states that nurse-patient communication (teaching) can be effective if it relates what the patient needs and wants to know [17]. Boyle and Jahns define the term "need" as a "condition that exists between what is and what should be, or what is and that which is more desirable" [11]. They go on to say that a need is the key initiator of behavior, since humans will become motivated to fill the need or find a substitute "so that equilibrium between what is and what should be is restored" [11].

Any change (such as disease or injury) that happens to a person arouses tension and stress. The person then acts to reduce this tension and to attach some meaning to the event. Gibson strongly supports the patient's need to learn, therefore, since a "lack of knowledge of even elementary medical matters often sabotages our best efforts" in the patient's behalf [35].

Patients often worry in order to resolve problems. When a patient is excessively fearful, however, he has little energy left. The nurse must then use realistic, comfortable communication to lessen fears so that the work of worrying can be eased more effectively. Christman feels that "by explaining [to the patient] the general course of his illness and its possible outcomes, fears of the unknown and the consequences of his illness can be relieved to a considerable degree" [15].

Each patient's roles and relationships help to establish a sense of identity and bolster emotional stability. In a hospital the patient is isolated from his usual roles and relationships. This isolation entails a helpless, passive, dependent position for the patient. Miner, in his dramatic account of this helplessness, says, "In every day life . . . [the patient] wards off exposure of his body and its natural functions. Psychological shock results from the fact that body secrecy is suddenly lost. . . . naked bodies are subjected to the scrutiny, manipulation and prodding of the medicine men. . . . The daily ceremonies . . . involve discomfort and torture" [69].

Patient education enables the hospitalized person to cope with the sick role as well as to establish a new, adjusted lifestyle after discharge. Messages that the nurse gives to the patient demonstrate "when a particular behavior is inappropriate and tend to cause behavior that is more acceptable" [15]. This same educational program may alleviate fear and increase the patient's ability to cope with or to ward off feelings of helplessness. "Of special importance are those recommendations which help to build up a sense of *active* control by informing the person about overt actions he can execute . . . and about decisions that will be left up to him. . . " [46].

The hospitalized patient can be motivated to adapt to new conditions caused by illness. The patient, however, must have the support of those who are caring for him or her. Christman has said that one means of support is "careful information [which] will assist the patient to develop the new orientations to behavior made unavoidable by the physical modifications in his activities of daily living" [15].

Compliance with Posthospitalization Prescriptions

Some diseases are of short duration and do not impose long-term limitations on the patient's lifestyle. When the disease is chronic, however, the individual will almost always need to follow the physician's prescriptions for quite some time after diagnosis of the disease. There is a nationwide trend toward treating more and more patients in their own environment after they have recovered from the acute phase of their illness. Johannsen and others state that a successful outcome depends directly on the patient's acceptance of recommendations [47]. The degree of compliance with prescriptions is a critical factor, for example, in the recovery of cardiac patients [18].

Research in Compliance with Posthospitalization Prescriptions

One assumes that patients will follow the physician's prescriptions and benefit from that diagnostic acumen. While these assumptions seem reasonable, "prospective studies have indicated that patients frequently do not comply with the physician's directions. These studies have disclosed an alarming rate of medication errors and noncompliance with regard to drug taking by patient populations" [94].

Patterns of Compliance. "Compliance can be said to exist when the patient carries out his doctor's orders with regard to the medical regimen" [19]. The actual health behavior of most people falls short of what is known to be optimal. Published reports of compliance behavior show wide variations (from 4 percent to 100 percent) in the extent to which patients default [33, 59]. Based on a review of the literature, Davis estimates that approximately 30 to 35 percent of all patients fail to follow their physician's medical recommendations [20].

Marston, however, cautions that "it is usually misleading to compare compliance rates from different studies. This is due to the wide variations in operational definitions of compliance among investigators, the lack of truly objective measures of compliance with certain recommendations, such as special diets, and the loss of precision that enters into estimates of compliance based on several quite different medical recommendations" [63].

Objective measures, such as the presence of a drug or marker in the patient's urine, help to compare compliance rates, but operational definitions of compliance vary from one study to another. Some investigators, for example, base their compliance measure on a one-time urine test that they obtain at the time of the patient's visit to the outpatient department or in an unannounced home visit

[26, 54, 63, 81, 83, 89]. Others have based their estimates on several repeated measures of markers in the urine [8, 14, 62, 102].

The investigators, however, have judged compliance by varying standards. When the number of urine specimens that were negative for isoniazid approached 50 percent, for example, Morrow and Rabin classified their patient as noncompliant; conversely, patients with 50 percent or more positive tests were classified as compliant [71]. Classifying 50 percent positive results as indicative of compliance allows the patient a fairly large amount of deviation. In contrast, Wynn-Williams and Arris, who also used repeated measures, categorized patients with only one negative test as noncompliant [105].

Measures other than urine tests have been used to estimate the amount of compliance. These measures include pill counts [31, 57, 77], observation of the patient [100], and patient's reports [9, 70, 78]. Varying levels of noncompliance were again found.

Even though the data in the various studies may be misleading, Marston states that "It is clear . . . that the problem of noncompliance with medical recommendations is a substantial one, and there is much we need to learn concerning the factors involved in helping people to take care of their health when they are not under the direct surveillance of professional caretakers, such as physicians and nurses" [63].

Correlates of Compliance. An overview of the literature produces conflicting conclusions concerning the correlates of medical compliance. Many factors have been studied in an attempt to find who complies and who does not comply with physicians' orders, but the studies have not been conducted consistently, and the results may not be conclusive. Some demographic attributes seem to characterize a noncompliant patient. Females appear somewhat more likely to default than males [26, 59, 71, 105], and older patients [16, 21, 88], patients in lower socioeconomic status groups [27, 40, 47, 61, 64, 82, 101], and patients with little education [21, 82] are least likely to follow doctors' orders.

Patients are most likely to comply with easy medical regimens [21], and patients with severe disabilities are more likely to comply with a medical regimen than those with a less serious illness [27]. In contradiction, Davis found that patients with serious illnesses are less likely to follow their medical regimens than those with less severe ailments. Consequently, Davis speculated that the more elaborate medical regimens of the more seriously ill patients may account for their greater noncompliance [22].

Knowledge of the disease and of its treatment is usually associated with increased compliance [29, 41, 43, 50, 103]. Time may also be a factor in compliant behavior. Davis found that patients exhibit more compliance over time, and if they change their initial behavior, it is less likely to be in the direction of noncompliant behavior [19].

A few investigators examined personality correlates of compliance. Ley and Spelman found that patients with an average level of anxiety remember more of what they are told in an outpatient department than do those with a low or a high level of anxiety [55]. Stunkard and McClaren-Hume examined levels of anxiety with respect to weight loss. They found that obese persons show significantly greater anxiety than individuals of normal weight, but there is no relationship between anxiety scores and subsequent success at weight loss [97]. Marston found no relationship between willingness to take risks and noncompliance, or between belief in personal control over what happens to the individual and subsequent compliant behavior [63]. Bille found that patients who report a higher body cathexis score (and thus a higher degree of satisfaction with the parts or functions of the body) also achieve a higher compliance with physicians' orders. Body image was found thus to be significantly related to compliance [9].

REFERENCES

1. Abdellah, F., and Levine, M.   Polling patients and personnel. I: What patients say about their nursing care. *Hospitals,* 40 : 76, 1966.
2. Alt, R.   Patient education program answers many unanswered questions. *Hospitals,* 40 : 76, 1966.
3. American Hospital Association.   *A Patient's Bill of Rights.* Chicago: The Association, 1972.
4. American Nurses Association.   *Standards of Nursing Practice.* Kansas City: The Association, 1973.
5. American Nurses Association.   *Standards of Cardiovascular Nursing Practice.* Kansas City: The Association, 1975.
6. Bane, C. L.   The lecture versus the class discussion method of college teaching. *School and Society,* 21 : 300, 1925.
7. Bartz, W., and Darby, C.   A study of supervised and nonsupervised programmed instruction in the university setting. *Journal of Educational Research,* 58 : 208, 1970.
8. Bergman, A. B., and Werner, R. J.   Failure of children to receive penicillin by mouth. *New England Journal of Medicine,* 268 : 1334, 1963.
9. Bille, D. A.   Patients' knowledge and compliance with post-hospitalization prescriptions as related to body image and teaching format. Ph.D. dissertation, University of Wisconsin—Madison, 1975.
10. Bovard, E. W.   The psychology of classroom instruction. *Journal of Educational Research,* 45 : 215, 1951.
11. Boyle, P. G., and Jahns, I. R.   Program Development and Evaluation. In R. M. Smith, G. F. Aker, and J. R. Kidd (Eds.), *Handbook of Adult Education,* New York: MacMillan, 1970. P. 61.
12. Brown, E. L.   The social sciences and improvement of nursing care. *American Journal of Nursing,* 56 : 1148, 1956.
13. Carlson, C. R.   A study of the relative effectiveness of lecture and directed discussion methods of teaching tests and measurements to prospective air force instructors. *Dissertation Abstracts,* 8 : 1112, 1953.
14. Charney, E., et al.   How well do patients take oral penicillin? A collaborative study in private practice. *Pediatrics,* 40 : 188, 1967.
15. Christman, L.   Assisting the patient to learn the "patient role." *Journal of Nursing Education,* 6 : 20, 1967.
16. Cobb, B., et al.   Patient-responsible delay of treatment in cancer. *Cancer,* 7 : 920, 1954.
17. Couture, N. A.   Communication with patients: Approach and content used by nurses. Ph.D. dissertation, St. Louis University, 1967.
18. Croog, S. H., et al.   The heart patient and the recovery process: A review of the

directions of research on social and psychological factors. *Social Science and Medicine,* 2 : 111, 1968.
19. Davis, M.   Predicting non-compliant behavior. *Journal of Health and Social Behavior,* 8 : 265, 1967.
20. Davis, M.   Variations in patients' compliance with doctors' orders: Analysis of congruence between survey responses and results of empirical investigations. *Journal of Medical Education,* 41 : 1037, 1966.
21. Davis, M., and Eichhorn, R.   Compliance with medical regimens: A panel study. *Journal of Health and Human Behavior,* 4 : 240, 1963.
22. Davis, M.   Physiologic, psychological and demographic factors in patient compliance with doctors' orders. *Medical Care,* 6 : 115, 1968.
23. Davis, R. et al.   Interaction of individual differences with modes of presenting programmed instruction. *Journal of Educational Psychology,* 61 : 198, 1970.
24. Deutsch, M.   Social relations in the classroom and grading procedures. *Journal of Educational Research,* 45 : 145, 1951.
25. Di Vesta, F. J.   Instructor-centered and student-centered approaches in teaching a human relations course. *Journal of Applied Psychology,* 38 : 329, 1954.
26. Dixon, W., Stradling, P., and Wooton, I.   Outpatient P.A.S. therapy. *Lancet,* 273 : 871, 1957.
27. Donabedian, A., and Rosenfeld, L.   Patients do not do what doctor says. *Public Health Reports,* 79 : 228, 1964.
28. Eglash, A.   A group discussion method of teaching psychology. *Journal of Educational Psychology,* 45 : 257, 1954.
29. Elling, R., Whittemore, R., and Green, M.   Patient participation in a pediatric program. *Journal of Health and Human Behavior,* 4 : 166, 1963.
30. Epstein, R. L., and Benson, D. J.   The patient's right to know. *Hospitals,* 47 : 47, 1973.
31. Feinstein, A. R., et al.   A controlled study of three methods of prophylaxis against streptococcal infection in a population of rheumatic children. *New England Journal of Medicine,* 260 : 697, 1959.
32. Fisher, S.   *Body Consciousness: You Are What You Feel.* Englewood Cliffs, N.J.: Prentice Hall, 1973. Pp. 5–6.
33. Fox, W. Problem of self-administration of drugs, with particular reference to pulmonary tuberculosis. *Tubercle,* 39 : 269, 1958.
34. Gerberich, J. R., and Warner, K. O.   Relative instructional efficiencies of the lecture and discussion methods in a university course in american national government. *Journal of Educational Research,* 29 : 574, 1936.
35. Gibson, W. B.   But who teaches the patient? *Archives of Dermatology,* 88 : 935, 1963.
36. Gibb, L. M., and Gibb, J. R.   The effects of the use of "participative action" groups in a course in general psychology. *American Psychologist,* 7 : 247, 1952.
37. Haar, D. J.   Improved phenylketonuric diet control through group education of mothers. *Nursing Clinics of North America,* 1 : 715, 1966.
38. Haigh, G. V., and Schmidt, W.   The learning of subject matter in teacher-centered and group-centered classes. *Journal of Educational Psychology,* 47 : 295, 1956.
39. Hall, L. E.   Nursing—what is it? *Canadian Nurse,* 60 : 150, 1964.
40. Hardy, M.   Psychologic aspects of pediatrics: Parent resistance to need for remedial and preventive services. *Journal of Pediatrics,* 48 : 104, 1956.
41. Hecht, A.   Improving medical compliance by teaching outpatients. *Nursing Forum,* 13 : 112, 1974.
42. Hegyvary, S. T., and Haussmann, R. K. D.   Monitoring nursing care quality. *Journal of Nursing Administration,* 5 : 17, 1975.
43. Heinzelmann, F.   Factors in prophylaxis behavior in treating rheumatic fever: An exploratory study. *Journal of Health and Human Behavior,* 3 : 73, 1962.
44. Henderson, V.   The nature of nursing. *American Journal of Nursing,* 64 : 62, 1964.

45. Hurst, J. G.   The relationship between teaching methods and course objectives in educational psychology. *Journal of Educational Research,* 57 : 147, 1963.
46. Janis, I. L.   *Psychological Stress: Psychoanalytic and Behavioral Studies of Surgical Patients.* New York: Wiley, 1958. P. 384.
47. Johannsen, W., Hellmuth, G., and Sorauf, T.   On accepting medical recommendations. *Archives of Environmental Health,* 12 : 63, 1966.
48. Joint Commission for Accreditation of Hospitals.   *Accreditation Manual for Hospitals.* Chicago: The Commission, 1979. P. 106.
49. Joint Commission for Accreditation of Hospitals.   *Hospital Survey Profile.* Chicago: The Association, 1977.
50. Kegeles, S.   Why people seek dental care: A test of a conceptual formulation. *Journal of Health and Human Behavior,* 4 : 166, 1963.
51. Knowles, M. S.   *Informal Adult Education.* New York: Association Press, 1950. P. 47.
52. Kreuter, F. R.   What is good nursing care? *Nursing Outlook,* 5 : 302, 1957.
53. Lambertsen, E. C.   Nursing definition and philosophy precede nursing goal development. *Modern Hospitals,* 103 : 136, 1964.
54. Leggat, P.   P.A.S. and the patient. *Lancet,* 273 : 1283, 1957.
55. Ley, P., and Spelman, M.   Communications in an outpatient setting. *British Journal of Social and Clinical Psychology,* 4 : 115, 1965.
56. Lineham, D. T.   What does the patient want to know? *American Journal of Nursing,* 66 : 1066, 1966.
57. Lipman, R. S., et al.   Neurotics who fail to take their drugs. *British Journal of Psychiatry,* 111 : 1043, 1965.
58. Longstaff, H. P.   Analysis of some factors conditioning learning in general psychology. *Journal of Applied Psychology,* 16 : 9, 1932.
59. Luntz, G., and Austin, R.   New stick test for P.A.S. in urine. *British Journal of Medicine,* 1 : 1679, 1960.
60. MacArthur, C.   We teach—do our patients learn? *Canadian Nurse,* 55 : 205, 1959.
61. MacDonald, M., Hagberg, J., and Grossman, B.   Social factors in relation to participation in follow-up care of rheumatic fever. *Journal of Pediatrics,* 62 : 503, 1963.
62. Maddock, R. K.   Patient cooperation in taking medicines: A study involving isoniazid and aminosalicylic acid. *Journal of the American Medical Association,* 199 : 169, 1967.
63. Marston, M. V.   Compliance with medical regimens: A review of the literature. *Nursing Research,* 19 : 312, 1970.
64. Mather, W.   Social and economic factors in relation to correction of school discovered medical and dental defects. *Pennsylvania Medical Journal,* 62 : 983, 1954.
65. McDaniel, E., and Filiatreau, W. K.   A comparison of television and conventional instruction as determinants of attitude change. *Journal of Educational Research,* 58 : 293, 1965.
66. McKeachie, W. J.   Individual conformity to attitudes of classroom groups. *Journal of Abnormal Social Psychology,* 49 : 282, 1954.
67. Mezzanotte, E. J.   Group instruction in preparation for surgery. *American Journal of Nursing,* 70 : 89, 1970.
68. Miller, J. W.   An experimental comparison of two approaches to teaching multiplication of fractions. *Journal of Educational Research,* 57 : 468, 1964.
69. Miner, H. M.   Body ritual among the nacirema. *American Anthropologist,* 58 : 503, 1956.
70. Mohler, D. N., Wallin, D. G., and Dreyfuss, E. G.   Studies in the home treatment of streptococcal disease, Part I: Failure of patients to take penicillin by mouth as prescribed. *New England Journal of Medicine,* 252 : 1116, 1955.

71. Morrow, R., and Rabin, D.   Reliability in self-medication with isoniazid. *Clinical Research,* 14 : 362, 1966.
72. Newman, M.   Identifying and meeting patients' needs in short-span, nurse-patient relationships. *Nursing Forum,* 5 : 76, 1966.
73. Nite, G., and Willis, F.   *The Coronary Patient: Hospital Care and Rehabilitation.* New York: MacMillan, 1964.
74. *NLNE: Standard Curriculum for Schools of Nursing.* National League for Nursing Education, Baltimore: Waverly, 1918. P. 6.
75. *NLNE: A Curriculum Guide for Schools of Nursing.* New York: The League, 1937.
76. *NLNE: Nursing Organization Curriculum Conference.* Glen Garden, New Jersey: Libertarian Press, 1950.
77. Nugent, C. A., et al.   Glucocorticoid toxicity: Single contrasted with divided daily doses of prednisolone. *Journal of Chronic Diseases,* 18 : 323, 1965.
78. Park, L. C., and Lipman, R. S.   A comparison of patient dosage deviation reports with pill counts. *Psychopharmacologia,* 6 : 299, 1964.
79. Parsons, T.   *The Social System.* New York: Free Press, 1951.
80. Peplau, H. E.   *Interpersonal Relations in Nursing.* New York: Putnam, 1952.
81. Pitman, E. R., Benzier, E., and Katz, M.   Clinic experience with a urine P.A.S. test. *Diseases of the Chest,* 36 : 1, 1959.
82. Pragoff, H.   Adjustment of tuberculosis patients one year after hospital discharge. *Public Health Reports,* 77 : 671, 1962.
83. Preston, D. F., and Miller, F. L.   The tuberculosis outpatient's defection from therapy. *American Journal of the Medical Sciences,* 247 : 21, 1964.
84. Rambousek, E.   Teaching the Patient After Hospital Discharge. In F. Storlie (Ed.), *Patient Teaching in Critical Care.* New York: Appleton-Century-Crofts, 1975. P. 146.
85. Redman, B. K.   *The Process of Patient Teaching in Nursing* (2nd ed.). St. Louis: Mosby, 1972.
86. Rosenstock, I. M.   What research in motivation suggests for public health. *American Journal of Public Health,* 50 : 295, 1960.
87. Safford, B. J., and Schlotfeldt, R.   Nursing service staffing and quality of nursing care. *Nursing Research,* 9 : 149, 1960.
88. Schwartz, D., et al.   Medication errors made by elderly, chronically ill patients. *American Journal of Public Health,* 52 : 2018, 1962.
89. Simpson, J. M.   Simple tests for the detection of urinary P.A.S. *Tubercle,* 37 : 333, 1956.
90. Skipper, J. K., Tagliacozzo, D., and Mauksch, H.   What communication means to patients. *American Journal of Nursing,* 64 : 101, 1964.
91. Skipper, J. K.   Communications and the hospitalized patient. In J. K. Skipper and R. C. Leonard (Eds.), *Social Interaction and Patient Care.* Philadelphia: Lippincott, 1965.
92. Smith, N. H.   The teaching of elementary statistics by two conventional classroom methods versus the method of programmed instruction. *Journal of Educational Research,* 55 : 417, 1962.
93. Solomon, D., Bezdek, W., and Rosenberg, L.   *Teaching Styles and Learning.* Chicago: Center for the Study of Liberal Education for Adults, 1963. P. 1.
94. Stewart, R. B., and Cluff, L. E.   A review of medication errors and compliance in ambulant patients. *Clinical Pharmacology and Therapeutics,* 13 : 463, 1972.
95. Storlie, F.   Some latent meanings of teaching of patients. *Heart and Lung,* 2 : 506, 1973.
96. Streeter, V.   The nurse's responsibility for teaching patients. *American Journal of Nursing,* 53 : 818, 1953.
97. Stunkard, A., and McClaren-Hume, M.   The results of treatment for obesity: A review of the literature and report of a series. *Archives of Internal Medicine,* 103 : 79, 1959.

98. Travelbee, J.   *Interpersonal Aspects of Nursing.* Philadelphia: Davis, 1971.
99. Wandelt, M. A., and Ager, J. W.   *Quality Patient Care Scale.* New York: Appleton-Century-Crofts, 1974. P. 22.
100. Watkins, J.   Observation of medication errors made by diabetic patients in the home. *Diabetes,* 16 : 229, 1966.
101. Watts, D. D.   Factors related to the acceptance of modern medicine. *American Journal of Public Health,* 56 : 1205, 1966.
102. Willcox, D., Gillan, R., and Hare, H. H.   Do psychiatric outpatients take their drugs? *British Medical Journal,* 2 : 790, 1965.
103. Williams, T. F., et al.   The clinical picture of diabetic control studied in four settings. *American Journal of Public Health,* 57 : 441, 1967.
104. Wispe, L. G.   Evaluating section teaching methods in the introductory course. *Journal of Educational Research,* 45 : 161, 1951.
105. Wynn-Williams, N., and Arris, M.   On omitting P.A.S. *Tubercle,* 39 : 138, 1958.
106. Zimmer, M. J., Lang, N. M., and Miller, D. I.   Development of sets of patient health outcome criteria by panels of nurse experts. Wisconsin Regional Medical Program, Jan. 1–June 30, 1974.

A Comprehensive System of Patient Education

guidelines for development

Where do I begin?
What do I need to know before initiating a patient education program?
Where can I go for help?

Health-care organizations are examining their role in educating the many clients they serve. This self-examination may be initiated by consumer demands, by new or more stringent standards of care, or by attempts to remain competitive in hiring staff or maintaining occupancy rates. The results of self-examination may point to the need to reorganize current patient education programming or the need to initiate entirely new programs. The organization or reorganization of patient education programming requires careful planning to achieve an overall, systematized approach. The following chapter describes a methodology for developing an organized system of patient education in a health-care setting. Data requirements in inpatient, outpatient, and community settings are described. Support systems and inservice education needs are identified, and strategies for sustaining a patient education program are identified.

The information in this chapter should help the reader to

1. *List types of data that need to be collected when developing an individualized, organized system of patient education*
2. *Identify resources available to assist in planning and providing patient education programs*
3. *Describe support systems that are necessary for development of a patient education system*
4. *List strategies for developing an overall, systematic patient education program for an organization*

5. List elements to be included in staff development programs that prepare personnel for the teaching role
6. Identify strategies for assuring success of a patient education system

Patient education is not a new field in health care today. There is, however, greater emphasis on delivering organized, systematic patient education as an integral entity within the health-care system rather than as a haphazard, episodic, fragmented occurrence [6, 14]. Previously, there was no guarantee that patients or consumers would receive the education they need and rightly deserve. Providers of health care are now developing organized patient education programs so that patients with an expressed or perceived need for education will receive it as a routine component of their care. "There is significant evidence that education of patients to understand the nature of their illness and what they can do to help themselves, and education of the public to use new methods of health service delivery could reduce the cost of health care" [20].

Patient education can be defined as a systematic, planned, learning experience, based on an individual's needs that results in a change of behavior with the goal of promotion and maintenance of optimal health. Community-based health education is composed primarily of health awareness, health promotion, and disease prevention programs for a large group of people.

To develop an organized system of patient education in a health-care setting requires research, planning, implementation, and evaluation on the part of the providers of health care. No two patient education programs can be exactly identical because no two settings are identical. Each area has different needs, characteristics, resources, and budgets. What may be feasible for one hospital or clinic may be totally unworkable in another hospital or clinic. All too often health professionals planning patient education programs become frustrated with this fact because they want someone to give them exact instructions that they can implement. Developing a program takes both individual and group effort by the providers to design the ideal patient education program for their individual setting.

The guidelines set out in the succeeding pages can be used to assist each group of health-care providers in developing an organized system of patient education individualized for their own setting. Many of the steps are the same for an inpatient, outpatient, and community setting; however, the approach to these steps might be different. It is imperative that all providers be aware of the delivery systems and models used in the settings developed by the other providers so that all people can learn. Before a plan of action can be developed, it is essential that data be gathered by each group to determine the characteristics of each setting for synchronization of teaching efforts.

One of the first tasks in planning a patient education program for a hospital, a clinic, or a community health program is the collection of data. First, it is essential that the patient educator know the characteristics of the population he or she intends to educate. Program planners must try to determine the average age, educational level, and socioeconomic level of the local population. They should investigate whether the predominate lifestyle, the recreational activities, or the industrial environment, have significant health effects on the population.

Second, the patient education program planners must survey the facilities and resources available for the program. The physical limitations of the hospital or clinic setting must be determined, and the community health program must determine what buildings (schools, churches, motel conference rooms, shopping malls, or other public buildings) are available for use. Program planners must determine what personnel are available and interested in planning, implementing, and evaluating the program. Teaching aids and equipment should be inventoried; often a supply of projectors and other audiovisual equipment will already be available, either within the institution or accessible somewhere else in the community.

Finally, planners must ascertain what support is available for the patient education program. The administration of the hospital, clinic, or community health organization should commit itself in writing to both moral and budgetary support for the program. The overall policy of the institution must support the principles of patient education. Planners should investigate the possibilities of outside funding for the program if necessary. Existing patient education programs (perhaps some exist even within the same institution) must be investigated and mined for ideas, materials, and methods. Experts in various fields should be identified as resource persons who may be able to support and help the program at some time. Not until all this information has been gathered can the patient education program planning continue.

RESOURCES

The provider should determine what resources are available to assist in planning and providing the patient education program. Many patient education coordinators have used great creativity and ingenuity in utilizing these resources for the programs. One coordinator, for example, borrowed the videotape playback machine from the local university. The coordinator then solicited money from a local television merchant for purchasing the videotapes for the program. An outline of resources available for all settings follows.

Program development and implementation support
    Health professionals from inpatient, outpatient, clinics, and community settings
    Peer pressure among staff, department heads, physicians, and community groups
    Already established patient education programs
    Past patients
    Clergy
    Auxiliaries of service organizations, hospitals, etc.
    Boards of directors
    American Hospital Association
    American Group Practice Association

    Professional organizations
Educational materials
    Pharmaceutical companies
    Voluntary health organizations
    State Department of Health
    National Institutes of Health
    Public Health Service
    Commercial audiovisual companies
    Libraries
    Government Printing Office
    Governmental extension agencies
Funding or service
    Welfare departments
    Division of Vocational Rehabilitation
    Crippled Children's Service
    Third party payers
    Local merchants
    United Way
    Chambers of Commerce
    Service organizations
    Community volunteer organizations
    Charitable foundations, grants, endowments
Settings for patient teaching and health education
    Health care facilities
    Day care centers
    Nursery schools
    Head start programs
    Community educational institutions
    Senior citizens centers

Using the information gained from this initial database and the identification of resources, the plan of action for the patient education system can be developed. The following areas relate to both an inpatient and outpatient or clinic setting.

SUPPORT

The most integral part of developing a patient education system is to have strong support from the power people and policy makers in the organization: administrators, department heads, and physicians. All too often a patient education program developed through great individual effort on the part of the staff has dissolved due to lack of support from these influential people in the organization. In soliciting this support, it is essential to request not only verbal support, but also a written policy statement indicating the philosophy of patient education in that setting. Time allocation needs to be defined for the staff to assist in developing the programs and implementing them. Budgetary allotments for the development of the programs, the gathering of materials needed, and ultimately a person designated as a Patient Education Coordinator constitutes a vital phase of planning. The most successful patient education programs have been in health-care facilities in which a person was given the overall responsibility for coordinating the patient education activities in the institution. Depending on the size of the health-care facility and its needs, the patient education coordinator may be a full- or part-time position [2]. This position should be recognized on the organizational chart. The person selected as coordinator should be a dynamic, creative, and innovative person who has good rapport with people at all levels in the organization, has good organizational ability, and is committed to the concept of patient education.

Salesmanship is an asset in soliciting support for patient education. The coordinator must point out the needs as identified in the initial data gathering; relate patient, staff, and physician interest in patient education; discuss the trends in the nation towards patient education, the Patient's Bill of Rights, professional policy statements, and legal and accreditation ramifications [4]; and present a logical plan for developing the patient education program. One must be realistic in developing the patient education program and set some long and short range goals with time limits. *Example:* The ultimate goal is to develop an overall, systematic patient education program for the hospital. To accomplish this, the initial goals are:

1. Within one month develop a policy statement on patient education supported by the administration indicating the hospital's philosophy
2. Develop an interdisciplinary Patient Education Advisory Committee within one month
3. This Advisory Committee will identify the characteristics, needs, and resources in the hospital within six months
4. This Advisory Committee will develop a plan of action to meet those needs within eight months
5. Upon completion of each goal, the Patient Education Coordinator will communicate the progress to the administrator of the hospital

Patient Education Advisory Committee

The patient education advisory committee should be an interdisciplinary committee composed of representatives from each department involved in patient education [2]. To enhance the decision making and policy setting function of the committee, the members should be not only staff representatives but also department heads, administrators, and physicians. Consumer representation on the committee is becoming more common. The committee should be responsible for planning, organizing, developing, and evaluating the total system of patient education. The Patient Education Coordinator chairs the committee, thus enhancing communication and continuity. The committee should have the following functions:

1. Preview the characteristics of the setting
2. Determine the needs in patient education
3. Prioritize the needs and make recommendations

4. Delegate responsibility to a Patient Education Program Subcommittee to develop an individual program to meet each identified need
5. Approve individual programs as they are developed
6. Identify the approach of the educational delivery system: one-to-one teaching, group teaching, self-instructional programs, or a combination
7. Identify who will be teaching the patient: staff, clinical specialists, teaching teams, or a combination of these
8. Communicate information regarding patient education programming between the committee and the respective departments and vice-versa
9. Evaluate the overall patient education system

Patient Education Program Subcommittee

With the recommendations from the patient education advisory committee as to the needs, staff responsibility, and approach of the program, the patient education program subcommittee develops the format for an individual patient education program, such as the diabetes, postcoronary, respiratory, or prenatal program [16]. A subcommittee may be formed for each identified program need. Each program designed should have the following basic components:

1. An interview form or assessment sheet that the educators can use to determine the patient's education needs
2. A teaching plan to document the patient's education needs
3. A teaching manual for the educators to use with guidelines for teaching the patient [12]. *Example:* A teaching manual can divide all the content information regarding a certain disease into single concept modules with these areas delineated in each module:
   a. Learning objectives for the patient
   b. Teaching materials to use
   c. Content to be taught
4. A method of documenting what the patient was taught and his response to the content. This could be in the form of progress notes or a patient education documentation form

Besides using the patient learning objectives as an evaluation tool through observation, return demonstration, or return explanation, other evaluation tools such as pretests and posttests, situation problem-solving, and physical parameters (weight, blood pressure, blood sugar, or frequency of respiratory problems) could be developed.

AUDIOVISUAL MATERIALS

At various times, the advisory committee, the subcommittee members, and the Patient Education Coordinator will determine what aduiovisual aids should be used in the individual and overall programs. It is best to use the Adopt-Adapt-Produce process. This process begins by reviewing what other companies and programs are using. If that material meets the needs of the program, it can be adopted. If only a part of the material meets identified needs, it can be adapted by blending materials from several areas with those at hand. If after these steps needs are still neglected, then a process of producing materials in their entirety on a local level becomes necessary. Such a process can save both time and money.

There are a myriad of audiovisual materials available today: pamphlets, booklets, flip charts, posters, audiocassette tapes, slides, filmstrips, movies, videotapes, and many others. These products must be evaluated carefully since one audiovisual aid will not be suitable for all situations. A variety of aids may be needed. Not all audiovisual materials need be costly: a simple diagram drawn on a sheet of paper or blackboard can be just as effective a teaching tool as a videotape on closed circuit television [3].

STAFF TRAINING

Before implementing an individual patient education program, the people involved in delivering the program must be well trained. Their role and responsibility should be clearly delineated and presented in an inservice training program. A frequent comment from staff regarding patient education is that they do not know what to teach or how to teach and do not view themselves as educators. The manuals that contain the guidelines for teaching the content information of the particular disease can be the basis for the training program. To assist in learning patient education techniques, these steps in the education process should be integrated into the inservice sessions:

1. Interview patient to determine knowledge, skills, and lifestyle
2. Assess the patient's knowledge and skills
3. Determine the patient's education needs
4. Establish a teaching plan to meet the patient's education needs
5. Implement the teaching plan and do the teaching
6. Evaluate the patient's response to the teaching
7. Revise the teaching plan as needed
8. Provide ongoing follow-up and support of the patient
9. Cooperate with other health team members and communicate the patient's status to them
10. Chart the patient's education progress

Other patient education content areas could be: teaching-learning principles, stages of adaptation to chronic illness, effective use of audiovisual materials, and interviewing, assessment, listening, communication, motivation, and evaluation skills [18, 22]. Positive reinforcement from the Patient Education Coordinator and supervisors for the staff's efforts in patient education should be prevalent at all times. Through this reinforcement the staff's perception of their roles as educators will improve. This component is just as important for the success of the patient education program as the initial staff training.

TESTING THE PROGRAM

When implementing each individual patient education program, the coordinator should test it initially in a small area for a period of time. For example, the diabetes education program could be implemented on one medical station for six months. During this trial period, the program can be evaluated, "debugged," revised, and improved before implementing it throughout the health-care facility. This will ensure that the program is effectively designed for optimal efficiency.

EVALUATION

In evaluating the overall system of patient education, the coordinator must evaluate not only each individual program but also the interaction of all programs within the total system. How effective are the programs? Which programs are functioning more efficiently than others and why? Are the programs meeting the needs that were initially identified? Is the designed delivery system functioning efficiently? This data can be gathered in a variety of ways: patients, staff members, administrators, and physicians can be polled through interviews, letters, or questionnaires to determine their perception of the patient education programs; the number of hospital admissions or out patient department visits before, during, and after education can be tabulated; records can be kept of the number of patients seen in the patient education center or group class; auditing charts can determine the prevalence of patient education as an integral component of the patient's care; and feedback from other health professionals working with the patient, such as public health nurses, can indicate knowledge gained, retention of learning and application of information by the patient. Through constant follow-up, health professionals can continuously evaluate the effectiveness of a patient education program on a patient's behavior. A combination of these tools should be utilized to evaluate the patient education system.

TIPS FOR A SUCCESSFUL PATIENT EDUCATION SYSTEM

Involvement. By involving as many people as possible (physicians, administrators, department heads, supervisors, staff, and representatives from all departments doing patient education), communication will be more open and effective, support and commitment to patient education will be increased, and potential problem areas will be identified and resolved before they become problems.

Expectation. The philosophy, policy, or expectation of providing quality patient education that is fostered throughout the health-care facility will create a climate for the staff to be motivated to implement patient education. This expectation can be promulgated by a policy statement from administration for patient education, patient education functions integrated into job descriptions for the staffs, each staff member's patient education performance evaluated during annual salary review, teaching manuals and inservice training on what to teach and how to teach provided to the staff and ongoing support and positive reinforcement given to the staff by their supervisors and the Patient Education Coordinator for their patient education efforts.

Ease of implementation. Each patient education program should be designed so that it is very easy for the staff to integrate it into their everyday care of the patient rather than being a cumbersome extra responsibility. Patient education materials and teaching aids should be centrally located and easily accessible for the staff for the efficient utilization of time.

Communication. Effective channels for open communication about the patient education programming should be developed among the health professionals, departments, and committees involved. Fostering an openness to new ideas and a willingness to try will create new, innovative approaches to patient education. Information regarding patient education programs in the inpatient, outpatient/clinic, and community settings should be communicated to the other departments.

Parallelism. When a total patient education system is composed of many individual patient education programs, keeping the design of the programs parallel eliminates confusion. *Example:* An overall patient education system may have forty different patient education programs, but each program should have a teaching manual with guidelines for the educator as to his or her role and responsibility in that program, the content to be taught, the interview form, and documentation format. Thus, the educators will always know where to go for reference and guidance.

Coordination. All the patient education programs should be coordinated through a central person or department, that is, the Patient Education Coordinator or Education Department.

Educational phases. Because each patient's acceptance of his health problem, readiness to learn, and motivation is different, the educational program and teaching should be staged to accommodate the optimal learning time. *Example:* A diabetic patient should receive only beginning information while hospitalized during the initial diagnosis. A brief definition of diabetes, the techniques for urine testing and insulin injection, treatment of hypoglycemia, and the basic diabetic diet will be enough. After discharge and utilizing this information at home for a few weeks, the patient can return as an outpatient for individual or group instruction to reinforce initial learning and learn the remaining aspects of diabetes management. At each visit to the doctor thereafter, the patient should have one aspect of his or her management reviewed, thus providing continuing education and updating. For continuity of care, a report of the educational encounter in each setting should be documented and forwarded to the health professional responsible for the patient's education in the other settings [8, 11].

PATIENT EDUCATION IN THE COMMUNITY

The same general principles described previously can be extrapolated to the community setting. The main difference is that the members of the various committees would be health professionals, business personnel, consumers, and others from a cross section of community organizations rather than an internal organization. Involving many groups in coordinated planning is an asset to avoid duplication of services. Besides verbal support, each group will need to provide a commitment of time for people working on the program, physical facilities, or media for presenting the program, publicity, and funding. Because a community-based program does not have a captive audience as in the inpatient or outpatient/clinic setting, extensive publicity is needed to inform community members of the health education program. This can be done through the newspapers, radio, television, brochures, flyers, posters, billboards, community newsletters, church bulletins, or bill enclosures. The extent of the publicity will greatly affect the impact of the health education program.

Using these guidelines, health-care providers can develop organized systems of patient education in an inpatient, outpatient/clinic, or community setting. Other guidelines published can also be used for reference [2, 11, 13, 15, 16, 17, 21]. An extensive amount of information is available from the American Hospital Association based on the outcome of their 1975 Survey on Inpatient Education Programs [1, 2, 3, 4]. Through this contact with the Bureau of Health Education, a coordinated effort to organize hospital-based patient education in the United States has been accomplished.

Because of these efforts and those of health-care providers, patient education has become an accepted component of health care today. "Quality health care can only be achieved by informed patients cooperating with interested and knowledgeable health professionals" [11].

REFERENCES

1. American Hospital Association. *Hospital Inpatient Education: Survey Findings and Analysis, 1975.* U.S. Department of Health, Education and Welfare, 1977.
2. American Hospital Association. *Implementing Patient Education in the Hospital.* Chicago: The Association, 1978.
3. American Hospital Association. *Media Handbook: A Guide to Selecting, Producing, and Using Media for Patient Education Programs.* Chicago: The Association, 1978.
4. American Hospital Association. *Professional, Accreditation, and Legal Statements Supporting Patient Education.* Chicago: The Association, 1977.
5. Bell, D. F.   Assessing educational needs: Advantages and disadvantages of eighteen techniques. *Nurse Educator,* 3 : 15, 1978.
6. Breckon, D. J.   Highlights in the evolution of hospital-based patient education programs. *Journal of Allied Health,* 5 : 35, 1976.
7. Committee on Educational Tasks in Chronic Illness, Public Health Education Section, American Public Health Association.   *A Model for Planning Patient Education.* Rockville, Md.: Health Services and Mental Health Administration, n.d.
8. Etzwiler, D.   Education of the patient with diabetes. *Medical Clinics of North America,* 62 : 857, 1978.

9. Fralic, J. F.   Developing a viable inpatient education program—a nursing director's perspective. *Journal of Nursing Administration,* 6 : 30, 1976.
10. Fylling, C. P.   The Nurse Educator In A Health Maintenance Organization: Developing And Implementing An Educational Program For Diabetic Patients. In J. T. Bailey, and K. E. Claus, (Eds.), *Decision Making in Nursing: Tools for Change,* St. Louis: Mosby, 1975.
11. Fylling, C. P., Griffin, J. A., and Findley, D. E.   Education of the diabetic patient. *Minnesota Medicine,* 58 : 789, 1976.
12. Gusfa, A., Christoff, V., and Headley, L.   Patient teaching: One approach. *Supervisor Nurse,* 6 : 17, 1975.
13. Kucha, D.   The health education of patients: Development of a system, Parts 1 and 2. *Supervisor Nurse,* 5 : 8, May and June 1974.
14. Lee, E. A., and Garvey, J. L.   How is inpatient education being managed? *Hospitals,* 51 : 75, 1977.
15. Maryland Hospital Education Institute.   *Organizing and Implementing an Inpatient Education Program.* Lutherville, Md.: The Institute, 1977.
16. Pritchett, S.   *Patient, Family and Community Health Education: Design and Management of Hospital Based Programs.* Atlanta: Pritchett-Hull Associates, 1977.
17. Professional Research, Inc.   *Blueprint: A Patient Education Program for the Hospital.* Los Angeles: Professional Research, 1978.
18. Redman, B. K.   *The Process of Patient Teaching in Nursing* (2nd ed.). St. Louis: Mosby, 1972.
19. Richards, R. F., and Kalmer, H.   Patient education. *Health Education Monograph,* 2, Spring 1974.
20. Roccella, E. J.   Potential for reducing health care costs by public and patient education. *Public Health Reports,* 91 : 112, 1976.
21. Special Issue: Patient Education, *Journal of Biocommunication* 5 : 3–23, 1978.
22. Storlie, F.   *Patient Teaching in Critical Care.* New York: Appleton-Century-Crofts, 1975.

Donald A. Bille

Developing a Philosophy
of Patient Teaching

How does learning occur?
Why are adult learners different from younger learners?
What can I do to promote the adult's learning?

Principles of teaching and learning have been known for many years. Current research, however, indicates that principles appropriate for teaching children may not be appropriate for teaching adults, especially the adult who must also adapt to being a patient. This chapter describes a philosophy of adult education, and how that philosophy changes once the adult enters the health-care system as a patient and client. Approaches for enhancing the effectiveness of teaching and learning are described.
    The information in this chapter should help the reader to

1. *List four assumptions about why adult learners are different*
2. *Describe implications of adult education theory for the patient educator*
3. *Formulate a personal philosophy appropriate to patient education*

The activities performed in patient education programs derive from the basic assumptions and beliefs the educator holds. These assumptions and beliefs form the educator's philosophy of education. The tenets of this philosophy have a profound effect on the success of the teaching. Therefore, it is useful for patient educators to examine their own beliefs and assumptions—their own philosophy—about how their patients learn. In some cases it may be necessary to adapt some of these beliefs and assumptions to accord with recent findings about how adults (especially patients) learn.

A sound philosophy of education should stem from scientific theories of learning. This requirement poses some problems, since "all of the scientific theories of learning have been derived from the study of learning by animals and children" [4]. These theories that form the framework for philosophies of pedagogy, may not always be best for the teaching of adults. Within the past few decades, some educational theorists have turned to studying the adult as a learner, and have formulated a theory of adult education, or *andragogy*. One such theorist is Knowles [5], who points out that adults learn differently from children for at least four reasons:

. . . 1. his self-concept moves from one of being a dependent personality toward one of being a self-directing human being; 2. he accumulates a growing reservoir of experience that becomes an increasing resource for learning; 3. his readiness to learn becomes oriented increasingly to the developmental tasks of his social roles; and, 4. his time perspective changes from one of postponed application of knowledge to immediacy of application, and accordingly his orientation toward learning shifts from one of subject-centeredness to one of problem-centeredness.

All educational theorists take their theoretic framework from research on the healthy learner. Illness and injury change certain psychologic processes that an individual calls upon during the learning process [1, 2, 7, 9]. Thus theories of both pedagogy and andragogy must be adapted to the learners who find themselves clients somewhere in the health-care system. In this chapter, each of Knowles's assumptions about the adult learner will be described. Adaptations of andragogic theory to the situation of patients and implications for the patient educator will be explored.

SELF CONCEPT

As an individual moves from childhood to adulthood, he also moves from complete dependency through various stages toward greater self-direction and independence. During this development of independence the adult also defines his role in life for example, as breadwinner, spouse, or homemaker. The healthy adult makes his own decisions and has learned to accept the consequences of a wrong decision. Thus the adult is self-responsible and self-directing. He believes that he can run his own life. Adults "tend to avoid, resist and resent being placed in situations in which they feel they are treated like children—told what to do and what not to do, talked down to, embarrassed, punished, judged" [6].

When the adult suffers an illness (whether in the hospital or not) he or she frequently indulges in some dependence on others. This may range from simply the dependence on a nurse to bring the medication at the proper moment to total dependence while critically ill. Hospitalization itself may threaten the adult's self-concept, because of institutional policies that mandate such normally self-controlled activities as mealtimes, bedtime, visiting regulations, and at what time of day personal hygiene measures are to be carried out.

Implications. Adults resist learning under conditions incongruent with their self-concept as autonomous individuals [6]. Virginia Henderson defined nursing as assisting the individual to perform health activities he would do unaided if he only possessed the strength, will, or knowledge to do so [3]. A philosophy of teaching adults, especially hospitalized adults, suggests then that certain elements be present to create the optimal learning environment.

First, a climate of mutual respect between the patient and his teacher must be created. The teacher must support rather than judge. The interactions between teacher and patient should be friendly and informal.

Second, patients can be helped to diagnose their own needs for learning. Through discussion and observation patients can discover for themselves what they most need to learn. The patient knows his own environment outside the hospital better than any other person. Thus, the patient will best identify what learning needs exist in order to cope more effectively with that environment after discharge.

Third, patients' learning needs that are diagnosed by the teacher do have a place in patient education, but they are not to be imposed on the patient with a "you have to do this" attitude. These needs are negotiated with the patient in the spirit of mutual respect.

Fourth, the patient needs to feel some responsibility for his or her own learning. Although the teacher is usually the content expert, the patient must feel that responsibility is shared between teacher and learner. One such responsibility is working with the teacher on translating diagnosed learning needs into specific educational objectives, and then designing learning experiences to achieve those objectives.

Fifth, the patient can evaluate the progress toward individualized learning objectives. Since the evaluation process involves judgment, the teacher should not be set up as the patient's judge, but rather should help the patient see the progress being made toward the objectives of the patient teaching program.

EXPERIENCE

Every adult has had a variety of experiences throughout life. These experiences may include travel, work, marriage, parenthood, and countless others. The adult defines who he or she is in terms of the experiences he or she has had, and therefore values these experiences highly.

Hospitalization is one experience that few humans learn to prepare for or cope with until it is too late to do so. New concepts can usually be grasped more easily when they relate to past experiences. This poses a problem for the patient who has never been hospitalized before, but it may also be a problem for the patient who has been hospitalized many times. Each stay in the hospital can reveal new needs, anxieties, and insights into the patient's personality.

Because of past experience, the patient may have fixed habits or thoughts. It will be more difficult, for instance, to achieve dietary changes when the patient experienced a satisfying life with a preferred diet. It will be more difficult to stop smoking when the patient has a higher pack-year history of smoking.

Reliance on experience and habit may hinder new learning, especially when the learning involves change of one's lifestyle. A great deal of encouragement and support will be required not only during hospitalization but also for several months following discharge, while the new knowledge or practice becomes a habit.

Implications. During hospitalization, as well as throughout the patient's exposure to the health-care system, it may seem easier for the teacher simply to put together a teaching program based on the textbook or on some standardized, diagnosis-based teaching plan. To do so, however, ignores or minimizes the importance of the adult's experience. The patient may feel that if you reject his experience, you reject him.

Since only the adult can tell the educator about personal experiences, a philosophy of teaching adults suggests that certain techniques will promote a feeling of acceptance between patient and teacher.

First, the adult needs a chance to be an active participant in all activities surrounding the educational program. Thus a lecture method of teaching is not as likely to be successful for the adult learner as an open, two-way discussion. Other techniques useful in the hospital include analysis of critical incidents, simulation exercises, and actual laboratory training.

Second, the life experiences must be taken into consideration when new concepts are illustrated. For instance, this author, while teaching a farmer about his arteriosclerotic heart disease (ASHD) learned that the farmer was adept at repairing his own tractor engine. In teaching about coronary circulation the author compared the tractor engine's oil pump to the coronary arteries. It was then much easier for the patient to realize the effects on the heart's chambers (cylinders) when they received no fresh blood (oil bath).

The experiences of many adults include a number of dissatisfying events throughout their earlier education. They may remember sitting in a long row of desks, getting rapped on the knuckles for each misbehavior, or standing in the corner as punishment for not learning the lesson well enough. Thus the patient educator must always be cognizant of the patient's feelings, yet at the same time provide objective, realistic, and nonthreatening feedback on the patient's performance. Above all, the patient must be involved in his own diagnosis of learning needs and goals.

READINESS TO LEARN

Children learn when they are physiologically and mentally mature enough to do so. For instance, children learn to walk when they are strong enough and have learned to crawl. Walking becomes a developmental task, and the child learns to walk only when it becomes a *personal* developmental task. The adult, on the other hand, learns primarily through the evolution of social roles. One learns how to fill the role of worker by first getting a job and then learning all about the job. One learns how to be a spouse by getting married and learning such skills as sharing and communicating. The patient cannot learn what it means to be a patient, then, until faced with illness or hospitalization. What may be even more frustrating for the hospital-based patient educator, is the fact that the patient will best perceive a need to learn about the posthospitalization concerns only after discharge.

Implications. The patient is ready to learn when he or she is faced with a concern that needs to be answered. Thus a patient educator should begin the program by eliciting those concerns the patient is dealing with at the moment. A philosophy of patient education would suggest several important points necessary to maximize the patient's readiness to learn.

First, the patient will be faced with many concerns about how lifestyle must change due to illness. Unless these concerns are dealt with first, the patient may not be ready to listen to anything else his teacher has to say to him. For instance, before beginning the standardized information given to every patient going into surgery, it is necessary to ask what the patient is concerned with or wondering about in light of the impending operation.

Second, when a patient faces any procedure, treatment, or medication, there will be information that he or she will want in order to participate fully in the decision of whether or not to go ahead with the procedure or treatment. By explaining each task before it is done, the teacher will help the patient learn about that task at the teachable moment—the time it is needed, before it is done.

Third, the patient will usually not have a realistic idea of what life will be like after returning home. The patient educator will need to listen carefully, therefore, to the patient's description of his or her usual life patterns before illness. This will assist the patient educator in providing a careful explanation of how that lifestyle has been changed by disease. Once the patient is aware of the need to learn about the altered lifestyle, it will be easier to learn what is needed to adapt to those changes.

TIME PERSPECTIVE

Throughout a person's childhood (during the time he is subjected to a pedagogic philosophy), his or her learning is traditionally organized around certain subjects such as history, English, and the sciences. The child learner is primarily accumulating facts and has a subject-centered focus. He is also more or less willing to postpone the use of learning until some future date. The adult, on the other hand, needs to feel that the skill or knowledge to be learned has immediate applicability. Learning has come to be a means of coping with life's problems; it has a problem-centered focus.

Implications. The teachable moment for the adult arrives when he recognizes that a problem needs to be solved. A philosophy of patient education needs approaches that are problem-centered.

First, the starting point of the patient's educational program should be the problems and concerns that exist at the beginning of the interaction with the teacher. It will be useful if the patient educator asks the patient about his questions and concerns before beginning any teaching interaction. A question such as "Your doctor wants you to be on a low-salt diet when you go home. What questions or concerns does this raise in your mind?" will be useful in starting the diagnosis of learning needs.

Second, the patient educator may have other objectives for the patient's learning that he or she expects to deal with, but these objectives should only be introduced after the patient's own questions have been answered. Thus, the patient who is facing a biopsy should be asked what concerns he or she has about the procedure before the educator tells anything else about the biopsy procedure. At times, the patient may reply, "I don't know anything about the procedure and don't know what to ask." At least this patient has been shown the respect that is due him or her before embarking on a more structured teaching program.

Third, the patient needs to recognize that a health problem exists before he or she will learn how to solve that problem. The patient needs to understand, for example, that heart damage exists before he or she will be willing to learn about how to change lifestyle because of that damage. When the patient denies that anything is wrong, it will do more harm than good to teach about the thing that is being denied. The result of teaching about a concept the patient is denying is that the patient may feel an even greater need to continue the denial.

Fourth, the patient educator needs to become known and trusted by the patient so that the patient will feel free to share those things that are of real concern. Realistically, the patient educator cannot expect to learn all about the patient and his or her concerns in the first few interactions. Trust and rapport take time to develop.

The foregoing beliefs and assumptions, based on how adults (especially patients) differ from children, form a basic philosophy of patient education; they help to place patient education into a certain perspective in which the patient is the focus.

The patient has made decisions about his own life for some time. This autonomy needs to continue if feelings of usefulness and cooperation are to be maintained. Patients should be included in planning their own patient education programs and allowed to make decisions about what they are to learn. Rosenberg [8] says

The use of an educational process that involves patient participation in the decision-making is the sine qua non for effective programming. Asked to provide a definition of patient education, I would say it would be the educational experiences planned with and for the patient by professional personnel as a component of his total care. Health care professionals must not forget that the physician no longer makes decisions once he or she has prescribed. It is the patient's decision to take the medication properly, to adhere to a diet, to maintain a proper exercise regimen. To put it another way, the physician makes the decision regarding therapy. The patient makes decisions regarding adherence, and in order for him to correctly make his decisions, he needs to know not only what and how, but why, what if, what if not, etc.

REFERENCES

1. Bille, D. A.   Patients' knowledge and compliance with posthospitalization prescriptions as related to body image and teaching format. Ph.D. dissertation, University of Wisconsin—Madison, 1975.
2. Crate, M. A.   Nursing functions in adaptation to chronic illness. *American Journal of Nursing,* 65 : 72, 1965.
3. Henderson, V.   The nature of nursing. *American Journal of Nursing,* 64 : 62, 1964.
4. Knowles, M.   *The Adult Learner: A Neglected Species* (2nd ed.). Houston: Gulf Publishing, 1973. P. 11.
5. Knowles, M.   *The Modern Practice of Adult Education: Andragogy Versus Pedagogy.* New York: Association Press, 1970. Pp. 39ff.
6. Knowles, M.   Program planning for adults as learners. *Adult Leadership,* 16 : 267, 1967.
7. Lederer, H. D.   How the sick view their world. *Journal of Social Issues,* 8 : 4, 1952.
8. Rosenberg, S. G.   Patient Education: An Educator's View. In A. R. Somers (Ed.), *Promoting Health: Consumer Education and National Policy.* Germantown, Maryland: Aspen Systems, 1976. Pp. 94–95.
9. Suchman, E. A.   Stages of illness and medical care. *Journal of Health and Human Behavior,* 6 : 114, 1965.

William H. Roach, Jr.

4

The Patient's Right to Know

What information must I give my patients?
How do the patient's rights intertwine with my responsibilities to teach?
What if I disagree with another health care team member, especially the physician?

Consumer rights, accountability of staff, and malpractice litigation are topics that should be of concern to every health care professional. Merely touching the patient or client involves each practitioner with certain rights and responsibilities—as well as potential litigation. The following chapter describes the doctrine of informed consent and the responsibility of doctors and nurses to assist patients and clients in reaching an informed choice. Current literature seems to minimize the role of the nurse in obtaining informed consent for nursing procedures. This chapter points out that nurses do need to teach, document teaching-learning outcomes, and (perhaps most important) communicate with the physician about the patient's teaching program. The nurse does not necessarily have to gain the physician's permission to teach, but rather facilitate communication so that all care providers have an accurate picture of the patient's care and teaching plans. It is likely that future litigation will more often involve nurses and result in more clearly defined regulations in the role of the nurse as patient educator.

The information in this chapter should help the reader to

1. *Define informed consent*
2. *List the basic elements of information necessary to informed consent*
3. *Describe situations in which information may be withheld from patients*
4. *Describe the legal ramifications of A Patient's Bill of Rights*
5. *Describe the nurse's duty to inform*

6. Describe the nurse's authority to inform
7. Describe actions to resolve conflicting judgments between a physician and a nurse

Traditional legal theories of patient consent provide a sound base for patient teaching. Well-established principles of battery and negligence law require physicians and nurses to give their patients certain information about proposed treatment, and, although practitioners are not legally required to *educate* their patients concerning illness and treatment, the legal advantages of formal teaching are readily apparent. This chapter discusses the legal principles underlying the practitioner's duty to inform and the relevance of these principles to formal methods of patient education.

THE DUTY TO INFORM THE PATIENT

It is a general rule that physicians must give their patients sufficient information upon which to make intelligent judgments as to whether to proceed with proposed medical treatment. Arising from traditional principles of the law of battery and modern theories of negligence law, this rule has been codified in recent years in some state statutes that require health care practitioners to give certain information to their patients before rendering treatment. Federal regulations now specify the kind of information physicians must give their patients before certain federally funded treatment may be performed. Moreover, the private health care industry, in response to consumer demands for greater sensitivity among health care personnel toward patients as people, has published A Patient's Bill of Rights that includes the right to receive information about proposed treatment. Thus, although the authorities may disagree about exactly what and how much information one must provide a patient, most agree that the patient should receive enough information concerning proposed treatment to make a reasoned, informed choice to accept or reject the care recommended.

Consent to Treatment

The duty to inform grows out of the traditional law of battery that holds that a person has the right to be free from unwarranted and unauthorized physical interference. This fundamental principle was applied in a medical care setting as early as 1905 in the Illinois case of *Pratt* v. *Davis* [1], and in the 1914 New York case of *Schoendorff* v. *New York Hospital* [2]. The holding in *Schoendorff*, written by the eminent Justice Cardozo, and quoted in every treatise on informed consent, is still sound law today [3]:

Every human being of adult years and sound mind has a right to determine what shall be done with his own body; and a surgeon who performs an operation without his patient's consent commits an assault, for which he is liable in damages.

Performing a medical procedure upon a patient without proper consent constitutes a battery and renders the treating party liable in damages even though the patient may have suffered no injuries. Actual bodily contact with the patient is not necessary for a battery to occur. It is sufficient if the touching occurs through the use of some instrument, such as x-rays, sound waves, medication, or other treatment methods under the control of the treating practitioner.

The consent or authorization of the person who is touched (the patient in the medical care setting) provides a complete defense to an action in battery. The patient who has given valid consent to treatment cannot be heard to complain of the touching that necessarily accompanied the treatment, even though the patient may have suffered actual harm. However, a consent obtained through misrepresentation, fraud, or duress is invalid, as are a consent given by one who had no authority to give it and a consent to perform an unlawful act.

A patient's consent may be express or implied. Express consent is a verbal or written authorization to perform a specified procedure or render certain treatment. The patient's statement, "Yes, you may give me an injection of penicillin," and his signature on a hospital's printed Consent to Surgery form both are examples of express consent to treatment upon which physicians and nurses routinely rely.

In certain circumstances consent may be implied from the patient's own behavior and by application of law. A patient who voluntarily submits himself for treatment may by his own conduct give rise to an implication that he has consented to such treatment, even though he has not given his express consent. In *O'Brien* v. *Cunard Steamship Company* [4], an 1891 Massachusetts case, the plaintiff, a passenger on an ocean steamer, observed a man in a white coat giving injections to persons as they reached the front of a line which had formed on deck. The plaintiff joined the line and in due course received an injection. When he sued the steamship company, alleging battery by its employed physician, the court held that the plaintiff had implied consent to the injection by voluntarily presenting himself for treatment, and that, therefore, no battery had occurred.

The implication of consent from voluntary submission is not unlimited, however. The courts require that, for such consent to be valid, the patient have some understanding of the nature of the treatment involved and the common risks associated with it and have an opportunity to withdraw from the treatment. Implied consent will not likely arise, therefore, if the treatment is a highly complex medical procedure involving a multiplicity of risks or if the patient is unable to stop the treatment and withdraw.

Patient consent may also be implied by application of law in certain fact situations. Generally, the courts will find the patient's consent implied when the patient is suffering from an emergent condition [5]. The courts assume that the patient would expressly authorize treatment necessary to protect his health or life if he could and, therefore, as a matter of law find that the emergency condition implies the patient's consent. For consent to be implied by the patient's condition, the proposed treatment must be for the patient's benefit, a true emergency must exist, and neither the patient nor someone authorized to act on the patient's behalf is able to give express consent [6]. An emergency is a condition in which there is an immediate threat to the life, person, or health of the patient and the hazard to the patient will increase if treatment is delayed [7].

The courts will also find implied consent by application of a statute. For example, the statutes of several states declare that a person who operates a motor vehicle on the public streets in the state automatically consents to a test to determine the alcoholic content of his blood [8]. Where such a statute is applicable, the practitioner need not obtain the patient's express consent because it is implied as a matter of law.

When consent may be implied, there is no *legal* duty to obtain express consent and therefore no legal duty to give the patient information about the proposed treatment. Although it is advisable not to treat a patient without giving the patient an explanation of the proposed treatment, in these situations such an explanation may be useless (as in an emergency or when testing the blood alcohol of an inebriate) or unnecessary (as when the patient has voluntarily submitted himself for a routine procedure).

Informed Consent

Unlike the traditional theories of consent to treatment that are grounded in the law of battery, the doctrine of informed consent generally applies to the law of negligence and concerns a physician's negligent failure to disclose adequate information to a patient about to undergo medical treatment. *Informed consent* means just what it suggests: giving the patient sufficient information upon which to make a reasoned, informed decision about the proposed treatment and the patient's authorization to treat. The doctrine arose from court decisions that held the traditional theories of battery to be inadequate or inappropriate when applied to cases in which the patient gave consent to treatment but was not advised of all the risks associated with such treatment and was injured when one of the undisclosed risks materialized. The courts found that, whereas an uninformed consent might be sufficient to defeat an action in battery, a physician may be liable in negligence if the information he disclosed to the patient failed to meet the applicable standard of disclosure.

Although there is still some debate in the legal literature as to whether informed consent is based upon battery or negligence, most courts agree that negligence is the proper theory of liability when the physician has failed to disclose adequate information about a proposed treatment [9]. However, battery may still be the appropriate theory of liability in cases in which the patient consents to one procedure, but the physician (1) performs an entirely different procedure, (2) fails to disclose a contingency that is certain to occur if the patient undergoes the proposed nonemergency treatment, or (3) fails to disclose that the procedure performed was experimental in nature [10].

The major problem in applying the doctrine of informed consent is determining what information the practitioner must disclose to a patient. There are primarily two standards of disclosure applied by the courts of the various states: the professional standard and the material risk standard.

The courts in a majority of states measure the physician's duty to disclose by the professional standard, that is, the customary disclosure practices of other physicians [11]. Most of these courts require a physician to disclose what a reasonable physician would disclose when practicing under the same or similar circumstances [12]. Other courts following the majority rule have held that a physician must inform the patient in accordance with "prevailing medical practice" [13] or consistent with disclosures of other physicians in the same or similar community [14]. And in *Ridinger v. Colburn* [15] the court held that the physician's duty of disclosure is measured by the disclosure practices of physicians in the community, but that when relatively complicated surgery is involved the physician must disclose known risks of death or serious bodily injury. In the jurisdictions following the professional standards rule, the plaintiff has the burden of proving through expert testimony that the defendant physician failed to meet the applicable standard of disclosure [16].

The trend in the United States is represented by a minority of states, in which the courts have adopted the more stringent material risk standard of disclosure. In *Wilkinson v. Vesey* [17] the Rhode Island Supreme Court stated that the patient's right to do with his body as he wills "should not be delegated to a local medical group." The court held that a physician must disclose all facts that a reasonable person would consider material in view of the severity of risk associated with the proposed treatment and the likelihood of its occurrence—the more serious or likely the danger, the more probable that it will be perceived by a reasonable person as material [18]. Likewise, the California Supreme Court, in *Cobbs v. Grant* [19], rejected the professional standard as overbroad and nebulous and declared that a physician must disclose known risks of death or serious bodily harm and any other information that would be material to the patient's decision concerning the proposed treatment. The court stated that although a physician is not required to give the patient "a minicourse in medical science," the physician should disclose the nature and purpose of the proposed procedure, the risks and benefits reasonably to be expected and the alternative methods of treatment, if any [20]. The court in *Canterbury v. Spence* [21] agreed that requiring physicians to disclose every possible risk would be "obviously prohibitive and unrealistic" and that a physician must disclose only information material to the patient's decision of whether to accept the proposed treatment [22]. In states that have adopted the material risk standard, the plaintiff does not need expert testimony to prove the defendant physician failed to meet the standard of disclosure, since the courts will allow the jury to determine what information was "material." Expert testimony may still be required to show the nature of the procedure and risks involved and the causal relationship between the defendant's failure to disclose and the plaintiff's injury.

Who Must Give Consent?

The general rule is that the patient, if a competent adult, must consent to proposed treatment. Incompetent patients and minor patients, however, constitute notable exceptions to this rule.

The courts consider a patient who is so incapacitated by illness or injury as to be unable to understand the nature and consequences of his conduct to be incompetent to give consent [23]. The incompetent patient's physician must obtain an informed consent, sometimes referred to as *substituted consent,* from the patient's authorized representative, who may be a court appointed guardian or conservator if the patient has been adjudicated to be incompetent, or the patient's closest known relative. The patient's representative stands in the place of the patient and has the same rights as the patient would have if he were competent to consent to information concerning the proposed treatment. Failure to disclose information to the incompetent patient's representative consistent with the applicable standard of disclosure will subject the physician to liability for failure to obtain an informed consent.

Minors are persons who have not reached the age of majority in the state in which they reside and are considered legally incompetent to consent to their own medical care. As a general rule, therefore, one may not treat a minor without first obtaining the informed consent of the minor's parent or legal guardian. This rule is shot through with exceptions, however. Most states have enacted legislation that allows certain categories of minors to consent to their own medical care, including pregnant minors, married minors, minors in need of birth control services, minors suffering from drug abuse or venereal disease, and minors requiring emergency care. In addition, the courts of some states confer authority to consent to medical care on an emancipated minor, one who is living apart from his parents and conducting and supporting his own affairs. As the laws governing minors' consent vary from state to state, one should not undertake to treat a minor patient without a thorough understanding of applicable consent rules.

If a minor patient does not fall into one of the categories of minors who may consent to their own care, the patient's parent or legal guardian must consent to proposed treatment. The general rules of informed consent requiring adequate disclosure apply, and the practitioner who fails to give sufficient information to the patient's parent or guardian will be liable for injuries that occur as a result.

Statutorily Mandated Consent

In response to documented and well-publicized abuses of patient rights by some medical researchers and physicians, the federal government has issued regulations that govern the consents of persons who participate as subjects of drug research [24] or medical research supported by federal funds [25] and the consents of persons undergoing sterilizations paid for by federal funds [26]. These regulations spell out in detail the type of information to be given patients and the manner in which such information must be presented.

Before a practitioner may engage in research that would place human subjects at risk, as defined by the regulations, the practitioner must obtain the subject's informed consent that is defined quite specifically as follows [27]:

"Informed consent" means the knowing consent of an individual or his legally authorized representative, so situated as to be able to exercise free power of choice, without undue inducement or any element of force, fraud, deceit, duress, or other form of constraint or coercion. The basic elements of information necessary to such consent include:

1. A fair explanation of the procedures to be followed and their purposes, including identification of any procedures which are experimental;
2. A description of any attendant discomforts and risks reasonably to be expected;
3. A description of any benefits reasonably to be expected;
4. A disclosure of any appropriate alternative procedures that might be advantageous for the subject;
5. An offer to answer any inquiries concerning the procedures; and
6. An instruction that the person is free to withdraw his consent and to discontinue participation in the project or activity at any time without prejudice to the subject.

The regulations further specify the format the subject's consent form must take and require the form to be approved prior to use by an approved institutional review board of a hospital or facility that is authorized to conduct federally funded medical research.

Regulations issued by the (then) United States Department of Health, Education, and Welfare pursuant to the Food, Drug, and Cosmetic Act [28] require an investigator using investigational, that is, experimental, drugs to certify that

he will inform any patients or any persons used as controls, or their representatives, that drugs are being used for investigational purposes, and will obtain the consent of the subjects, or their representatives, except where this is not feasible or, in the investigator's professional judgment, is contrary to the best interests of the subjects.

These regulations [29] define *consent* to mean

that the person involved has legal capacity to give consent, is so situated as to be able to exercise free power of choice, and is provided with a fair explanation of pertinent information concerning the investigational drug, and/or possible use of a control, as to enable him to make a decision on his willingness to receive said investigational drug. This latter element means that before the acceptance of an affirmative decision by such person the investigator should carefully consider and make known to him (taking into consideration such person's well-being and his ability to understand) the nature, expected duration, and purpose of the administration of said investigational drug; the method and means by which it is to be administered; the hazards involved; the existence of alternative forms of therapy, if any, and the beneficial effects upon his health or person that may possibly come from the administration of the investigational drug.

This consent is required in all cases in which an investigational drug is administered "primarily for the accumulation of scientific knowledge" or is administered to patients who are otherwise receiving medical care [30].

Federal regulations governing sterilizations prohibit nonemergency sterilizations upon any patient in a program supported by federal funds administered by the United States Public Health Service or whose care is paid for by Medicaid unless, among other things, the phyisician first obtains the patient's informed consent on forms prescribed by the regulations [31]. Informed consent in sterilization procedures is described as follows [32]:

1. Advice that the individual is free to withhold or withdraw consent to the procedure any time before the sterilization without affecting his or her right to future care or treatment and without loss or withdrawal of any federally funded program benefits to which the individual might be otherwise entitled;
2. A description of available alternative methods of family planning and birth control;
3. Advice that the sterilization procedure is considered to be irreversible;
4. A thorough explanation of the specific sterilization procedure to be performed;
5. A full description of the discomforts and risks that may accompany or follow the performing of the procedure, including an explanation of the type and possible effects of any anesthetic to be used;
6. A full description of the benefits or advantages that may be expected as a result of the sterilization; and
7. Advice that the sterilization will not be performed for at least 30 days except under the circumstances specified [elsewhere in the regulations].

The regulations also specify the exact wording of the consent form and the manner in which it must be presented and witnessed.

In addition, some states have enacted statutes that define a practitioner's duty to obtain patients' consent to proposed treatment [33]. A few statutes set forth the information a practitioner must give the patient [34] and declare that a signed document attesting that the information was given constitutes conclusive evidence that the patient gave informed consent to treatment. Other statutes codify the professional standard of disclosure and establish a cause of action against the practitioner who fails to meet the standard [35].

Additional Disclosure Requirements

The physician's duty to inform his patient is not limited merely to disclosing information that might be material to the patient's decision concerning proposed treatment. In most cases, a physician must also advise the patient of the diagnosis he has formed and give the patient adequate instructions to enable the patient to care for himself properly.

It is generally recognized that a physician has a duty to inform his patient of the diagnosis he has formed [36]. When a physician fails to advise the patient of the diagnosis or the results of a diagnostic test, the physician will be liable in negligence for any injuries the patient suffers as a result [37]. However, in *Sinkey* v. *Surgical Associates* [38], the court stated that a physician's duty to inform the patient of an unfavorable diagnosis does not extend to a disclosure of all diagnoses that might arise from the patient's condition. A physician is not required to disclose a speculative or indefinite diagnosis. However, when the physician makes a reasonable effort to inform the patient of important test results but is unable to do so because the patient gave misleading information concerning his address and telephone number, the physician will not be held liable for damages the patient may incur due to his failure to receive the test results [39]. Finally, if the patient is not injured as a result of the physician's failure to disclose a diagnosis or test result, the physician will not be found negligent for such nondisclosure. The failure to inform must have caused an injury before liability will attach [40].

A physician also has a duty to give the patient or the patient's family all necessary instructions as to the care to be given the patient and the cautions to be observed in attending the patient; failure to give such instructions will render the physician liable for resulting injury [41]. In *Barnes v. Bovenmeyer* [42] the defendant physician failed to remove a splinter of steel from the patient's eye, even though the object was clearly visible upon x-ray examination, and failed to give the patient instructions as to how and where he should seek treatment for its removal. As a result, the patient did not receive necessary surgery soon enough, and lost the eye to infection. The court states: "It is a duty of a physician taking charge of a case to follow the case and to give proper instructions to the patient as to his future acts and conduct" [43]. When the patient is unable to care for himself properly and is discharged in the care of a friend, the physician must instruct the friend concerning the patient's continued treatment. In *Batemen v. Rosenberg* [44] the physician discharged an adult patient following a tonsillectomy without giving the patient's neighbor who accompanied the patient to her home instructions as to how to position the patient so as to prevent blood from collecting in the patient's airway. The neighbor, who had no nursing experience, put the patient to bed in such a way that she died of strangulation from blood in her bronchial tree. The court held that the jury could find the physician liable for failing to ascertain whether the patient would be adequately supervised and to give sufficient instructions for the patient's care [45]. If the patient is a minor, the physician has a duty to instruct the patient's parents or guardian concerning the patient's care [46]. Likewise, the physician must inform an incompetent patient's representative of the need for providing medical care or treatment to the patient [47].

A physician also may have a duty to disclose to the patient the identity and status of the persons who will be treating the patient. Although no cases have been reported that hold a physician liable for failing to identify a practitioner as a student, there is opinion that such failure may create exposure both for the physician and the institution in which the student is practicing [48]. Similarly, the practice in some teaching hospitals of allowing resident physicians to operate on a patient without informing the patient that surgery will be performed by a surgical team, including such residents, has been criticized [49]. Although the courts have not as yet recognized specifically the duty to identify students and resident physicians, disclosing the identity of the professional staff who will be treating the patient is advisable.

THE PHYSICIAN'S PRIVILEGE TO WITHHOLD INFORMATION

There is a well-recognized exception to the general rules of disclosure that excuses a physician's withholding information from a patient. This *therapeutic privilege* is allowed to protect a patient from disclosure that might be unhealthful to the patient. In *Cornfeldt v. Tongen* [50] the court stated that, for the therapeutic privilege to apply, the physician must determine that disclosure of the information would complicate or hinder treatment, cause such emotional distress as to preclude a rational decision by the patient concerning the proposed treatment, or cause psychologic harm to the patient. It is clear, however, that a physician may not remain silent simply because disclosure of information about the proposed care would prompt the patient to forego treatment [51]. If the physician determines that in view of the patient's condition, nondisclosure is warranted, the physician should obtain the informed consent of a close relative of the patient who can act on the patient's behalf [52]. As the burden of proof in most cases will be upon the physician to show that the prerequisites for application of the therapeutic privilege have been met, it is extremely important for the physician to be able to show, on the basis of the patient's record and other evidence that may be available to document the patient's condition, that disclosure of information was contraindicated.

A PATIENT'S BILL OF RIGHTS

During the past two decades consumer interest in the health care industry has increased markedly and has resulted in a closer examination of industry practices by patient advocacy and other consumer groups. Partly in response to the demands of these organizations, the American Hospital Association (AHA) published its Patient's Bill of Rights in 1972 as a guide for hospitals to use in treating their patients. The AHA Bill of Rights states explicitly that the patient should receive adequate information about his case [53]:

2. The patient has the right to obtain from his physician complete current information concerning his diagnosis, treatment, and prognosis in terms the patient can be reasonably expected to understand. When it is not medically advisable to give such information to the patient, the information should be made available to an appropriate person in his behalf. He has the right to know by name the physician responsible for coordinating his care.
3. The patient has the right to receive from his physician information necessary to give informed consent prior to the start of any procedure and/or treatment. Except in emergencies, such information for informed consent should include but not necessarily be limited to the specific procedure and/or treatment, the medically significant risks involved, and the probable duration of incapacitation. Where medically significant alternatives for care or treatment exist, or when the patient requests information concerning medical alternatives, the patient has the right to such information. The patient also has the right to know the name of the person responsible for the procedures and/or treatment.
4. The patient has the right to refuse treatment to the extent permitted by law, and to be informed of the medical consequences of his action.

. . . . .

8. The patient has the right to obtain information as to any relationship of his hospital to other health care and educational institutions insofar as his care is concerned. The patient has the right to obtain information as to the existence of any professional relationships among individuals, by name, who are treating him.
9. The patient has the right to be advised if the hospital proposes to engage in or perform human experimentation affecting his care or treatment. The patient has the right to refuse to participate in such research projects.

Since the publication of the AHA Bill of Rights, other organizations have created similar documents pertaining to specific categories of patients: elderly patients, minor patients, pregnant patients, dying patients, handicapped patients, mentally ill patients. All of these pronouncements include some provision for disclosing information that may be material to the patient's choice of treatment [54]. In most states a patient's bill of rights has no force and effect of law; rather, it is a statement of policy or a set of guidelines that its authors hope will be used by hospitals and practitioners in treating patients.

In at least two situations, however, a patient's bill of rights can create an affirmative duty to adhere to the code of conduct it prescribes. When a state has included all or a portion of the AHA Bill of Rights in a statute, failure to comply with it will constitute a violation of law. For example, Minnesota incorporated the AHA document almost verbatim into a state statute that includes stiff enforcement provisions [55]. In addition, some hospitals and other institutions have adopted the AHA Bill of Rights as official institutional policy. Inasmuch as failure to follow hospital policy in many states can subject the hospital, a nurse, or a physician to liability in negligence for any resulting injuries to the patient, practitioners working in an institution that has adopted the AHA Bill of Rights as official policy must afford its patients all of the rights described in the policy, including disclosure of information. Clearly, a hospital should not adopt the AHA Bill of Rights as institutional policy without careful consideration of its effect upon medical and nursing staff.

THE NURSE'S DUTY TO PROVIDE INFORMATION

As a general rule, the theories of disclosure of information and of informed consent that have been enunciated in terms of the physician's duty are applicable to nurses practicing in a clinical setting. Although the primary responsibility for informing the patient lies with the patient's physician and although the author has found no cases reported that hold a nurse liable for nondisclosure of information, there is little doubt that nurses attending the patient must advise the patient about the nursing care that has been ordered or that is proposed. The same rules of patient consent apply to nursing and medical treatment, and a nurse's failure to obtain the patient's consent to a nursing procedure will create liability in the nurse for any injury that may result. A nurse should have the patient's express or implied consent to any touching by the nurse and the patient's informed consent to proposed nursing procedures, especially those that involve high risk or are particularly complex.

It is not clear whether a professional nurse has a therapeutic privilege to withhold otherwise necessary information from the patient. If nurses are considered competent to determine what nursing care the patient requires, it follows that nurses should be able to determine whether the patient's condition indicates that withholding information would be in the patient's best interest. Given the strong consumer interest in disclosure of information to patients, however, and the trend in some states to a broader standard of disclosure, a professional nurse who believes disclosure would be harmful to the patient should consult with the patient's physician before remaining silent. In view of the cases decided on the question of therapeutic privilege, the courts will likely look to the physician for a determination on the appropriateness of disclosure. If the physician agrees that the patient should not receive information about the proposed treatment, the nurse and the physician are less likely to be attacked successfully for failure to inform.

A nurse's duty to inform does not end with disclosure of information about proposed nursing care. Nurses employed by a hospital to perform clinical nursing functions also have a duty to advise their patients concerning the policies, rules, and regulations of the hospital. Policies regarding visitation, medications, smoking, bed-rails, preoperative procedures, and use of equipment can significantly affect the patient's well-being. In most institutions it is the nurse's responsibility to see that patients understand the rules. Clearly, a nurse's failure to inform a patient concerning an important policy, such as use of bed-rails, could result in serious injury to the patient and substantial liability for the nurse and the hospital.

Professional nurses may acquire responsibility for informing and instructing patients concerning *medical* treatment. In some clinical settings and for certain procedures, it is customary for physicians to delegate this function to professional nursing staff. In some states, for example, nurses who have received advanced training in obstetrical care may be authorized by statute to act as nurse-midwives [56], and in so doing acquire the duty to inform their patients consistent with the medical standard of disclosure in their states. Where no enabling statute exists, physicians still may delegate to nurses the task of informing patients about certain proposed medical treatments. However, this delegation can be extremely hazardous for nurses inasmuch as a nurse legally has no "physician judgment" to rely upon in determining what information a patient should receive and may have insufficient knowledge of the proposed treatment to advise the patient properly. Therefore, nurses should accept such delegation only when (1) they are thoroughly familiar with the procedure or treatment involved, and (2) there are specific written guidelines approved by a licensed physician that describe what information is to be given to the patient or a written statement approved by a licensed physician that includes the information the patient will require and that the nurse may use in her communication with the patient. Delegation of disclosure duties is common in clinics where the same procedures are performed routinely (for example, prenatal and family planning clinics) and, if these safeguards are in place, is perfectly acceptable.

The courts have not yet held specifically that a physician or a nurse has a duty to *educate* patients. To the extent patient instruction is necessary to advise a patient of the nature of proposed treatment or how to care for himself, physicians and nurses have a duty to provide it, but extensive, general patient teaching is not required by law. Nevertheless, patient education is widely recognized as an important part of health care and may be provided by a variety of professional health personnel working in coordination with their patients' physicians.

In many cases documentation of information given to patients is essential. When the information provided is necessary to enable the patient to care for himself or to make an informed decision concerning proposed treatment, practitioners should make a permanent record of the information given. In hospitals and other institutions a standard consent form may be used to document the information the patient received. The patient's medical record, whether in a hospital or physician's private office, can be used to record instructions given to the patient. Some hospitals give their patients preprinted discharge instructions concerning their follow-up care or symptoms to look for after they leave the hospital. Specific documentation provides a better record of the physician's or nurse's disclosure, but a summary of the information given will usually suffice. A good record of information provided patients will often prevent a patient from successfully bringing a legal action against a hospital or practitioner for injuries allegedly resulting from a failure to provide information.

The Nurse's Authority to Provide Information

What acts a professional nurse legally may perform as a nurse are set forth in the definition of "professional nursing" contained in the nurse practice act of each state. The definition varies from state to state, and no nurse should engage in clinical nursing without a thorough understanding of the nurse practice act of the state in which he or she practices.

The nurse practice acts of some states specifically authorize professional nurses to teach their patients. The Connecticut statute [57], for example, states that the practice of nursing means

the process of diagnosing human responses to actual or potential health problems, providing supportive and restorative care, *health counseling and teaching,* case finding and referral, collaborating in the implementation of the total health care regimen and executing the medical regimen under the direction of a licensed physician or dentist. [Emphasis added.]

New York and New Jersey practice acts have similar provisions [58]. In states that specifically define the practice of nursing to include teaching, nurses are statutorily authorized to instruct their patients concerning health problems.

In other states, licensure laws have failed to keep pace with customary nursing practice and have not specifically authorized nurses to teach patients. In Illinois [59], for example, *professional nursing* is defined as

the performance for compensation of any nursing act (a) in the observation, care and counsel of the ill, injured, or infirm; or (b) in the maintenance of health or prevention of illness of others; or (c) the administration of medications and treatments as prescribed by a licensed physician or dentist; or (d) any act in the supervision or teaching of nursing; any of which requires substantial specialized judgment and skill and the proper performance of which is based on knowledge and application of the principles of biological, physical and social science acquired by means of a completed course in an approved school of professional nursing. The foregoing shall not be deemed to include those acts of medical diagnosis or prescription of therapeutic or corrective measures which are properly performed only by physicians licensed in the State of Illinois.

Here the statute gives no clear direction concerning patient teaching; therefore, teaching patients about their medical care may be legally hazardous for a nurse, unless the nurse's instruction is part of a treatment regimen or plan of care approved by the patient's physician.

In states where patient teaching is not clearly authorized by statute, a teaching program may be authorized by physician order. Seen as part of the patient's overall treatment, teaching prescribed by a physician is within the scope of licensure for professional nurses in all states. When health care is a team effort, all professional personnel involved can provide patient education under the guidance of the patient's physician. If the patient is under the care of a physician and a primary nurse, the nurse will often provide extensive patient teaching coordinated with the patient's medical care provided by the physician. The expanding use of programmed teaching aids and sophisiticated intrahospital video instruction, often developed by physician-nurse teams, has created a growing demand for patient education, and physicians have increasingly looked to nursing personnel to provide it.

A physician need not order teaching for the patient in each individual case. An institutionalized program established as a routine procedure and supported either by a standing physician order or by guidelines describing the general patient education effort and approved by a physician will protect nurses providing patient training in accordance with the accepted program from allegations of improper practice.

Conflict Between Nurse and Physician

A nurse who provides unauthorized patient teaching or instruction or who improperly discloses information to a patient or the patient's family may incur, at best, the strong disapproval of his or her colleagues and, at worst, exposure to legal liability. Providing information that may be harmful to the patient will likely subject the nurse to liability in negligence for any injuries that result, if it can be shown that a competent nurse would not have provided such information under the same or similar circumstances. If the patient's physician in the proper exercise of the therapeutic privilege has directed the nursing staff to refrain from disclosing information to the patient, a nurse who violates the order will likely be liable for resulting injuries to the patient. Regardless of the nurse's beliefs concerning the "right" to teach patients, the nurse must avoid conduct that a court would consider inconsistent with the standard of care of professional nurses in the community. Failure to meet such a standard, whether by improperly performing a nursing task or by improperly disclosing information to a patient, will subject the nurse to liability in negligence for injuries that result.

Improper disclosure of information may also be grounds for revocation or suspension of a nurse's license to practice, as shown by a recent case in which the Idaho State Board of Nursing suspended a nurse's license for six months after a physician complained that she had inappropriately discussed treatment alternatives with his patient [60]. The nurse's unauthorized discussion of laetrile as an alternative to the cancer therapy prescribed by the patient's physician delayed the patient's prescribed treatment. The Board's Hearing Officer found that the nurse asked the patient not to tell the physician that she had discussed laetrile and advised the patient that, although laetrile was an illegal drug in Idaho, it could be obtained. Testimony showed that the nurse realized the information presented to the patient was of an illegal and unethical nature [61]. The decision of the Idaho State Board of Nursing does not indicate that a nurse does not have a responsibility to teach patients; it demonstrates that state licensing authorities may not tolerate patient instruction that includes inappropriate information or that conflicts with the attending physician's treatment.

The nurse appealed the Board's action to the Idaho District Court which upheld the Board's six-month license suspension order. However, the Idaho Supreme Court reversed the District Court and struck down the Board's action on the grounds that it had failed to give the nurse adequate due process. It is important to note that the court *did not* hold that a nurse has a right to educate her patient, but held that the Idaho Board of Nursing may not declare as "unprofessional conduct" activities that the Board has not specifically proscribed in its rules and regulations [62].

The importance of the Idaho case is that it demonstrates the difficulties that can develop when a nurse undertakes to instruct a patient without coordinating her effort with the patient's physician. But what should a nurse do when the physician prohibits teaching that the nurse believes, based upon his or her experience and professional judgment, is necessary for the patient's well-being? There are no reported cases that address this precise question, but the few decisions that discuss a nurse's duty to seek intervention when the patient needs care or when a physician's order is unclear or contraindicated are instructive.

In *Toth* v. *Community Hospital at Glen Cove* [63] the court held that the primary duty of a hospital staff nurse is to follow the physician's orders, except when the nurse knows that the physician's orders are so clearly contraindicated by normal practice that ordinary prudence requires inquiry into the correctness of such orders. In the more recent case of *Carlsen* v. *Javurek* [64] the court stated that, when a nurse anesthetist disagreed with the patient's physician as to the type of anesthetic to use during surgery, she had a duty to discuss the anesthetic order with the physician and, if no agreement could be reached, to seek cancellation of the operation [65]. In the important case of *Norton* v. *Argonaut Insurance Company* [66] the court held a nurse liable in negligence for failing to know the different methods of administering a dangerous drug and for failing to seek clarification of the physician's drug order. The court stated [67] that

not only was [the nurse] unfamiliar with the medicine in question, but she also violated what has been shown to be the rule generally practiced by the members of the nursing profession in the community . . . namely, the practice of calling the prescribing physician when in doubt about an order for medication.

The ordering physician also was held liable for his failure to write an explicit medication order. Finally, in *Goff* v. *Doctors General Hospital of San Jose* [68] the defendant hospital was found liable for the patient's death resulting from the hospital nurse's failure to seek the assistance of the patient's physician. Although the patient's obstetrician had instructed the nurse to telephone him if his patient's postpartum bleeding was excessive, the nurse failed to do so because she disagreed with the physician's treatment methods, and, as a result, the patient died of hemorrhage.

The rules of these cases are applicable when a nurse and physician disagree over whether the nurse should engage in patient teaching or should inform the patient about proposed treatment or treatment alternatives. If a nurse, in his or her professional judgment, believes the patient should receive information that the physician refuses to give or to authorize the nurse to give, the nurse should first advise the physician that he or she disagrees and why and, if agreement cannot be reached, seek the intervention of a nursing, medical, or administrative superior in the institution. The nurse must seek the help of a decision-maker to resolve the matter in a rational manner, for the law will not likely support a nurse who erroneously violates the orders of the patient's physician. Each case of disagreement requires the exercise of sound professional judgment and diplomacy. The nurse must determine, given the circumstances of each case, how far he or she must go to resolve the controversy.

REFERENCES

1. 118 Ill. App. 161 (1905), *aff'd,* 224 Ill. 300, 79 N.E. 562 (1906).
2. 211 N.Y. 125, 105 N.E. 92 (1914), *overruled on other grounds,* Bing v. Thunig, 2 N.Y. 2d 656, 143 N.E. 2d 3, 163 N.Y.S.2d 3 (1957).
3. 211 N.Y. at 126, 105 N.E. at 93.
4. 154 Mass. 272, 28 N.E. 266 (1891).
5. 61 AM. JUR. 2d "Physicians and Surgeons" §159 (1972).
6. Tabor v. Scobee, 254 S.W.2d 474 (Ct. App. Ky. 1952); Jackovach v. Yocom, 212 Iowa 914, 237 N.W. 444 (1931); Luka v. Lowrie, 171 Mich. 122, 136 N.W. 1106 (1912).
7. Luka v. Lowrie, 171 Mich. 122, 136 N.W. 1106 (1912).
8. See, for example, Ill. Ann. Stat. ch. 95 1/2 §11-501.1 (Smith-Hurd Supp. 1978).
9. Annot., 88 A.L.R.3d 1008 (1978); See Note, Informed Consent Liability, 26 DRAKE L. REV. 696 (1977).
10. Fiorentino v. Wenger, 19 N.Y.2d 407, 227 N.E.2d 296 (1967); Bang v. Charles T. Miller Hospital, 251 Minn. 427, 88 N.W. 2d 188 (1958).
11. Annot., 88 A.L.R. 3d 1008 (1978).
12. Moore v. Underwood Memorial Hospital, 147 N.J. Super. 252, 371 A.2d 105 (1977); Hood v. Phillips, 554 S.W. 2d 160 (Tex. 1977); Thomas v. Berrios, 348 So. 2d 905 (Fla. App. 1977); Miceikis v. Field, 37 Ill. App. 3d 763, 347 N.E.2d 320 (1976); Nishi v. Hartwell, 52 Hawaii 188, 473 P.2d 116 (1970).
13. Riedisser v. Nelson, 111 Ariz. 542, 534 P.2d 1052 (1975).
14. Butler v. Berkely, 25 N.C. App. 325, 213 S.E.2d 571 (1975).
15. 361 F. Supp. 1073 (D.C. Idaho 1973).
16. Annot., 52 A.L.R.3d 1084 (1973).
17. 110 R.I. 606, 295 A.2d 676 (1972).
18. See also Cornfeldt v. Tongen, 262 N.W.2d 684 (1977).
19. 8 Cal. 3d 229, 502 P.2d 1, 104 Cal. Rptr. 505 (1972).
20. *Id.* at 244, 502 P.2d at 11, 104 Cal Rptr. at 515.
21. 464 F.2d 772 (D.C. Cir. 1972).
22. *Id.* at 786.
23. See Grannum v. Berard, 70 Wash. 2d 304, 422 P.2d 812 (1967).

24. 21 U.S.C.A. §321 et seq. (1972); 21 C.F.R. §310.102 and 312.1 (1978).
25. 45 C.F.R. §46.101 et seq. (1978).
26. 43 Fed. Reg. 52146 et seq. (1978).
27. 45 C.F.R. §46.103(c) (1978). On November 3, 1978, the Department of Health, Education, and Welfare issued interim final regulations which add the following paragraph to the definition of "informed consent" effective January 2, 1979:

> (7) with respect to biomedical or behavioral research which may result in physical injury, and explanation as to whether compensation and medical treatment is available if physical injury occurs and, if so, what it consists of or where further information may be obtained. This subparagraph will apply to research conducted abroad in collaboration with foreign governments or international organizations absent the explicit nonconcurrence of those governments or organizations. 43 Fed. Reg. 51559 (1978).

28. 21 C.F.R. §312.1(a)(13) (1978).
29. 21 C.F.R. §310.102(h) (1978).
30. 21 C.F.R. §310.102(b) and (c) (1978).
31. 43 Fed. Reg. 52165-75 (1978).
32. Id. at 52166 and 52172.
33. See, for example, Alaska Stat. §09.55.556 (Supp. 1978); Iowa Code Ann. §147.137 (Supp. 1978); Pa. Stat. Ann. Tit. 40, §1301.103 (Supp. 1977).
34. See Idaho Code §39-4304 (Supp. 1978); Iowa Code Ann. §147.137 (Supp. 1978); Nev. Rev. Stat. §41A.100 (1975); Ohio Rev. Code Ann. §2317.54(c) (1978).
35. Alaska Stat. §09.55.556 (Supp. 1978); Del. Code Ann. Tit. 18, §6852 (1976).
36. Annot., 49 A.L.R. 3d 501 (1973).
37. Martisek v. Ainsworth, 459 S.W. 2d 679 (Tex. 1970); Vigil v. Herman, 102 Ariz. 31, 424 P.2d 159, later app., 11 Ariz. App. 282, 464 P.2d 353 (1967); United States v. Reid, 251 F.2d 691 (5th Cir. 1958).
38. 186 N.W. 2d 658 (Iowa 1971).
39. Ray v. Wagner, 286 Minn. 354, 176 N.W. 2d 101 (1970).
40. Edwards v. Wiggins, 65 Ohio L. Abs. 292, 114 N.E. 2d 504 (1953); Cady v. Fraser, 122 Colo. 252, 222 P.2d 422 (1950).
41. Christy v. Salitermann, 288 Minn. 144, 179 N.W. 2d 288 (1970).
42. 255 Iowa 220, 122 N.W. 2d 312 (1963).
43. Id. at 227, 122 N.W. 2d at 315.
44. 525 S.W. 2d 753 (Mo. Ct. App. 1975).
45. Id. at 757.
46. Vann v. Harden, 187 Va. 555, 47 S.E. 2d 314 (1948).
47. Steele v. Woods, 327 S.W.2d 187 (Mo. 1959).
48. LUDLAM, INFORMED CONSENT 10 (1978); Hirsh, Which Physicians Are Students?: The Patient Has A Right to Know. THE HOSPITAL MEDICAL STAFF, Dec. 1978; Annas and Healey, The Patients' Rights Advocate—Redefining the Doctor-Patient Relationship in the Hospital Context, 27 VAND. L. REV. 243 (1974); Stulberg, The Legal Status of Medical Students in the State of Michigan, 36 U. MICH. J. 77 (1970); Employment of Medical Students as Externs, 196 JOURNAL OF THE AMERICAN MEDICAL ASSOCIATION 327 (1966).
49. CBS Television Network Transcript, "Ghost Surgery," 60 Minutes, Vol. IX, No. 23 (Feb. 27, 1977).
50. 262 N.W. 2d 684 (1977).
51. Canterbury v. Spence, 464 F.2d 772 (D.C. Cir. 1972).
52. See also Watson v. Clutts, 262 N.C. 153, 136 S.E. 2d 617 (1964); Roberts v. Wood, 206 F. Supp. 579 (S.D. Ala. 1962); Lester v. Aetna Cas. & Sur. Co., 240 F.2d 676 (5th Cir. 1957); Smith, Therapeutic Privilege to Withhold Diagnosis From Patient Sick with Serious or Fatal Illness, 19 TENN. L. REV. 349 (1946); Waltz and Scheuneman, Informed Consent to Therapy, 64 N.W.U.L. REV. 628 (1969).
53. American Hospital Association, A Patient's Bill of Rights (1972).

54. See, for example, *The Dying Person's Bill of Rights*, 75 AMERICAN JOURNAL OF NURSING (1975).
55. Minn. Stat. Ann. §144.651 and 144.652 (Supp. 1978). See also Ohio Rev. Code Ann. §3721.13 (1978).
56. Col. Rev. Stat. §12-37-101 (1974); Ky. Rev. Stat. §211.180 (Supp. 1978); N.Y. Public Health Law §2560 (McKinney 1977); Tenn. Code Ann. §63-608 (1976).
57. Conn. Gen. Stat. Ann. §20-87a (Supp. 1978).
58. See N.J. Stat. Ann. §45:11-23 (1978); N.Y. Education Law §6091 (McKinney Supp. 1979).
59. Ill. Ann. Stat. ch. 111 §3405 (Smith-Hurd 1978).
60. *In the Matter of Tuma*, Idaho Bd. of Nursing, Aug. 24, 1976. See *More on the Tuma Case*, NURSING OUTLOOK 8 (Jan. 1978); *Professional Misconduct*, NURSING OUTLOOK 546, 561 (Sept. 1977); *Feedback: On "The Right to Inform,"* NURSING OUTLOOK 738 (Dec. 1977).
61. Tuma v. Board of Nursing of the State of Idaho, No. 12587 (S.Ct. Idaho Apr. 17, 1979).
62. *Id.*
63. 22 N.Y. 2d 255, 239 N.E. 2d 368, 292 N.Y.S. 2d 440 (1968).
64. 526 F.2d 202 (8th Cir. 1975).
65. *Id.* at 208.
66. 144 So. 2d 249 (Ct. App. La. 1962).
67. *Id.* at 260.
68. 166 Cal. App. 2d 314, 333 P.2d 29 (1958).

Resource Materials

SUGGESTED READINGS

Creighton, M. *Law Every Nurse Should Know* (3rd ed.). Philadelphia: Saunders, 1975.

Helmelt, M. D., and Mackert, M. E. *Dynamics of Law in Nursing and Health Care.* Reston, Va.: Reston Publishing Co., 1978.

Holder, A. R. *Medical Malpractice Law.* New York: Wiley, 1975.

Hospital Law Manual. Rockville, Md.: Aspen Systems Corporation, 1978.

Ludlam, J. E. *Informed Consent.* Chicago: American Hospital Association, 1978.

Murchison, I. A. *Legal Accountability in the Nursing Process.* St. Louis: Mosby, 1978.

Rothman, D. A., and Rothman, L. R. *The Professional Nurse and the Law.* Boston: Little, Brown, 1977.

Streiff, C. J., ed. *Nursing and the Law* (2nd ed.). Rockville, Md.: Aspen Systems Corporation, 1975.

Donald A. Bille

5

The Teaching-Learning Process

How can I best organize material to aid the patient's learning?
Is teaching a separate function, or can I integrate it into the rest of the patient's care?

Patient education can be a very time consuming task, especially if not well planned in advance. The teaching-learning process is a means of structuring teaching-learning activities for both the teacher and the learner. This structured approach, however, does not mean that patients can simply be told what they must learn. Each patient's individualized learning needs must be accurately assessed. Then these individualized needs can be set into the structure of the five steps of the teaching-learning process. This structure helps to achieve the efficiency and effectiveness too often lacking in teaching-learning interactions. The following chapter describes each step of the teaching-learning process and provides examples of how to apply the information in the patient care setting. An adult education focus is maintained throughout the chapter, stressing the need to individualize each patient's teaching-learning program.

The information in this chapter should help the reader to

1. Define the teaching-learning process
2. List five steps in the teaching-learning process
3. ·Describe each step in the teaching-learning process
4. Write measurable objectives for the patient's learning
5. Evaluate the extent of the patient's learning
6. Document outcomes of the teaching-learning process

The Joint Commission on Accreditation of Hospitals (JCAH), in its Standards for Nursing Service (April 1979), states that "A brief and pertinent written nursing care plan should be developed for each patient. . . . It may include . . . patient and family teaching programs and the sociopsychological needs of the patient" [5].

The JCAH and others describe the nursing process as encompassing the steps of assessment, planning, intervention (implementation), and evaluation [5, 7]. Communication among health care professionals, as well as legal requirements for a record of care given and the satisfaction of accreditation standards, mandates that the plan of care must also be documented. This chapter will examine the teaching-learning process, then, and define the actions of assessment, planning, intervention or implementation, evaluation, and documentation.

THE TEACHING-LEARNING PROCESS

The lack of an organized approach to the planning and implementation of patient teaching programs has been documented in some of the older literature [3, 9]. This author has found that the situation has not improved significantly since those articles were published [2]. Patient teaching programs sometimes seem to take a shotgun approach: some of the shot (information to be taught) hits the target (the patient), but a large portion of the shot scatters around the target and is wasted. Because of a lack of organization, efforts at patient teaching may take too much of the practitioner's valuable time and may not always produce the optimum learning.

Organizing teaching-learning activities into a particular framework, then, may actually save time for the patient educator, and may ultimately achieve a higher degree of success in getting the patient to learn what he needs to learn.

The patient's teaching-learning process will be defined, then, as a set of activities organized and structured to maximize the results for the patient and family (in terms of new knowledge, skills, or attitudes) and to minimize the amount of time and effort on the part of the health care practitioner.

Assessment

In patient teaching *assessment* is the activity of gathering facts and information that assist the patient's teacher in meeting the patient's or the family's needs for learning. Assessment is a vital component in an organized patient education program, since it will serve many purposes for the teaching. It will identify what the patient wants to learn, allow therapeutic seeding, establish a point of reference in learning, identify incorrect knowledge, establish a base of data for evaluation, build trust and rapport, and provide for family involvement.

Purposes of Educational Assessment

Identify What the Patient Wants to Learn.   An adult learns best those things that are related to identified problems. If the adult does not yet recognize a problem, it is unlikely that a significant amount of learning will occur. It is impossible to *make* the adult learn. The educator can teach, but unless the patient identifies the need to learn, efforts to teach may fail.

Assessing what the patient wants to learn is often no more difficult than asking something like "What concerns you?" Or "As a result of your hospitalization what questions do you have?" Once the patient expresses a concern or question, the *need* to learn is clearly identified, and learning can take place efficiently and effectively.

Allow Therapeutic Seeding. Anyone who has ever tried to teach patients probably realizes that patients often will not express questions or concerns, thus making the teaching-learning process more difficult. At such times the teacher cannot *make* the patient learn. A technique that this author calls therapeutic seeding, however, can be utilized to plant ideas in the patient's mind. After the patient has had a chance to think about the idea, needs for learning may be more easily identified and satisfied through teaching-learning.

The process of therapeutic seeding may seem to take an inordinate amount of the busy practitioner's time. When one examines the amount of time wasted in the past trying to make the patient learn, however, therapeutic seeding becomes a big time saver. Consider the following examples.

Mrs. George is a 40-year-old woman who is recovering from surgery for gallbladder removal. Conversations with the nurse have already indicated that Mrs. George has not identified any learning needs. The nurse's therapeutic seeding would consist of statements such as, "Mrs. George, many women who have had their gallbladder removed express concerns about how this may affect their diet. What concerns do you have about your diet?"

The patient teacher should note that externally generated objectives (those thought of by the caregiver, not the patient) can be inserted into the teaching program. The patient hears the fact that other patients have problems and can feel comfortable with the fact that he or she too can have problems.

If the patient states, "Oh, I'm not concerned with that," he or she may really be saying "I'm not ready to learn about that yet." The teacher should not become discouraged if the patient is not ready to identify concerns the first time a subject is approached. A day later, the teacher can say, "Mrs. George, remember we were talking about concerns you may have regarding your diet? Now that you've had a chance to think about it, what concerns have you come up with?"

When used with patience and persistence, this technique proves to be more successful than does simply teaching those things the nurse feels the patient must learn. Therapeutic seeding lets the patient make some decisions about his teaching program.

Establish a Point of Reference for Learning. It is much easier to learn something when the new information can be related to preexisting knowledge. Thus, another purpose of assessment is to find out what the patient already knows.

Some time and effort will be required during the assessment phase to identify the patient's knowledge level. The knowledge may or may not be in a subject directly related to what the patient wants to learn. For instance, when teaching about signs and symptoms of an impending myocardial infarction, the teacher might ask the patient what signs and symptoms brought him or her to seek medical attention. In this case, the preexisting knowledge will be directly related to the learning objective. On the other hand, the patient who is learning about colostomy irrigation may have never seen a colostomy before, but will have an indirect point of reference in having given or observed an enema.

Identify Incorrect Knowledge. Gibson has stated that the patient's knowledge "is a hodge-podge of folklore, handed-down family experience, hearsay, bits of advertising, much misinformation, [and] many misconceptions" [4].

The mass media conveys a great deal of health-related information every day. Information gained from the media or even from friends and relatives may be factual but irrelevant to the patient's current illness. It is often difficult for patients to make this discrimination, however, and they may be inclined to believe something because they heard it on television or from a relative.

During the teaching-learning process the patient's teacher must identify any incorrect information (including superstitions and folklore) and dispel this as incorrect *before* the process of teaching the correct information begins.

Identify a Baseline of Data for Evaluation. Evaluation may be conducted for many reasons. Two of the most common reasons for evaluation, however, are to prove that the patient has learned (by measuring the individual patient's knowledge) and to justify the existence of the overall patient teaching program (by examining the results of measurements of all patients who have been taught).

The patient should be asked specific questions prior to teaching each objective. This technique is called pretesting. The same question may again be asked after the teaching has been done (posttesting), and the answers are then compared to determine the change in the patient's knowledge level. Educators may ask, "But if I ask the same question on the pretest as I do on the posttest, won't the patient learn to answer just that question?" Patients may indeed learn to answer just the posttest questions, but if the educator is asking the right questions—questions based on learning objectives—this is exactly what is desired.

The administration of a pretest is another means of performing therapeutic seeding, since patients are able to see the types and the amount of information they do not know. Once the pretest results are shown to the patient, a greater degree of motivation to learn may appear, since the patient is now more aware of the need to learn.

When the pretests of all patients are compared with their posttests, the overall success of the patient education program can be seen. If many patients are showing little or no increase in knowledge between the pretest and posttest, it is time to examine the patient teaching program in detail.

Build Trust and Rapport. One of the most important factors in achieving successful teaching-learning outcomes is establishing trust and rapport: a situation of mutual respect between the patient and the teacher [1]. The teacher's approach to the patient will not only determine to a large degree the amount of information the patient receives, but, what is more important, may even affect the accuracy of this information. When the patient senses an attitude of sincerity, integrity, and warmth in the care giver, the freedom to discuss all matters relating to health is more likely to exist, regardless of how personal those matters may be [8]. Patients will reveal their inner feelings only when they perceive that the teacher accepts them unconditionally. This does not mean that the teacher has to agree with the patient, but rather that the teacher refrain from making moral judgments about the actions or beliefs of the patient. "The establishment of rapport or lack of it explains why one examiner may elicit a significant history from a patient when another fails to obtain clear-cut information from the same person" [8].

Provide for Family Involvement. The learning needs of the family, like those of the patient, are essential in promoting the optimum outcome of the patient's health care (see Chapter 8). Ignoring or minimizing the family's input to the patient teaching program will ultimately result in less than the optimum teaching-learning outcomes [1]. It is essential, then, that the family be involved in the assessment phase as well as in the remainder of the teaching-learning process.

The effective patient teacher will determine the family's needs for learning as well as the family's perceptions of the patient's needs. The family can also provide information about the home environment and the resources they can provide to ease the patient's transition from hospital to home. These resources may be personal (assisting the patient with procedures, cooking, dressing), material (providing finances or equipment), or architectural (moving the patient's bedroom to the first floor).

Assessment of the teaching-learning process takes place throughout the entire program. Information is obtained during each teacher-learner contact. Even the most ideal situation will not yield a complete picture of the patient's learning needs during one encounter, especially the initial contact. As additional information is gained, the patient's teaching-care plan should be revised accordingly.

Conducting the Educational Assessment

Assessing the patient's and family's educational needs is done through a good interview, conducted in much the same way as history taking. Prior and Silberstein list the three components of history taking as listening and questioning, observation, and integration [8].

Listening and Questioning. Interviewing depends partly on the ability to ask pertinent questions. Once the question is asked, however, the ability to listen becomes the most important skill. The teacher must listen, not only to the words the patient is saying, but also to what the patient says between the lines or by hidden meaning in those words.

The best type of question is phrased in such a way as not to be answered by a "yes" or "no." This is called an open-ended question, since the words in the question require the patient to answer with several words or sentences and the question does not imply an answer that the teacher would like to hear. Examples of open-ended questions include: "When did you first notice that you were not feeling well?" "What is your usual day of activities like?" or "Tell me about the foods you normally eat in one day." Compare these open-ended questions with their closed-ended counterparts: "Was it about a month ago that you first became ill?" "Do you usually have a physically active day?" "Do you normally eat lots of spicy foods?"

A closed-ended question, then, elicits less information and is often answered with one or two words. In some situations, such as when the patient is dyspneic or very weak, questions ought to be of the closed-ended type to conserve the patient's strength or energy. It is important to judge the patient's condition when deciding how to phrase questions.

When the question has been asked, the teacher must listen attentively to what the patient is saying in his or her answer. When the patient stops talking, it is helpful to reflect or restate the answer. For instance, when the patient states "I have had pain for several months now," the restatement "You have had pain for several months now" or the reflection, "You have been experiencing pain for quite a while" will encourage the patient to elaborate further on the original statement. Reflection and restatement also move the assessment to greater depth, since the patient realizes that the nurse has accurately heard what was being said. At times, reflection and restatement allow patients to hear their own words, and thus to think again about what they have just said.

When the patient has finished answering the first question, the next question should cover the same or a similar topic more specifically. For example, building on the questions asked previously, further questioning would include: "What were you doing when you first noticed your symptoms?" "How far do you normally walk in one day?" and "Which of the foods you normally eat seems to cause the most problems for you?"

Observation.   Interviewing and questioning provide a great deal of information. If this information is taken in isolation, however, the interview will not be complete. Nonverbal communication is often as important to the true meaning of a communication as the words themselves.

The patient's actions while talking should be observed. Nervousness, looking away from the interviewer, and hesitancy in speech add to the total of information being collected.

Integration.   Verbal information given by the patient and observations made by the practitioner must be combined to give a total picture of the patient, the patient's illness, the patient's reaction to the illness, and finally, the learning needs recognized by the patient.

Planning

The next step of the teaching-learning process begins as soon as a learning need has been identified by the patient. A teaching-learning plan must be focused on the patient's need to learn. This plan will contain objectives for the patient's learning. The learning objectives are goals, ends, or outcomes desired from the teaching-learning interactions and are written in terms of those things the patient *should* be able to do after the teaching-learning interactions have occurred.

Purposes of Learning Objectives

The writing of learning objectives is probably one of the most difficult aspects of the teaching-learning process, especially for the beginning teacher. It is also one of the most time-consuming aspects. With time, practice, and experience, however, the writing of objectives becomes easier and more meaningful.

The usefulness of learning objectives far outweighs the effort needed to write them, since the objectives not only clarify what is to be taught (providing for continuity of the teaching-learning process), but they also clarify what is to be learned, what (and how) to evaluate, and what to document.

Objectives Clarify What is to be Taught.   Many different practitioners interact with each patient every day. A written teaching-care plan, then, containing objectives for the patient's learning, aims at achieving continuity of all teaching efforts toward specific goals. In the absence of this type of organized teaching plan, the patient is more likely to experience frustration as different personnel teach different concepts, or perhaps the same concept with different interpretations.

Objectives Clarify What is to be Learned.   Just as objectives for nursing care should be planned in conjunction with the patient and family [5], objectives for the patient's teaching-learning process should be established together with the patient and the family. Once learning needs are identified, these needs should be discussed and the planning of objectives (and the learning experiences that follow) should become a mutual undertaking between the learner and the teacher.

Mutual teacher-learner planning fits into the philosophy of adult education (see Chapter 3). "In traditional education the learning activity is structured by the teacher and the institution. The learner is told what objectives he is to work toward, what resources he is to use and how (and when) he is to use them, and how his accomplishment of the objectives will be evaluated. This imposed structure conflicts with the adult's deep psychological need to be self-directing and may induce resistance, apathy or withdrawal" [6].

The mutual planning of objectives is sometimes called a *learning contract*. Although this technique has seldom been used in those hospitals visited by this author, the technique is a vital component of a successful patient education program, since through this methqd, "the learner develops a sense of ownership of (and commitment to) the plan" [6].

Objectives Clarify What (and How) to Evaluate. At the time an educational plan is written out, the patient and his teacher agree on what he should be able to do after he has learned. Evaluation (somewhat oversimplified) is the determining of whether or not the patient has learned adequately to satisfy the objective. A well-written objective, then, tells what the patient will be able to do. It specifies the particular behavior that will demonstrate that learning has occurred. For instance, one typical objective for learning for a patient with ulcerative colitis is "List stress factors in your own lifestyle that aggravate ulcerative colitis." Evaluation of this objective would be accomplished by having the patient write or verbalize a list of the various life stressors that increase the symptoms of ulcerative colitis.

Objectives Clarify What to Document. Documentation of the patient's learning outcomes is problematic for many practitioners. As a result, few medical records have adequate documentation of teaching-learning outcomes [2]. This author, during many workshops conducted on the subject of patient teaching, has heard practitioners from all health-care disciplines complain that they simply do not know what is important to document. A well-written objective assists the practitioner in documentation as well as in evaluation. Documentation of the objective for the ulcerative colitis patient, for instance, might simply be "Accurately listed those stress factors in own lifestyle that aggravate ulcerative colitis."

The Process of Writing Objectives

At first, writing objectives (for nursing care or for the teaching-learning process) is difficult for most practitioners. With practice, however, and attention to the following points, the process of writing objectives becomes easier and less time-consuming.

The Components of an Objective. Each objective for patient teaching must contain two important components: a verb and the content.

The first part of each learning objective should contain a *verb* or *action word* (a word that describes an observable behavior) that states what the learner is to do to demonstrate achievement of the objective. Verbs, such as "know," "understand," or "comprehend," although frequently used in some objectives, are poor terms because they are neither observable nor easily interpreted. On the other hand, terms such as "identify," "list," "state," "plan," and "define" relate to more easily observed actions, have fewer interpretations, and thus are more useful to the patient's learning program. An extensive list of acceptable verbs follows.

Acceptable Verbs for Patient Teaching Objectives

analyze	distinguish	paraphrase
arrange	estimate	perform
apply	explain	plan
categorize	express	point out
choose	find	predict
combine	generalize	prepare
compare	give	produce
compile	help	recall
compose	identify	recognize
compute	illustrate	relate
conclude	indicate	report
construct	infer	reproduce
contrast	interpret	revise
convert	label	rewrite
create	list	select
criticize	listen	separate
defend	match	solve
define	modify	state
demonstrate	name	summarize
describe	observe	support
diagram	operate	take
differentiate	organize	translate
discriminate	outline	use

The second part of each objective is the content (in terms of knowledge, attitudes, or skills) that the patient will learn and subsequently demonstrate the ability to act upon. The content is the substance of the objective that meets the assessed learning need. Examples of the content part of objectives include: "contributing factors in coronary artery disease," "signs and symptoms of postoperative infection," "rationale for low residue diet," "1800-calorie diabetic diet for 24 hours," and "peptic ulcer." By combining the two components (the verb and the content), complete, observable objectives are written, for example:

Identify contributing factors in coronary artery disease.
List signs and symptoms of postoperative infection.
State rationale for low residue diet.
Plan 1800 calorie diabetic diet for 24 hours.
Define *peptic ulcer.*

The Utility of an Objective.   Once an objective has been written, it must be examined for four qualities in order to certify its usefulness to the patient's teaching-learning program. Objectives must be specific, inclusive, measurable, and realistic.

An objective is *specific* if it contains a singular idea. Although combining similar ideas into one objective (i.e., "list signs and symptoms of hypoglycemia *and* hyperglycemia") may make a shorter list of objectives, it encumbers the teaching and evaluation stages, making more work for the teacher later on.

The amount of information contained in an objective may also make it more *inclusive*. For instance, if all persons involved in teaching the patient about the signs and symptoms of hypoglycemia know and agree what those signs and symptoms are, there is no need to list them in the objective. However, if one or more persons disagree, then the content portion of the objective should be expanded to include the information the patient should learn. The more inclusive objective now becomes "List signs and symptoms of hypoglycemia, including headache, nervousness, sweating, tiredness, thirst, hunger, numbness, and blurred vision."

An objective becomes more easily *measurable* if the number of items in the content portion is mentioned. For instance, "List the four E's contributing to a heart attack."*

An objective is *realistic* only if it can be attained by the patient. This quality can be ascertained by assessing with the patient his or her ability to perform the objective. At times, an objective that is not realistic for the patient may need to be taught to a member of the family. (For example, "Give 40 units of NPH insulin daily" may not be realistic for the patient who has crippling rheumatoid arthritis, but might be managed by a family member.)

Implementation

Once a learning need has been identified and an objective agreed upon by the teacher and learner the most difficult parts of the teaching-learning process have been accomplished. Implementation of the learning objectives can be accomplished by communicating information about specific objectives to the patient.

This author firmly believes that skill in the art of teaching is not the result of an advanced college education but the result of actual practice. Thus, the lack of a college diploma should not be an excuse for not teaching. Knowledge of what is to be taught, the ability to communicate that knowledge to others, and the sensitive observation of the patient's or family's reactions will likely promote successful outcomes of *most* teaching-learning interactions. Even an "expert" educator will not always achieve success in *every* teaching-learning interaction. This concept will be described in greater detail in Chapter 6.

Before beginning the actual communication of knowledge, the patient's teacher should examine his or her own philosophy of education (see Chapter 3). Then, armed with this philosophy, the teacher must examine the content to be presented to the patient.

---

*The four E's are emotion, eating, exercise, and exposure to cold.

Examine Content to be Taught

Ideas are more easily understood if they are organized in a logical sequence. The teacher must analyze all the material to be presented before beginning. Does the patient need background information prior to teaching towards a specific objective? Is there a logical progression inherent in the material itself?

One of the greatest fears expressed by nurses who are about to teach is that of not knowing all there is to know about what they are teaching. Thus, they fear that a patient may ask a question for which they may not know the answer. Undoubtedly, this situation does occur, but can best be handled by saying something like, "That's a very good question, and I don't know the answer—but, I'll find out for you." Thus, both patient and nurse have learned new information.

Examine Method of Presentation

During the past decade the field of audiovisual education has proliferated. This proliferation has spilled over into the field of patient education, and many educators now rely heavily on mediated presentations. The rationale behind mediated instruction is sound; humans *do* learn better when more than one of their body's senses is involved in the learning process.

Hearing, when used alone, is one of the most passive activiites we can undertake—it requires no muscular movement. A teacher who relies solely on the hearing of the learner (by using only a lecture) does not encourage the optimum of learning experiences. For each sense that is added, in addition to the hearing, the learning process becomes not only more active but also more and more efficient (see Figure 5-1).

The teacher can involve the patient's senses by teaching while performing a procedure. For instance, while giving foot care to a diabetic, the teacher can explain the procedure to the patient; the procedure can then be *seen* and *felt* by the patient. If an infection is present, the sense of *smell* may enter into the teaching-learning process. Four senses will then have been combined into one teaching-learning interaction, making it more effective, and more efficient.

All five senses can be involved, for example, by teaching about a therapeutic diet while the patient is eating. The patient will be able to *hear* the explanation, *see, smell,* and *taste* the food, and may even learn useful information by *touching* the food. For instance, if the patient requires a low residue diet, the concept of the effect of food residue on the lining of the gastrointestinal tract can better be understood if samples of high and low residue foods can be felt at the same time. When the patient senses the difference in consistency between the two types of foods, he or she will be able to understand how residue affects the lining of the intestines.

Audiovisual materials, such as motion pictures, slides, and television, are useful *supplements* to the human teacher. Whereas audiovisual materials may be able to convey all of the information needed in a high school or college

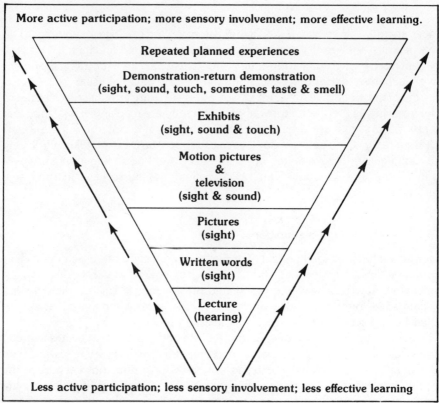

More active participation; more sensory involvement; more effective learning.

Repeated planned experiences

Demonstration-return demonstration
(sight, sound, touch, sometimes taste & smell)

Exhibits
(sight, sound & touch)

Motion pictures
&
television
(sight & sound)

Pictures
(sight)

Written words
(sight)

Lecture
(hearing)

Less active participation; less sensory involvement; less effective learning

Figure 1. *Diagram for estimating the effectiveness of learning experiences.*

course, thus replacing the human teacher, patient education will always require live human interactions because of the psychosocial adjustments the patient undergoes.

Observe Patient's Reactions to Teaching-Learning Interactions

Throughout the teaching-learning interactions the teacher should be sensitive to the patient's reactions. Observation can uncover such things as the patient's lack of acceptance of illness, the patient's lack of understanding, or the patient's short attention span.

Evaluation

The process of evaluation, or determining whether the patient has achieved the learning objectives, is easy once the objectives have been written. The objectives tell what the patient will be able to do and specify the particular behavior that demonstrates that learning has occurred.

Evaluation of the patient's learning can be illustrated by using those objectives developed earlier in this chapter. For instance, the objective "Identify contributing factors in coronary artery disease" can be evaluated by asking the patient to talk about the various things that probably cause narrowing of the coronary arteries. "List signs and symptoms of postoperative infection" can be evaluated by saying, "Tell me what things you should look for around your incision," or "What would you notice if your incision was becoming infected?" The objective "State rationale for low residue diet" can be evaluated by asking "Why has your doctor placed you on your special diet?" Or, "Why are you supposed to avoid foods with high residue?" The objective "Plan 1800-calorie diabetic diet for 24 hours" can be evaluated in several ways: the patient can be asked to plan a menu for one day, listing the types and amounts of food to be included; the patient could be given a 24-hour menu from the hospital and be asked to choose the types and amounts of foods to be included; or the patient could be given a typical restaurant menu and be asked to select a meal that would fit in with the remainder of the day's dietary intake.

Finally, the objective "Define *peptic ulcer*" can be evaluated by asking the patient "What does the term *peptic ulcer* mean?" Once the teacher is sure the patient knows the correct answer, a chance not only to reevaluate the patient's learning but also to raise the patient's self-esteem occurs when the patient is asked to explain or define the term to a family member. During this brief period the patient is allowed to step out of the sick role and into the role of teacher.

Documentation

Once the teaching-learning interaction has occurred, the outcome must be recorded in the medical record. This documentation has at least three purposes: it provides valuable communication to all other members of the health-care team, it serves as a legal record of what happened to the patient during hospitalization, and it helps to satisfy accreditation standards of the JCAH. Documentation, however, is often not sufficient by itself to meet any of these purposes [2].

Documentation of the patient's learning outcomes can be simplified and streamlined to a point where it becomes less difficult for the busy practitioner to remember what to chart and to decide how extensive the charting should be. Documentation of the patient's learning program will be adequate if two components are present: notations on how well the patient achieved the learning objectives, and notations on the patient's reactions to the teaching-learning situation and content being taught.

Note Patient Achievement

Each time a teaching-learning interaction occurs, especially those times when an objective is achieved, a notation should be made in the patient's medical record. The learning objective can be used as a basis for the information to be documented simply by adding a qualitative description of how well the patient achieved the objective to the objective itself. For instance, the documentation of the objectives developed earlier might read something like the following: "*Accurately* identified contributing factors in coronary artery disease"; "Listed four signs and symptoms of postoperative infection; will reteach *swelling* and *heat*"; "Stated correct rationale for low residue diet"; "Planned 1800-calorie diet for 24 hours to within 100 calories; needs to pay more attention to distribution of calories among the three meals"; and "Correctly defined *peptic ulcer*."

Note Patient Reactions

Observation of the patient is an ongoing task for each member of the health-care team. The teaching-learning process also requires particular observations throughout each interaction. The teacher needs to be alert to subtle cues that the patient does not understand information being taught or does not accept the information or the condition itself. This observation is also sometimes helpful in predicting how closely the patient will follow posthospitalization prescriptions as well as in deciding how much or what kind of follow-up is needed by other health-care agencies when the patient leaves the hospital.

Observations should be recorded as they are seen or heard, without subjective information or opinions. For instance, to say that the patient is denying or appears to be denying the disease or condition is a subjective, opinionated statement. It would be better to document exactly what the patient said or did that gave the impression of denial and leave formulation of the opinion to the reader of the chart. For example, if the patient who was to learn how to plan a diabetic diet expressed some doubt about his or her will to follow the diet, documentation might resemble the following: "Accurately planned 1800-calorie diabetic diet, but stated 'I doubt that I will follow this diet! It sounds too difficult for me!' "

Documentation, once completed, also completes the chain of events known as the teaching-learning process. At this point, the chain of events may start all over again, as further assessment is carried out. Has the patient reached the objective, or is some reteaching required? Has the new knowledge, skill, or attitude brought to mind any other learning needs for the patient? This new chain of events, then, cycles the patient and teacher through another teaching-learning interaction.

REFERENCES

1. Bille, D. A.   Patients' knowledge and compliance with post-hospitalization prescriptions as related to body image and teaching format. Ph.D. dissertation, University of Wisconsin—Madison, 1975.
2. Bille, D. A.   Personal conversations with Joint Commission on Accreditation of Hospitals Nurse Surveyors, May 21, 1979.
3. Brown, E. L.   The social sciences and improvement of nursing care. *American Journal of Nursing*, 56 : 1148, 1956.

4. Gibson, W. B.   But who teaches the patient? *Archives of Dermatology,* 88 : 935, 1963.
5. Joint Commission on Accreditation of Hospitals.   *Accreditation Manual for Hospitals.* Chicago: The Commission, 1979.
6. Knowles, M.   *The Adult Learner: A Neglected Species* (2nd ed.). Houston: Gulf Publishing Co., 1973. Pp. 198–199.
7. Marriner, A.   *The Nursing Process: A Scientific Approach to Nursing Care.* St. Louis: Mosby, 1975.
8. Prior, J. A. and Silberstein, J. S.   *Physical Diagnosis: The History and Examination of the Patient* (4th ed.). St. Louis: Mosby, 1973. Pp. 2–5.
9. Streeter, V.   The nurse's responsibility for teaching patients. *American Journal of Nursing,* 53 : 818, 1953.

6

Barriers to the Teaching-Learning Process

Where did I go wrong?
Why can't that patient remember what I told him?

The teaching-learning process, even when carried out exactly as described in Chapter 5, may not result in a very high level of learning. Factors exist in any teaching-learning interaction that minimize or even prevent learning. The following chapter describes factors that interfere with the teaching and learning processes. Suggestions are presented that help to break down some of the barriers, and encouragement is provided for the teacher who simply could not get through to the patient.
The information in this chapter should help the reader to

1. List at least seven barriers to teaching
2. Describe strategies for minimizing each barrier to teaching
3. List at least seven barriers to learning
4. Describe strategies for reducing each barrier to learning

A patient teaching program, even though it is based on a philosophy of adult education and utilizes all of the steps of the teaching-learning process appropriately, may not always be successful in achieving optimum learning. Certain factors in any teaching-learning interaction limit the degree of success attained in that interaction. These factors may be influenced by the nurse or other patient educator, or by the patient, family member, or significant other. This chapter will examine various factors that impose limitations on or even prevent the success of the teaching-learning interactions.

As discussed in Chapter 3, nearly all research on the teaching-learning process has been conducted on healthy humans or animals. Once the individual becomes a patient or client within the health-care system, however, research findings from a healthy population cannot be applied completely to a population that has to deal with illness and its concomitant psychologic stressors. In order to validate this perspective, the author conducted a survey during the presentation of several nursing education workshops. The results of this survey support beliefs about the existence of barriers to the teaching-learning process and also assist in developing recommendations for overcoming the barriers. The survey provides data to support the belief that some barriers to teaching-learning interactions are inherent in the teacher's role while others are inherent in the role of the patient as a learner.*

BARRIERS TO TEACHING

Textbooks on educational psychology and similar subjects describe somewhat idealistic classroom settings that enhance the student's ability to learn and the teacher's ability to teach. The busy health-care worker, however, can hardly identify with the ideal setting. Health-care professionals are faced with various situations that may limit their ability to teach. Some factors that are seen as limitations and thus barriers to teaching patients include time, communication, documentation, language, family involvement, continuity, and attitudes or values. Each of these barriers will be described in greater depth and suggestions will be offered for reducing the barrier's impact on teaching.

Time

"I don't have time!" is quickly volunteered by a majority of those professionals who are asked "What is the greatest barrier to your patient-teaching efforts?" When this barrier is examined more closely, however, at least five factors can be directly related to the lack of time, including the lack of know-how, the failure to see the importance of patient teaching, faulty definitions of teaching, the wrong source of objectives, and the attempts to teach too much material.

"I don't know how!" is what some people are really saying when they claim to lack the time to teach their patients. Lack of know-how is a legitimate problem that an organization must deal with *before* beginning concentrated efforts to establish and maintain effective patient education programming. The staff development department must assess the learning needs of all personnel who are involved in patient teaching and prepare to meet those needs at the same time that patient teaching is made a job expectation. One reason many practitioners feel they do not know how to teach is that they try to make patient teaching more difficult than it really needs to be. Knowledge or skill and the ability to communicate that knowledge or skill are all that is needed.

*The author wishes to express appreciation to the participants in the "Patient Teaching Workshop," Mercy Hospital and Medical Center, Chicago, Illinois, which met between April 1976 and August 1977.

"It's not important!" is a comment heard from many practitioners. The importance of patient education is occasionally given lip service by administrators, and yet the practice of patient teaching is not tied into the organization's performance appraisal system. Thus, personnel can still receive satisfactory performance evaluations and even merit raises and promotions without performing the important function of patient teaching. When embarking on an organized patient education program, then, the health care administrator of each discipline having patient-teaching responsibilities should revise job descriptions to include elements of patient education Once patient-teaching activities are seen as important for job success, a greater effort will be put forth in accomplishing them.

Faulty definitions of teaching are another source of trouble. Many people teach in the same way they were taught during their own school years. Thus, it is no surprise that a great deal of teaching is carried on through lecturing or talking to the patient in isolation of other activities, a method of teaching that is rarely efficient or effective. Chapter 5 proposed several methods of teaching that integrate patient education with routine nursing procedures. The patient educator who can redefine his or her teaching activity in this way will find that patient teaching will not take a great deal of *extra* time since the procedure has to be done anyway, and the patient will learn more quickly because he is more actively involved in the teaching process.

Drawing objectives from the wrong source can waste a large amount of time. An attempt to teach patients something that is not important to them is rarely successful. The patient cannot learn something when he or she does not recognize the need to learn. Objectives for the patient's teaching program must be *internally* generated. That is, they must come from the patient, not from the institution or the care-giver. Once the patient's needs are met, the externally generated or structured objectives can be approached with the patient's input and permission.

The attempt to teach too much can also waste time. Structured patient-teaching programs, generated for each medical diagnosis, are useful to patient teachers. The structure provides information as well as security for the teacher who feels less knowledgeable or less skilled at patient teaching. This same structure, however, may hinder the teaching-learning interaction if the educator thinks the content *must* be taught, regardless of the patient's ability or readiness to learn.

The amount of information to be taught is different for each individual. The teacher must be careful to teach no more than the patient can learn adequately and clearly. When the teacher identifies that a safe level of knowledge does not exist, especially when the patient is about to go home, he or she should refer the patient to another agency. This referral agency can then provide needed observation as well as further instructions when the patient is ready to learn.

Communication

The patient is exposed to many different members of the health-care team during each day of hospitalization. Each of these team members needs to be aware of the patient's learning status if the team is to work effectively together towards furthering the patient's knowledge.

One of the most frequent complaints heard from nurses is, "How can we teach the patient if we don't receive the doctor's order to begin teaching until a few hours before the patient is to be discharged?" The statement seems legitimate enough. If the nurses are waiting until discharge to begin patient teaching, however, it is unlikely that a significant amount of learning can occur. The complaint of not having an order to teach the patient before the discharge order is written, however, is not legitimate. Once a physician's order has been written for the patient's admission to the hospital, the momentum for patient teaching can begin. The patient needs to be taught about each of the elements of care to be administered. Once these facets of care have been learned, it will be easier for the patient to learn about the changes in his or her condition since admission and about how to carry on self-care after hospitalization has ended.

Communication with the physician, however, is not the only interaction that is required for effective patient teaching. Each person caring for the patient must communicate both verbally and in writing with every other member of the team. In this way the patient's progress in learning can be well known to those personnel who will subsequently be interacting with the patient. The patient's educational program (as well as his total care) can only benefit by adequate communication between the various members of the health-care team.

Documentation

Information documented in the medical record is useful for at least four reasons: (1) the record is a means of communicating to all other personnel on the health-care team; (2) the medical record provides a legal record of the events occurring during the patient's hospitalization; (3) the medical record provides input to the organization's quality assurance program; and (4) it provides evidence that accreditation standards are being met.

Documentation becomes a barrier to the teaching-learning process when the nurse states, "But I'm too busy to document everything I do for the patient." Significant interactions occur with the patient and are then forgotten by the nurse. One way to remember to document is to keep a piece of paper and pen readily available (in a pocket or on the medication tray) with which a short memo can be written. Then, sometime later, a short note can be written in the patient's record. The nurse is too busy *not* to document, since unless there is a written record of what occurred, the nurse will have to depend on memory, and the memory cannot always be depended on to last the length of time it takes for malpractice litigation to get to the stage of a jury trial.

Language Barrier

Medical terminology is very useful in helping the practitioner to communicate with coworkers. This same terminology, however, may sound like a foreign language to the patient who has not had the advantage of studying medical terminology.

A situation that illustrates the problem occurred a few years ago when this author was the charge nurse on a surgical unit. Mrs. Greene, a 43-year-old homemaker, had undergone surgery to construct a pedicle skin graft on her abdomen. The pedicle had been attached to her arm, and the arm was now restrained against her abdomen with an elastic bandage. On the third postoperative day, the surgeon inspected the graft site and stated, "It looks macerated," and soon left the room. A few minutes later, Mrs. Greene was found crying, obviously distraught. When she had been calmed enough to talk, she said she was upset because the doctor had said it "looked like a massacre!" *Massacre* was the only word she knew that sounded like *macerate*. When it was explained that the word the doctor used meant the same thing as "dishpan hands," Mrs. Greene could describe not only what the area looked like, but also how it came to be that way. By using words the patient can understand, the teacher will save a great deal of time (since further explanation may not be necessary) and a great deal of emotion (since the patient will not have to imagine meanings of words).

Family Involvement

In many cases the patient will need to have some assistance in making the transition from the hospital back to the home. The patient may also need assistance with treatment measures. This assistance can be provided by a family member if he or she has been taught what to do.

Lack of family involvement in the teaching-learning interactions can handicap the patient and be a hindrance to his or her care. Take, for example, the case of Mr. Smith, a 32-year-old highway construction worker who suffered a myocardial infarction. Throughout his hospitalization he learned easily and well. Upon discharge, however, he was confronted with a nearly unmanageable situation. His wife and two children demanded some of his energies and nearly every neighbor came over to pay a visit. He ate very little supper that first evening, smoked two packs of cigarettes, and drank at least a six-pack of beer. He stayed up late and got less rest than he should have. The next day he was readmitted with an extension of his myocardial infarction. An interview was conducted with Mr. Smith after the readmission. During this interview he related the feeling of helplessness; he knew there were things he should not be doing, but the circumstances were not completely within his control. He stated that his wife could not be of much help because she didn't know how to help. She had never been involved in any of the teaching-learning interactions. Lack of family involvement in Mr. Smith's patient education program may have contributed to his readmission.

Continuity

It has already been pointed out that many different personnel interact with the patient each day. Each professional may have his or her own idea of what the patient should learn or may approach the patient in a different way. The different interpretation of facts and different approaches can be confusing. The only way to achieve continuity and thus to achieve optimal teaching-learning outcomes is to write a teaching-care plan. Although the writing of this plan takes some time, it must be done. Once a teaching-care plan is written, however, a great deal of time will be saved for all people involved. The teaching-care plan easily identifies what is to be taught. It identifies for the patient and family what is to be learned. The plan also helps to evaluate and document the teaching-learning interactions.

Attitudes and Values

Each person, both patient and nurse, has his or her own set of values and beliefs that guide daily actions and behaviors. The nurse, however, must teach with the patient's values and beliefs in mind and not make a value judgment when conflicting value systems exist. Value judgments become a barrier to open communication, and work to break down trust and rapport. Each patient must be given respect and be taught with an open mind.

A dietitian described a frustrating situation to this author. Her patient was a 32-year-old man with chronic renal failure. He had learned how to plan his therapeutic diet perfectly but stated, "I'm not going to follow it." The dietitian said, "What can I do? I'm so frustrated with him!" Her frustration arose from the belief that she had failed. This was not true—the patient could plan the diet well; the dietitian had taught well. However, the patient had his reasons for not following the diet. When the dietitian realized where her frustration was coming from, she decided to work at maintaining communication with the patient. He later told her that since following the diet would not help him live any longer, he wanted to live whatever time he had left eating the foods that he liked and that made him happy. The dietitian felt more comfortable at this point and told the patient that she would be available anytime in the future if he needed dietary information. This future interaction would not have been possible if a value judgment had allowed attitudes and values to get in the way of open communication.

BARRIERS TO LEARNING

Patients, too, are faced with various situations that place limitations on the ability to learn. Bergevin, in writing about the *healthy* adult learner, states that adult learning is limited by two factors alone: the individual's intellectual capacity and the psychologic restrictions placed on the self [1]. When a person becomes sick, however, learning limitations may increase, and the amount of learning that can take place may decrease. Some factors that are viewed as barriers to the patient's ability to learn include the process of psychosocial adaptation, motivation, the hospital's daily routine, trust and rapport, physical condition, age, and socioeconomic factors. Each of these barriers will be described in greater depth, and suggestions will be offered for reducing the barrier's impact on learning.

Psychosocial Adaptation

Changes are sometimes difficult for even the healthiest adult. Habit patterns and the ease of functioning in the same way from day to day become a way of life. The adult is accustomed to being independent, self-sufficient, and self-directing. Hospitalization interrupts the patient's role in life and the way in which life is lived. The change involved just in taking on the role of patient is traumatic, not to mention the life-altering changes that occur as the result of disease or injury. The psychological restrictions the patient constructs during illness are probably not conscious. However, these restrictions do interfere with the ability to learn about and adapt to a diseased state.

Several theorists have written about the process of psychosocial adaptation [4, 6, 7, 8, 12]. A review of these various theories provides guidelines for understanding the patient's behavior as the stages of psychosocial adaptation—disbelief/denial, developing awareness, reorganization, resolution, identity change, and successful adaptation—unfold (see Table 1).

Disbelief/Denial

The shock of discovering that something is wrong may cause the patient to think "No! Not me! It can't be happening to me!" During denial, the patient believes that nothing is wrong.

Although it may have some psychologic benefits for the patient, unfortunately denial gets in the way of the patient's learning. The patient may think, "Why should I learn about that medication or diet or procedure? There's nothing wrong with me!" Teaching efforts during the time of denial must be supportive (without agreeing with the patient that nothing is wrong), and teaching will be more effective if a present tense focus is maintained. For instance, "I'm giving you this pill to take away that thumping sensation you have in your chest." Or "This special diet will help relieve the burning sensation in your stomach that brought you to see your doctor." No references should be made to the future while the patient is in the stage of denial. Comments like "You will need to do this for the rest of your life" will not only fall on deaf ears, but will also increase the patient's need to deny.

Developing Awareness

As the patient's denial mechanisms give way, he or she becomes aware that something definitely *is* wrong. Patients are heard to say "Why me?" during this stage. Feelings of guilt arise as the patient wonders "Why is God punishing me this way? If only I had done things differently, I wouldn't be sick today!" This guilt causes feelings of anger to arise. If the anger is channeled inward, the patient will be depressed and less responsive. If anger is channeled outward, however, expressions of hostility will be heard as the patient uses those personnel caring for him as a pressure relief valve.

Teaching efforts during this emotional time are likely to remind the patient

Table 1. *Psychosocial Adaptation and Patient Teaching*

Stage of Adaptation	Patient's Beliefs/Behaviors	Reducing the Barrier to Learning
Disbelief (Denial)	Patient's thoughts "There's nothing wrong with me." "It can't be happening to me!" Patient's actions Disregards activity or diet restrictions. Ignores nurse's attempts to teach about self-care measures to be done after discharge.	Provide careful orientation to hospital surroundings and unit policies affecting the patient. Teach with a present-tense focus. Provide careful explanation of each procedure while it is being done. Assure patient that he is safe. Teach family members about what is happening to the patient. Concentrate on a one-to-one relationship for teaching.
Developing Awareness	Patient's thoughts "Why is God punishing me?" "If only I had been more careful (not eaten so much, smoked so much, etc.) maybe I wouldn't be sick." Patient's actions Places blame for illness on self and/or others. Strikes out at others to relieve own pent-up hostilities.	Listen carefully to what the patient is saying. Continue to teach with a present-tense focus. Understand that hostility needs venting and it is not personally directed at the care giver. Avoid arguing with the patient.
Reorganization	Patient's thoughts "I wonder how my loved ones feel about me now?" "I'm beginning to see how my life is changing." Patient's actions Avoids bringing up subject of illness or life changes with family members.	Ask the patient how he/she feels about having this disease. Build communication between patient and family, especially in terms of working together towards problem solution. Provide increased reassurance for patient's family members. Begin to teach some material the patient will need to know in the future. Maintain one-to-one teacher-learner interactions.

Resolution	Patient's thoughts "I see how my life has changed." "I recognize that other people with this same condition are functioning well." Patient's actions Seeks out other patients with same condition. May be more likely to openly express emotions (especially crying).	Encourage expression of feelings. Allow patient to cry. Begin to use group instructional setting. Have a recovered patient visit this patient.
Identity Change	Patient's thoughts "I have changed and life is going to be different from now on." "There are limitations on my life because I have a disease." Patient's actions Actively seeks out information about his/her own disease (in the library, etc.) Seeks level of greater independence.	Concentrate teaching content on the future, but also continue to teach about what is presently happening. Allow the patient to become as independent as possible.
Successful Adaptation	Patient's thoughts "I resign myself to this change for the rest of my life." "I wonder which is more important, quality or quantity of life?" Patient's actions Chooses which of his physician's orders he/she is going to follow.	Refer the patient to an agency that can continue the teaching-learning interaction after discharge from the hospital. Allow patient to discuss alternatives of following or not following doctor's orders (as well as consequences of each alternative). Maintain open communication by avoiding value judgments.

Source: Titles of the stages of adaptation are taken from M. A. Crate, Nursing functions in adaptation to chronic illness. *American Journal of Nursing,* 65:72-76, 1965.

about being sick and may be met with increased hostility against the teacher. Realizing that the hostility comes from within the patient, the teacher should proceed with an attitude that care and teaching are necessary. Teaching should continue to focus on the short-term, present tense learning needs.

Reorganization

The patient has by this time developed an energy reserve that is adequate to deal with the flood of emotions resulting from illness. Reorganization of the self-concept begins at this point, and the patient is ready to learn about elements of care that are recognized as being needed and important. At this delicate time in the teaching-learning interactions, the nurse must be sure to teach what the patient wants to learn. This will help the patient achieve a successful reorganization of his psychologic structures.

Resolution

Expressions like "I give up," or "Why fight it; I know I'm sick!" may be heard at this time. Patients, however, also begin to understand that other people have the same condition and are managing their life functions quite well. This is the stage during which the mastectomy patient can accept and identify with the "Reach to Recovery" program, or the colostomy patient can identify with an ostomate club member.

By the stage of resolution the patient is ready to handle externally generated objectives for learning. At this stage the patient is also ready to experience instruction in a group setting. Group instruction is an effective, time-saving way to teach patients. The patient educator, however, should be sure that patients have had time to resolve internal psychologic processes before placing them in a situation in which they have to cope with other patients. Teaching can begin to focus more on the future and long-term needs at this point.

Identity Change

The patient at this stage is ready to see long-range changes and limits to the former self-concept. Readiness to learn also expands to being able to see the need to learn about elements of care that others suggest. Teaching can continue to focus on future, long-term needs for learning.

Successful Adaptation

Most patients eventually achieve the state of psychosocial adaptation that permits them to live comfortably, or at least resignedly, with their disease-imposed changes and limitations. During this last stage the patient is best able to learn about all that is needed to provide adequate, safe self-care. Unfortunately, however, this stage is seldomly reached while the patient is still in the hospital.

Nite and Willis found, for instance, that this stage of adaptation for the myocardial infarction patient may come as late as the fifth or sixth week after diagnosis [11]. Most patients will have returned home by that time.

Since most patients reach the stage of successful adaptation after going home, the nurse must be aware of at least two important facts. First, since patients cannot learn everything that is needed until the stage of successful adaptation, it is unlikely that patients can learn all they need to know while still in the hospital. The nurse should realize this as a limitation to the amount of information that can be taught. Second, the patient usually achieves adaptation after arriving at home. Since this will be the best time for learning, the nurse must arrange for some mechanism whereby the patient can maintain contact with continued learning experiences. Referrals to community health programs should be made whenever feasible. The doctor's office nurse and the outpatient clinic staff can be alerted to the patient's needs. The primary nurse can make a home visit periodically, or the patient can be given the telephone number of the clinical unit where questions can readily be answered. The patient must be provided with a means for continued learning of self-care measures.

The patient's family or significant others also go through the stages of psychosocial adaptation but not necessarily in the same order or at the same time as the patient experiences them. The nurse must listen to and observe the family and their interactions with the patient. Teaching-learning interactions must also be provided for the family as the need arises.

Not every person will successfully travel through the stages of psychosocial adaptation. In fact, some patients never get past the stage of denial. Attempts to jolt these patients back to reality only make denial more necessary. Teaching these patients will be extremely difficult. The nurse should realize that these patients' psychological restrictions in no way reflect on the nurse's ability to teach. Efforts to teach the denying patient should continue, along with careful documentation of patients' behavior and reactions to the teaching-learning interactions.

Motivation

Patients learn only what they want or are motivated to learn. Yet a common complaint heard from patient educators is "That patient is *not* motivated to learn!" What they are more likely saying, however, is "That patient is not motivated to learn what I *am* motivated to teach."

All mental processes are "caused by some tension or psychic energy . . . the individual's behavior is always governed by some intention to do one thing or another. In other words all behavior is motivated" [3]. Motivation is an internal phenomenon. Thus the nurse may not be able to motivate patients to learn when they are not already motivated to do so.

Abraham Maslow has described one system of human needs that motivates human behaviors [9]. In his hierarchy, Maslow describes physiological needs as being most basic. Safety, belongingness and love, esteem, and self-actualization

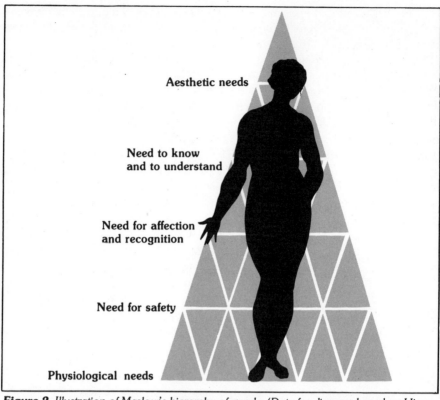

Figure 2. *Illustration of Maslow's hierarchy of needs. (Data for diagram based on Hierarchy of Needs in "A Theory of Human Motivation" in* Motivation and Personality *(2nd ed.) by Abraham H. Maslow. Copyright © 1970 by Abraham H. Maslow. Reprinted by permission of Harper & Row, Publishers, Inc.)*

are needs on the progressive steps of the hierarchy. The hierarchic arrangement of needs suggests that needs at the lower end of the hierarchy must be satisfied before the person can attend to those at the upper end (see Figure 2).

When a person has suffered a life-threatening disease, personal needs center on physiology and safety, the two lowest needs on the hierarchy. It may be difficult or impossible for the patient to think of learning about how to adjust to illness in the future, since this activity is most likely based in the esteem needs [10]. The patient at the earliest stages of hospitalization, then, is not motivated to learn about future self-care needs but is highly motivated to learn about physiologic and safety needs and how they are being met at that very moment.

Esteem needs and the motivation to learn are closely related. Therefore, motivation to learn may automatically increase as the patient's self-esteem increases. The nurse can help build the patient's self-esteem in at least two ways. First, open, two-way communication will help the patient express aspects of the self which may currently be responsible for the lowered self-image. Second, the nurse should provide opportunities for the patient to make decisions. These decisions *can* concern the patient's nursing care, and *should* concern the patient's teaching-care plan. The nurse must allow the patient to decide the content of the teaching program; the nurse must teach what the patient wants to learn.

Once the patient comes to believe that physical danger (such as death or worsening physical condition) is past, motivational levels begin to rise. The patient may then be better able to devote time and energy to learning about future care needs.

Hospital Daily Routine

The number of activities inflicted upon the patient each day may influence the ability to learn. A trend towards shorter lengths of stay demands that more care procedures be accomplished in a single day. When the patient is kept busy preparing for and going through one procedure after another, little time or energy may be left to carry out the intellectual functions of learning. The nurse's busy schedule may also detract from optimum teaching, since the patient may not be able to learn well at the moment the nurse is available to teach.

Breaking down this barrier requires at least two considerations. First, patients' activities should be organized in such a way as to provide rest periods as well as time for teaching-learning interactions. Without a rest period the patient may be too tired to learn. A second, perhaps more important, consideration has to do with the time when teaching-learning interactions are scheduled. If patient teaching efforts are to succeed, they must occur at the teachable moment—the time at which the patient is ready to learn. Not all patient teaching can occur on any one particular shift, and, therefore, mechanisms, such as staffing patterns, hours during which x-ray and laboratory procedures can be done and the like, may need to be examined to provide time for teaching-learning interactions. If patient teaching is to be done, and done successfully, planning must occur to arrange the hospital's daily routine around the needs of the patient.

Trust and Rapport

The level of the patient's learning may be related to the level of trust and rapport that exists between teacher and learner [2]. If the patient does not know or trust the teacher, a significant amount of learning may not occur. While the nurse is providing physical care to the patient, trust and rapport develop through their interactions. This trust transfers automatically to any other activity the nurse does for this patient, including teaching. When patient teaching is seen as a responsibility of someone else (for example, the patient education coordinator, staff development instructor, or group diabetes instructor), time must pass before trust can be built. Although other personnel can become trusted and effective teachers for this patient, time will be wasted in the process of developing this trust. Therefore, the best patient teacher, in terms of effectiveness and efficiency, will be the provider of personal care measures.

Physical Condition

Physiologic condition and physical health affect learning in various ways. Some patients are simply too sick to learn. The patient who is in a coma or the one who is experiencing the delirium tremens of alcohol withdrawal may not be able to retain information being taught. Explanations should still be provided, however, as a means of reassuring and comforting these patients.

Sensory impairment, such as poor vision or hearing, affect ability to take in information. Patients who wear glasses or hearing aids should have them on before teaching efforts begin. Good lighting and quiet places should be provided [6].

Pain, fever, or any other physiologic abnormality may also affect the ability to learn. Most often affected will be the attention span and the level at which the patient can understand. Special teaching efforts, with attention to teaching for shorter periods of time and at a lower level of difficulty, should be considered for the patient in poor health.

Age

Research is being done to determine the effect of aging on the learning process. When the person's aging process is accompanied by arteriosclerosis or other pathology, memory is often affected. Aging itself, with no other attendant pathology, does not affect *ability* (intellectual power) to learn. What does change is the speed or rate of learning. It may take the older adult a bit longer to learn the same amount of material than the younger patient. This age factor, however, is not always present, since the decline in rate of learning is likely to be minimized by continued use of the intellect [5].

Socioeconomic Status

"Socioeconomic circumstances are associated with values, demands, constraints and resources that can affect learning ability" [6]. The patient's income level may affect the ability to purchase and use medical equipment in the home. Religious beliefs, ethnic customs, folklore, and familial traditions must all be taken into consideration when planning the patient's teaching program. Through careful assessment the nurse can grow to understand each patient and his or her individual behaviors. The nurse must assess the patient adequately enough to discover the cause of health-related behaviors before those behaviors can be changed through teaching.

REFERENCES

1. Bergevin, P.   A Philosophy for Adult Education. New York: Seabury Press, 1967. P. 117.
2. Bille, D. A.   Patients' knowledge and compliance with post-hospitalization prescriptions as related to body image and teaching format. Ph.D. dissertation, University of Wisconsin—Madison, 1975.

3. Bolles, R. C. *Theory of Motivation*. New York: Harper & Row, 1967. P. 70.
4. Crate, M. A. Nursing functions in adaptation to chronic illness. *American Journal of Nursing*, 65 : 72, 1965.
5. Knowles, M. S. *The Modern Practice of Adult Education: Andragogy Versus Pedagogy* (2nd Ed.). New York: Association Press, 1975.
6. Knox, A. B. *Adult Development and Learning*. San Francisco: Jossey-Bass, 1977.
7. Kübler-Ross, E. *On Death and Dying*. New York: MacMillan, 1969.
8. Lederer, H. D. How the sick view their world. *Journal of Social Issues*, 8 : 4, 1952.
9. Maslow, A. *Motivation and Personality*. New York: Harper & Row, 1970. Pp. 35–47.
10. Maslow, A. A theory of human motivation. *Psychological Review*, 50 : 370–396, 1943.
11. Nite, G., and Willis, F. *The Coronary Patient: Hospital Care and Rehabilitation*. New York: MacMillan, 1964.
12. Suchman, E. A. Stages of illness and medical care. *Journal of Health and Human Behavior*, 6 : 114, 1955.

7

The Approach to Health Care
in Three American Minorities

How can I teach someone whose culture is different from mine?
How do cultural values affect the teaching-learning process?

Intercultural communication can be a barrier to the teaching-learning process. This barrier may arise from a lack of understanding of the differences in beliefs and values, or it may be due to value judgments made by the teacher or the learner. The following chapter describes three different minorities and some of their beliefs and values relative to health care. It would be impossible to describe all cultures and their beliefs in this text. Using these three minorities as an example, however, the patient educator can better understand how different beliefs affect the patient's perceptions of health care, the care-provider, and information the care-giver tries to teach.

The information in this chapter should help the reader to

1. *Develop awareness of cultural differences in the patient or client population*
2. *Relate cultural differences to the need for differing approaches to treatment and care*
3. *Describe how values affect day-to-day attitudes and behaviors for both teacher and learner*
4. *Describe strategies for minimizing the fears, doubts, and superstitions which hinder the teaching-learning process*

Like most other disciplines, the medical and health sciences emphasize closed curricula that are based on "precisely defined knowledge, technique, and procedures, all of which are discontinuous from ordinary social process" [13]. Unfortunately, the stress on scientific medicine has overshadowed traditional or folk health-care systems that are "*open* systems, accepting substantive input from—and thus capable of functionally contributing to—economic, familial, ritual, moral, and other institutional sectors" of society [17]. Folk health-care systems have been characterized as primitive and parochial, lacking both intuitive and scientific bases. However, such traditional medical beliefs and practices are not only usually soundly based but frequently complement and coexist with contemporary medical practices, attitudes, and services [14].

Health-care consumers in the United States have continued to seek medical advice and care from a variety of sometimes seemingly esoteric health practitioners. While some individuals purposefully avoid modern medical assistance because of their skeptical attitudes or fears, a far greater number of people persist in using folk medical therapies because of cultural, economic, or geographic accessibility. Other persons who utilize these traditional practices are from socially or culturally marginal minority groups; that is, they are persons who do not readily participate in mainstream American sociocultural institutions. Minority groups "maintain their medical traditions because [the traditions] affect undesirable biological states in expected ways, and because they are effective ways for dealing with disruptive events that cannot be allowed to persist" [25].

This chapter will discuss some of the traditional health-care beliefs and practices of three United States minority populations—Mexican-American, Navajo, and Southern Appalachian. An attempt will be made not only to illustrate the diversity of folk health-care systems in this country but also to demonstrate their compatibility with and utility to modern medicine and health-care education.

TRADITIONAL DISEASE ETIOLOGIES

Foster has characterized nonwestern medical system disease etiologies as either *personalistic* or *naturalistic* [4]. Though not mutually exclusive, each disease etiology consists of functionally different components which are governed by cultural factors. In the ethnographic profiles that follow, Foster's concepts are useful in understanding American folk health-care systems and patient-practitioner relationships.

The *personalistic* medical system is one in which there is little room for the accidental or chance occurrence of disease. Illness is thought to be derived from an *"active, purposeful intervention"* by an *"agent* who may be human (a witch or sorcerer), non-human (a ghost, an ancestor, an evil spirit), or supernatural (a deity or other powerful being)" [4]. This idea is consistent with the "common knowledge that in many cultures, ideas and practices relating to illness are for the most part inseparable from the domain of religious belief and practices" [4].

In the *naturalistic* medical system, on the other hand, death and disease are frequently felt to originate from impersonal *"natural forces or conditions"* like "an upset in the balance of the basic body elements" or humors [4]. Disease is considered unrelated to other misfortunes that might be at work on the individual and his family. In the naturalistic system, prevention of and responsibility for disease resides with the individual client, whereas in personalistic disease etiologies the whole community can in some way be part of either the cause or the cure necessary to overcome disease and illness.

In diagnostic and curative activities there are further distinctions between the two disease etiologies. In the personalistic system, a shaman, witch doctor, or other medicoreligious specialist usually diagnoses by divinatory techniques; the most well-known include bone-throwing, inducing trances, and magicoreligious rites like sacrifice. Medical practitioners in naturalistic systems are viewed primarily as curers, since diagnosis is usually performed by the patient himself, a relative, or a close member of the community.

In any event, the relationship between patient and practitioner in both disease etiologies is a social one and not merely "an interaction between two roles" [5] that is characteristic of much of modern American medicine. Furthermore, there is an inherent trust and confidence between client and healer in these medical systems; this creates a kind of symmetry or balance often foreign to institutionalized medicine.

Modern medical systems and disease etiologies frequently fail to take into account the various sociocultural forces which influence disease causation, prevention, and treatment in folk traditions. Moreover, the patient's world view—attitudes, beliefs, and values about the nature and order of the world—take on additional "significance when dealing with illness among ethnic or cultural minorities" [15]. The failure to learn about the primary beliefs of ethnic minorities can lead to faulty diagnosis or treatment, because that treatment can be "misunderstood, incongruous, meaningless, or contraindicated in the patient's world view" [15]. What could be misinterpreted as cultural resistance to modern medical practices could be, in fact, confusion rather than antagonism [22], "parochialism" rather than "cosmopolitanism" [23], and trauma rather than resistance [17].

THE MEXICAN-AMERICANS

By the mid-1970s, an estimated 6.6 million United States residents were of Mexican descent—the largest nonwhite minority after blacks. More than three-quarters of the Mexican-American population are urban dwellers. Many Mexican-Americans are fully integrated into mainstream American culture; but most, particularly the poor, are isolated by sociocultural, economic, and linguistic barriers and prejudices. As a consequence of sociocultural alienations, the health services available to Mexican-Americans are frequently underutilized [6]. When mental or physical health problems arise, traditional Mexican-American folk-healers, curanderos, are often consulted for diagnosis and treatment.

As a rule, preventive and curative medicine originates in the Mexican-American home under the supervision of a family member or an experienced neighbor [6]. The curandero is sought in more severe cases when home treatment has not sufficed. There are also a number of instances in which the aid of the curandero will be sought almost immediately, particularly in mental or emotional health problems. Since Mexican-Americans consider disease a social phenomenon as well as a unique personal experience, the role of the *curandero* must be clearly understood.

The popularity of this healer is not based solely on his relatively inexpensive services but on his ability to relate to his patients in culturally meaningful ways. The *curandero* does not confront his clients with unintelligible bureaucracies and medical practices; instead, he is usually a well-known community member who speaks a common language and shares the values and beliefs of the community at large.

According to Foster's characterizations of disease etiologies, that of the Mexican-Americans most closely resembles the naturalistic type. Here the concern is not with the *who* or *why* of illness, but with the *what*—that is, the means required to restore equilibrium in the client [4]. In essence this means that an attempt is made to strike a balance between the client's total environment and his or her well-being. In fact, Mexican-American concepts of disease have been likened to the "framework provided by the so-called Hippocratic system in which the body is visualized as healthy when sets of contrasting qualities . . . are balanced" [20]. For example, if the client is suffering from a respiratory disease—such as a cold or bronchitis—that is the result of "cold" *aires,* contrasting "hot" therapeutic procedures will be employed.

Although a variety of persons serve as *curanderos,* both male and female, the most significant are those who make medicine their full-time occupation and who are "theoretically now expected to be at the disposal of all who seek . . . assistance" [19]. Characteristically, the *curandero* is, like the majority of his clients, a religiously pious person whose talents are naturally acquired as gifts from God [8]. Like his patients, the *curandero* accepts life "as ordained by the divine will" [8] and considers the patient's plight not only a family but a community cause for concern. Suffering, whether physical or mental, is never an individual experience among traditional Mexican-Americans.

Good health in Mexican-American society means that there is a balance within the social and physical environment. However, "when traditional patterns of behavior are disrupted, the individual is more susceptible to the development of bad habits, conflict, and trouble" [8]. Diagnosis by the *curandero* takes into account not only the symptoms that have caused the client to seek medical help but also his social, domestic, and occupational life [24]. In other words, the life of the Mexican-American client is not segmented into neat divisions as is frequently the case with institutional American medicine.

Treatment may include a variety of practices—prayer, suggestion, practical advice, or hydro-therapy—depending on the particular malady. But the over-all emphasis in treatment is to unify the physical and spiritual well-being of the client and to restore the balance between him and his total environment. Therapy, thus, is frequently an attempt to reconcile "disturbed social relationships" [8], particularly in the case of mental disorders but also in the case of physical disorders.

The success or failure of the therapies of the *curandero* is couched in the "religious values of a family-centered, static agrarian society" [8]. Hence, when traditional values and norms have been violated, the Mexican-American patient is thought to be more susceptible to disease. Consequently, modernization and integration into American society—changing standards of morality, social roles and obligations, economic responsibilities, and values, to name a few—can affect the physical and psychological well-being of the client. "Those whose orientation is toward adoption of Anglo-American socio-cultural behavior . . . tend to disparage these concepts of illness as ingenuous beliefs, survivals of an unsophisticated past" [20]. Yet many middle-class, culturally integrated Mexican-Americans will seek the services of the *curandero* when scientific American medicine either fails to cure a client's particular disease or when the social distance between the client, his family, and the Anglo doctor has been stretched to its limits.

THE NAVAJO

Traditional Mexican-American folk medicine attempts to balance the physical and social welfare of the client; however, it is not as personalistic as the medicine practiced by the Navajo, the United States' most numerous native American population. Navajo theories of disease are complex. Illness results not only from biophysical disorders, but from social, cultural, and religious transgressions. Thus, disease may be caused not only by such factors as witchcraft or the breach of social intercourse, but by such things as ghosts, dreams, and supernatural powers [3, 9, 12]. As a consequence, the emphasis of Navajo diagnosis and treatment is on restoring the client's harmony with nature [11].

The act of diagnosis is usually performed by a hand-trembler, a medicine man who ascertains the cause of illness either by star-gazing, listening to the various sounds of the night, or by hand-trembling, that is, placing his hands over the affected body parts of the client. Like the *curandero,* the hand-trembler, as well as other Navajo medical personnel, never offers his services or solicits clients. Rather, he waits until he is sought by some intermediary who asks his aid. The selection of the diagnostician and, subsequently, the curer is based on such factors as relationship to the client, geographic proximity, or practical medical knowledge or skills for which the practitioner is known [11]. After the time, place, and fees for the curing ceremonial have been arranged, the hand-trembler begins his diagnostic procedures.

Although the diagnoses of the hand-trembler appear "patterned and . . . conditioned by the circumstances of the particular case" [10], the symptoms are not always consistent with the various agents of disease. Moreover, the Navajo themselves do not believe that it is necessary to have a one-to-one correlation between the cause, symptoms, and treatment of a specific malady [12]. For example, a disharmonious relationship with one's spiritual, physical, or social environment could result in a broken leg, a stroke, or some other malady.

After the hand-trembler has made his diagnosis, the client's family selects the curing ceremonial and then hires a singer or curer, both medicoreligious specialists or medicine men, to perform the specific curing activity, for example, chanting or preparing sand paintings. The Navajo curing ceremonials are explicitly aimed at helping the sick, as well as perpetuating the physical, social, and spiritual well-being of the community in general. As some Navajo scholars have indicated, the principal aim of the diagnostic and curing practices are to reassure the client, his family, and the community [12]. Those that attend a curing ceremonial are not "just a crowd . . . they are the living representatives of that race of chosen people to whom the patient belongs" [12]. This contrasts with the *curandero* who treats the client with the welfare of the family and community in mind.

Like the traditional American country doctor, the *curandero* and Navajo medicine man are familiar with the client's socioeconomic conditions, personal history, and current health. As a rule, they are both active in socially intimate environments conducive to the acceptance of practical medical therapies and treatments. Neither Mexican-American nor Navajo medical practitioners are very distant from the everyday, personal affairs of their clients.

The success or failure of a Navajo medical practitioner cannot be measured according to Western criteria. The failure of a hand-trembler to correctly diagnose a client's illness is, more often than not, attributed to his lack of knowledge or to other circumstantial factors. If one cure fails, one or several others may be attempted until some desired results have been achieved [2]. If, on the other hand, the failure to cure is thought to be the result of an inexperienced singer or curer, another might be sought, since the Navajo believe in gradations of therapeutic power among medical personnel [1].

The negative reactions of the Navajo to Western medicine, like those of the Mexican-Americans, focus on the loneliness and sameness of medical institutions, the impersonal behavior of medical personnel, and the cultural narrowness of medical diagnosis. Both minorities respond favorably to the personal and intimate relationships they have with their traditional medical practitioners, regardless of the outcome of treatment. For them, it is the moral support that the family and community offer as well as the belief in realigning with nature, that provide for better health and spiritual well-being.

SOUTHERN APPALACHIANS

Isolated by geography and traditional culture, the Southern Appalachians have maintained many of their traditional medical practices and beliefs. Their medicine is a unique synthesis of "European folk belief, American Indian therapeutic measures, and patent medicine advertising" [16] that falls somewhere between the naturalistic medicine of the Mexican-Americans and the personalistic medical practices and beliefs of the Navajo.

The supernatural, in the sense of "God's will" or "God's wrath," is interwoven with natural conditions and circumstances to form the basis of their beliefs. Consequently, many Southern Appalachians hold firm to their belief in faith-healing and the laying on of hands. Stekert observed that even migrants to the urban North maintain a strong adherence to faith healing in spite of the absence of religious behavior [21].

The traditional medical practitioner in the Appalachian region has been a wise or gifted older person—frequently a family member or neighbor—whose medical knowledge is based on the properties of local herbs, patent medicines, and home remedies. While Southern Appalachians may call a traditional medical doctor, it is usually a last resort [16, 21]; generally, "the way things were done back home in the past was far superior to the present" even for the many Appalachians who had migrated to the urban environment of Detroit [21].

The region's transmission of medical lore and practice has often been through women. Granny women still deliver many children and provide much of the pre- and postnatal care mothers receive [18]. However, with migration to the North, Appalachians' folk remedies and medical practices have been replaced or substituted with that which is available in the North. This does not mean, however, that Appalachians have turned to Western medical personnel for assistance. Rather, they have made the necessary adjustments in their beliefs and needs to provide for their well-being in a different environment.

As it is for the Navajo and Mexican-American, mainstream urban American culture is difficult for the Southern Appalachian to comprehend. Furthermore, it is difficult to maintain the close, supportive kin ties of the rural South in the urban North. The sense of community that is omnipresent in the South is generally absent from most Northern settings. Furthermore, the enduring Appalachian value of being "average" is defied in urban environments where the emphasis is on getting ahead and bettering one's neighbor. Consequently, the Appalachian migrant is often disarmed by urban competitiveness and the bureaucracies of everyday life. Where doctors and nurses are looked upon as more or less average people in Appalachia, they have an entirely different, almost unapproachable, status in the North. The social distance between medical personnel and migrant Appalachians is difficult to bridge, whether the context be social, cultural, or medical.

The emphasis in traditional Southern Appalachian medicine is on personal and close social relationships between the client and medical practitioner. Stekert describes these as "intense and reinforcing personal relationships" that are not one dimensional [21]; that is, the Appalachian client would be likely to interact with his doctor in a variety of settings and social contexts—for example, at church, school, business, and farm. Yet despite this interaction in the home community, a high value is placed on privacy and mutual respect.

While medical practices in Southern Appalachia are somewhat related to those of modern medicine, the underlying values of the people undermine their participation in scientific medicine. The emphasis on remuneration, punctuality and waiting, and physical immodesty in the health-care setting are all factors that keep Southern Appalachians away from medical personnel and keep them relying on herbal and patent medicine cures.

A Case Study

To illustrate some of the immediate and long-term results of intercultural communication and understanding in the health-care professions, the following recent case provides an excellent example of some health-care problems and their possible resolution.

An elderly Mexican-American migrant worker, whom we will call Señor Castillo, was brought to the emergency room of a rural Michigan hospital with complaints of abdominal pain. On admittance, the patient's blood pressure was 150/100. There were no observable problems. However, because Sr. Castillo was pointing to his left side and complaining of severe pain, the emergency room physician diagnosed a potential gall bladder problem. Films and serologic studies were scheduled for the next day, and the client was given Demerol with Vistaril for his discomfort.

The hospital had been unable to contact Sr. Castillo's immediate family, and the client was literally abandoned to a general ward. During the evening a student nurse approached the patient and, in the course of her routine duties, asked Sr. Castillo if he spoke Spanish. Though she had had only high-school Spanish, the student nurse was able to obtain the client's complete medical history, including the names of his previously prescribed antihypertension medications. The following morning a cholecystogram was performed and no gall bladder irregularities were observed. However, abnormalities in the serology and a blood pressure of 190/120 indicated other problems—namely, pancreatitis and complications due to hypertension. The patient was then treated properly and, after a short stay, was released in good health.

Difficulties in cross-cultural understanding can appear in all health-care environments. In this case, an inquisitive student nurse who used her basic foreign language skills was able to reveal many more dimensions of the client's personal medical history. In addition, the client's family, once they had been contacted, were able to provide the student nurse with an even more precise picture of Sr. Castillo's health. She discovered, for example, that the family believed that a *bruja*, a sorcerer, had been responsible for their father's declining health, but, since there had been no *curandero* in the worker's camp, no preventive medical action had been taken. Furthermore, the student nurse discovered that the family knew of neither their father's genuine health problems nor the medications that he had been taking. By the time the actual medical problem had been diagnosed, the nurse and staff had learned not only the particulars of Sr. Castillo's medical history but also something of the attitudes of Mexican-Americans towards scientific, institutional health care and of their attitudes towards illness in general.

As a lasting result of this incident, the hospital administration instituted a program in which all staff members who speak foreign languages were identified and then appropriately assigned to non-English-speaking patients. The program cost nothing to institute, and the services of the hospital were greatly augmented.

CULTURAL CONSIDERATIONS IN HEALTH-CARE DELIVERY

Although the specific treatments that these three minorities employ for disease differ, the underlying values that govern their medical behavior are similar in many ways. Foremost, there is an emphasis on reunifying the spiritual and physical well-being of the client and of the larger community. The health of the community is not just a biologic one; rather, the community can be deemed healthy when it is in working order physically, socially, and culturally. Modern medical personnel who have contact with any minority population have to be aware of sometimes small but always important differences in the approach to medical treatment and care. In the case of the Mexican-Americans and Navajo, language and culture can be primary obstacles in attempting to treat disease and to begin preventive medicine. For all three groups geographic accessibility and economic conditions can further inhibit the use of medical services and personnel. Most important and most sensitive, however, are the underlying values that minority populations maintain. Values form the basis of day-to-day attitudes and behaviors and must be respected by medical personnel. By sensitive, patient contact with minority clients, medical personnel—whether nurses, physicians, or technicians—must attempt to alleviate the fears, doubts, superstitions, and sense of isolation that minority patients often feel and that deter them from seeking concrete medical and health-care advice.

REFERENCES

1. Adair, J. The Indian health worker in the Cornell-Navaho project. *Human Organization,* 19 : 59, 1960.
2. Adair, J., and Deuschle, K. W. *The People's Health.* New York: Appleton-Century-Crofts, 1970.
3. Driver, H. E. *Indians of North America.* Chicago: University of Chicago Press, 1969.
4. Foster, G. M. Disease etiologies in nonwestern medical systems. *American Anthropologist,* 78 : 773, 1976.
5. Hayes-Bautista, D. E. Termination of the patient-practitioner relationship: Divorce, patient style. *Journal of Health and Social Behavior,* 17 : 12, 1976.
6. Hoppe, S. K., and Heller, P. Alienation, familism and the utilization of health services by Mexican-Americans. *Journal of Health and Social Behavior,* 16 : 304, 1975.
7. Ingham, J. M. On Mexican folk medicine. *American Anthropologist,* 72 : 76, 1970.
8. Kiev, A. *Curanderismo: Mexican-American Folk Psychiatry.* New York: Free Press, 1968.
9. Kluckhohn, C., and Leighton, D. *The Navaho.* New York: Doubleday, 1962.
10. Kluckhohn, R. (Ed.). *Culture and Behavior.* New York: Free Press, 1962.
11. Kniep-Hardy, M., and Burkhardt, M. Nursing the Navajo. *American Journal of Nursing,* 77 : 95, 1977.
12. Leighton, A., and Leighton, D. *The Navaho Door.* Cambridge, Mass.: Harvard University Press, 1944.
13. Manning, P. K., and Fabrega, H. F., Jr. The Experience of Self and Body: Health and Illness in the Ghipas Highlands. In George Psathas (Ed.), *Phenomenological Sociology.* New York: Wiley, 1973.
14. New, P. K. M. Traditional and modern health care: An appraisal of complementarity. *International Social Science Journal,* 29 : 483, 1977.
15. Nurge, E. Anthropological perspective for medical students. *Human Organization,* 34 : 345, 1975.
16. Pearsall, M. *Little Smokey Ridge.* Birmingham: University of Alabama Press, 1959.
17. Press, I. Urban folk medicine. *American Anthropologist,* 80 : 71, 1978.

18. Roberts, B., and Roberts, N.   *Where Time Stood Still.* London: Collier MacMillan, 1970.
19. Romano, O. I. V.   Charismatic medicine, folk-healing and folk-sainthood. *American Anthropologist,* 67 : 1151, 1965.
20. Rubel, A. J.   Concepts of disease in Mexican-American culture. *American Anthropologist,* 62 : 795, 1960.
21. Stekert, E.   Focus for conflict: Southern mountain medical beliefs in Detroit. *Journal of American Folklore,* 83 : 115, 1970.
22. Suchman, E. A.   Social factors in medical deprivation. *American Journal of Public Health,* 55 : 1725, 1965.
23. Suchman, E. A.   Social Patterns of Illness and Medical Care. In E. G. Jaco (Ed.), *Patients, Physicians and Illness.* New York: Free Press, 1972.
24. Weclew, R. V.   The nature, prevalence, and level of awareness of "curanderismo" and some of its implications for community mental health. *Community Mental Health Journal,* 11 : 145, 1975.
25. Young, A.   Some implications of medical beliefs and practices for social anthropology. *American Anthropologist,* 78 : 5, 1976.

Claire Gavin Meisenheimer

8

Family-Centered Teaching

Why do I need to involve the patient's family?
How can I use family resources to realize more effective teaching-learning outcomes?

Failure to involve a patient's family or significant others in the teaching plan may be a barrier to both teaching and learning. The family can provide crucial information in the assessment phase of the teaching-learning process. The family can also provide support and other resources that are essential not only to patient teaching but also to subsequent compliance with posthospitalization prescriptions. The following chapter describes family structures, roles, and relationships and their importance to patient education. Relationships within the patient's family structure are described, and a systematic process to assess family needs is presented as a means to create health-related change within the family system.
    The information in this chapter should help the reader to

1. Describe how the humanistic view of man relates to patient education
2. Define family as it relates to patient care
3. Describe family and health and how their interrelations affect learning
4. Use a Family Assessment Schema to promote effective learning
5. Design a teaching plan that encompasses family input as well as outcomes

"No man is an island, entire of itself; every
man is a piece of the continent, a part of the
main . . ." John Donne, *Devotions* XVII

This well-known passage as quoted by Anderson and Carter [1] provides the basis for the use of systems theory in the development of a family-centered teaching model. Family-centered care implies a systematic approach to the assessment and management of family health needs; it requires an environment conducive to therapeutic relationships. This approach also provides a clearer understanding of the complex hierarchy of man, families, communities, and society, and how they function to maintain their health.

This chapter will introduce and briefly discuss concepts of family theory as they relate to patient and family teaching and will provide an overall framework of health care, the family, and education. The primary emphasis will be on the multiple disciplines that provide patient education as they interface with each other, with patients, and with families. This systems perspective will provide the conceptual links between professionals and nonprofessionals that are necessary for a health-care team to achieve mutual goals with patients and their families. While this chapter is by no means an exhaustive study of families and health teaching, it does provide an overview of families, their structure, and roles as they interrelate with their subsystems and suprasystems.

THE FAMILY AS A SYSTEM

One distinct way of looking at family-centered teaching is the general systems model, as developed by Ludwig von Bertalanffy [2]. The systems view offers a perspective for looking at men and women and their environment as interacting wholes with integrated sets of characteristics and relationships.

Men and women, and therefore families, are living, open systems, comprised of elements interrelating with each other within a semipermeable boundary. The structure and functions or processes of the system regulate both the kind and rate of the flow of inputs and outputs to and from the system. These interactions and relationships bind the elements of the system together into a meaningful whole. The educators must be able to identify the significant relationships at the specific time. They must also be able to define the environment, that is, all the factors that influence or are influenced by the system. Arranged hierarchically, each system possesses a subsystem and a suprasystem. Therefore, it is the system and the environment that together comprise the total phenomenon.

The family is the single social unit in human society inextricably interwoven with all these other systems. The model of the systems concept for family-centered teaching (see Figure 3) depicts the structure in which the patient interfaces with his suprasystems while health education traverses all the systems. Input in the form of knowledge is taken into the systems and, through a complex

The author wishes to thank the Family Hospital Diabetic Education Committee for sharing their *Teaching Assessment Record* to aid in the writing of this chapter.

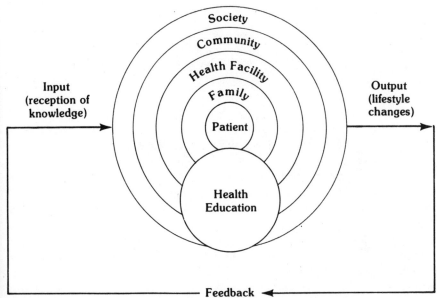

Figure 3. A model of the systems concept for family-centered teaching.

dynamic interaction of processes (throughput) and internal feedback, decisions to change lifestyles should be positive outputs. All of the concepts and principles of general systems theory are implied in this static, one-dimensional model. The following pages will discuss these processes.

Philosophy

The systems approach allows a humanistic view of people as holistic, goal-directed, self-maintaining, self-creating individuals of intrinsic worth, capable of reflection on their own uniqueness [3]. The individual is a total human being and a social creature who creates networks with others in hierarchically arranged human systems. From the level of the individual to the level of society, the person can be conceptualized as a patient or client, and can become the target for health education for all health professionals.

The systems perspective permits the organization of a vast number of theories and concepts into a meaningful frame of reference, and nurtures a significant philosophy of health care that recognizes values, attitudes, change, growth, and learning as possible because of the essential interrelatedness of all living systems. A philosophy of family-centered care implies the inclusion of all individuals—patient, family members, and health professionals and paraprofessionals—in the planning, implementing, and evaluating of health care.

The Family Defined

The family is a social system composed of family member subsystems, while the family itself functions as a subsystem within the larger suprasystem of health facilities, community, and society. The concept of family needs to be flexible and fluid. Customs vary widely by race, class, occupation, ethnic, and community background, and by religion.

Laws have defined family, including the rights and duties of all the members. The Federal Bureau of the Census defines a family as "a group of two or more persons related by marriage, blood, or adoption who reside together." Messer states the family "is an organization or social institution with continuity (past, present, and future), in which there are certain behaviors in common that affect each other; sharing of goals and identity, mutual concern for physical and emotional needs, and patterns or response that do not require the person to constantly be on guard" [5].

In light of changing social attitudes toward living arrangements involving new "family units," the definition of family must be changed to accommodate the increasing variety of nonprocreational forms of families, such as sibling families, communes, homosexual marriages, single parents, foster parents, and grand-parents. The definition adopted for this work is the following: the family is whoever is significant to the patient at a given point in time. A person's family consists of those with whom he or she interacts and performs the family functions. This definition will include the nuclear, the extended and sanguine, and the augmented family structures.

Family Processes: Adaptation, Integration, Communication, Decision-Making

In order to survive and grow, the family system requires adaptive, integrative, and decision-making processes. The family must respond to one another and to the environment as the situation demands. There must be flexibility of group structure and individual behavior. The process of family *adaptation* consists of the four boundary maintenance functions of obtaining, containing, retaining, and disposing [3]. During this process the family takes in certain products (knowledge) for its use (input); regulates admission to the system; keeps the appropriate matter, energy, and information; and disposes (output) either useful or waste products to the environment. Again, assessment of this process provides useful data in order to direct appropriate health-care intervention.

Family *integration* is the control of subsystem components through bonds of coherence and unity that run through family life, of which affection, common interests, common goals, and economic interdependence are of great importance. The family's ability to become integrated is strongly related to the manner in which it deals with bonding and values, norms and rules, roles, communication patterns, and transactional modes of its subsystems [3].

All transactional modes are carried out through *communication*. Communication determines the quality of life more than any other subprocesses of adaptation, integration, and decision-making. The giving and receiving of verbal and nonverbal messages between family members serves as the system's linkage mechanism. Decisions are made and family rules are established through this process. In a well-functioning family system, communication is meaningful, congruent with feelings and expectations, and growth-promoting. Communication in a family takes place through group structure. Members usually speak in terms of their prescribed roles, power, and status.

The overall goal of intervention is the promotion of rational *decision-making*. The appraisal of family dynamics in terms of roles, communication patterns, and transactional modes is vital to the health professional in assisting patients and their families to perform their adaptive, integrative, and decision-making tasks.

The family is a critical human system. It serves unique, although always changing, purposes for its subsystems—family members and combinations of family members—and suprasystems—society and parts of society. This systems approach to family and subsequently to family-centered teaching may concern those who have long been advocates of the holistic approach to understanding men and women as individuals. It must be quickly noted that this approach does not in any way negate the needs of the individual; rather it emphasizes that only through a concern for all can one insure that the individual will receive the care he or she needs. Only if individuals are viewed as interrelated, interacting, and interdependent parts of a significant social network can one understand them and help them achieve their maximum potential for health. Understanding the concepts of individual, self, and family role will assist the professional in developing a philosophy and a consistent practice.

HEALTH CARE AS A SYSTEM

It is an accepted fact that two societal subsystems, family and health care, affect each other. One of the principle functions of the family is to acknowledge the unique worth of individual members and to encourage their personal development and well-being. A major dimension of this basic family function is to protect health and to develop the unique physical capacities of individual members. Physical health is a resource that permits individuals to attain their goals and to achieve personal fulfillment. The family is a personal-care system within which health is molded and health care is mobilized organized, and executed.

The family's ability to perform its health function depends on its structure. It depends upon the extent and variety of interaction among family members, the extent of family links to other social systems, the extent of active coping effort by family members, the extent of freedom and responsiveness to individual members of the family, and the flexibility or rigidity of family role relationships [6].

King defines health as "a dynamic state in the life cycle of an organism which implies continuous adaptation to stresses in the internal and external environment through optimum use of one's resources to achieve maximum potential for daily living" [4].

Self-regulation is a characteristic of living, open systems. When the system can not cope with the stressors, then illness and disease may occur. The sick role affects both the relationship of the person assuming it and the other family members. Depending on the severity and length of the illness, role impairment or complete role disruption may become permanent. The impairment of any family role will require alteration of reciprocal roles. Such reorganization, although potentially stressful to individual family members, is essential to achieve a new equilibrium for the family organization. The process of reorganization involves all family members and can dramatically affect the patient and the outcome of his illness. The vulnerability of the family unit to a crisis is related to the ability of the family members to modify their respective roles, perform tasks essential for the continuity of family life, and redefine personal expectations and goals. The family's perception of the illness in terms of family relationships and goals, the resources available to the family, and reorganizational patterns chosen in any previous crisis are also important to assess.

Planning Change in the Family

Illness, generally, is perceived as a crisis-producing event. Illness demands that changes occur in the system. The concept of change is necessary to understand and utilize in intervention. Change is a phenomenon with which all individuals and social systems must deal since change occurs at all system levels. The ramifications of planned change need to be evaluated as integration of a change into a system is contingent upon positive reinforcement and the congruence with the existing value orientation. Crises can occur with any change if the demands upon a system are greater than the resources. Crises occur "when a person faces an obstacle to important life goals that is, for a time, insurmountable through the utilization of customary methods of problem solving. A period of disorganization ensues" [3]. A system that is in disequilibrium is emotionally vulnerable and receptive to crisis intervention (change) which should assist in establishing a new state of functioning. It should result in a system that learns new ways of behaving, ways that promote growth.

Providing Family-Centered Teaching

Health professionals must be able to assess the family's adaptive mechanisms to the crisis situation, their strengths, and their willingness and ability to change. They must know where the family places health in its value system in order to assist the family in changing to a new, more effective level of health practice.

Health professionals, by virtue of their position in society, usually have entry past the boundary of the family-unit system. Accessibility to the family's interpersonal system must then be negotiated. Effective use of their cognitive, interpersonal, and technical skills then depends upon their ability accurately to assess and meet the perceived needs of the family.

Family Assessment Schema

While the literature reflects several distinct approaches to family assessment (psychoanalytic, interactional, developmental, systems, and those of an eclectic nature), the development of an assessment tool suitable for collecting data describing the holistic nature of the family has been difficult [7]. While all members of the health team are responsible for assessment, the nurse, by virtue of her position at the bedside 24 hours a day, must initiate the data collection and coordinate the plan of care.

There are basically two methods of data collection: (1) interviewing for present and past information regarding health status, behavior, and feelings, and (2) observation of present condition, including congruencies and discrepancies between the various data sources. In order to design and evaluate a comprehensive plan of care, the following data must be collected.

Family Assessment Schema

I. Family membership
   A. Members living in household
      1. Name
      2. Date of birth
      3. Sex
      4. Race
      5. Religion
      6. Relationship to patient
      7. Occupation
   B. Members of family not living in household
   C. Roles and relationships of members
      (Who is responsible for various household tasks? Who will assume responsibilities of patient? Who usually makes major and minor decisions? How?)
   D. Activities of daily living
      1. Eating patterns
      2. Sleeping patterns
      3. Leisure activities
II. Health and medical history
   A. Present illnesses of patient
      (Duration, nature of onset, symptoms, precipitating issues, treatment of symptoms, outcomes)
   B. Illnesses of family members
   C. Past significant illnesses and accidents
   D. Special health regimens of patient/family
      1. Diet
      2. Medications (name, dosage, frequency, purpose)
      3. Physical activity

    E. Physical assessment
       1. Patient
       2. Family members
    F. Perceptions of health problem
       (Including perceived threat to family roles and relationships)
       1. Patient
       2. Family
       3. Nurse
       4. Physician
       5. Other disciplines
    G. Resources utilized in past to meet health needs
       1. Within family
       2. Community (public health, church, clubs, etc.)
III. Cultural and socioeconomic factors
    A. Education level (highest grade completed)
    B. Medical care financed
    C. Social relationships (outside family, church, clubs, community activities, etc.)
IV. Laboratory tests, X-rays and other diagnostic procedures
V. Summary
    A. Problem list (prioritized)
       1. Patient
       2. Family
       3. Nurse
       4. Physician
       5. Other disciplines

While sufficient data is seldom acquired during a single interview by one practitioner, the use of the Family Assessment Schema provides all disciplines the opportunity to assess, supplement, and refine information regarding the patient's health and family history. It prevents duplication, provides a systematic and comprehensive record, and commits all persons involved to meeting similar goals.

The problem list, developed by extracting all pertinent abnormalities and their projected consequences, reflects a synthesis of the data base. The listing of specific data relevant to each problem, along with an assessment of problem status and management plan, leads to the identification of education needs. Family roles and relationships, goals and values, communication patterns, resources within and outside of the family unit, and the family's potential for self-sufficiency should be determined during the assessment process. Who is the decision-maker? Who will be committed to the ill person? Who is physically and mentally capable of identifying needs and mobilizing resources? What needs can be met with patient education programming to create change within the family system?

Designing Family Teaching Programs

Recognizing the uniqueness of the patient and family, determined by biologic and psychologic makeup, social and physical environment, and past experiences, the patient educator must individualize the teaching plan. It must include knowledge of the disease or illness, treatment regimens, and resources with which the family can perceive ways to change behaviors.

The educational assessment should be planned using the expertise of all appropriate health professionals, the patient, and the family. Due to the specialization of knowledge, the multidisciplinary approach is necessary to provide comprehensive, coordinated, and continuous care. While there may be some overlap in the roles of the physician, nurse, social worker, physical therapist, dietitian, and other health professionals, each must contribute his or her unique knowledge and skills.

The *case conference* provides an opportunity for all persons involved to answer the question: "What do the patient and family know? What do the patient and family want to know? What do the patient and family need to know to change behaviors that will optimize their health outcomes?" This establishing of educational goals for the patient and family requires a mutual relationship built upon understanding and trust with involved health professionals. These goals must be communicated to all—patient, family, and professionals—and be understood and accepted if change is to occur.

The Teaching Assessment Record, as illustrated in the section entitled Resource Material: Sample Diabetic Teaching Assessment Record, should include the patient's and family's knowledge and skills relevant to (1) disease process, (2) symptom recognition, (3) symptom treatment and prevention, (4) diet, (5) medication, (6) exercise, and (7) good health practices. It should also include notations as to (1) receptivity to learning; (2) barriers/enhancers of learning (physical, emotional, intellectual, sociocultural, previous education); (3) effect of disease on work, finances, and environment; (4) strengths (coping abilities such as understanding and responding to health problems); and (5) teaching methods including visual aids.

This record is extremely important since it allows the individual team members to interact in the identification and solution of patient problems and allows each member of the team to know what has been done and why and allows assessment of significant information known about the patient. With the establishment of a specific body of knowledge individualized according to the particular learning needs of the patient and family, reinforcement can be done by all involved including those not on the formal team, at all times of the day and night. The degree of patient contact and scope of activity for any given member of the team will vary according to the nature of the patient's and family's problems.

Educational Methods

The educational methods chosen (individual, group, or a combination of both) again reflect the needs of the family. Criteria for selecting educational methods should include effectiveness, efficiency, adequacy, and appropriateness. The manpower, time, materials, and cost of the program are always issues to consider. Teaching-learning techniques such as demonstration, film, slides, discussions, role-playing, closed-circuit television, programmed instruction, and pamphlets and various reading materials should be chosen according to psychosocial, intellectual, and cultural needs.

Professionals are teaching all of the time, informally more often than formally. They must be available when the family is available. The family's life style must be considered when planning the program. If a skill needs to be mastered, demonstration and practice sessions must be provided for the patient and family when they are available. While families should be encouraged to participate in the treatment regimens, their schedules may not always coincide with the hospital routines. Alterations should be made to accommodate the supportive members of the family. For example, the dietitian may eat meals with the patient and family in the cafeteria, assisting them in selecting appropriate foods; a family member may come to the hospital before work to test the patient's urine and administer insulin in a site the patient is unable to reach; feeding techniques or other activities of daily living may be demonstrated and practiced before family members leave for work.

A less frequently utilized opportunity for assessment and teaching is the home visit prior to discharge. This visit provides the nurse with additional insights about the family as a resource in the maintenance or disruption of health needed to plan a total and frequently more realistic and holistic program for the family. Interacting with the family in their setting, where they can exert greater control over their own existence, will produce treatment regimens to meet immediate and long term goals. It is imperative to give the family opportunities to identify their own strengths and weaknesses, and to request specific experiences that they feel would facilitate their learning. Simulating the home environment in the hospital will ensure greater commitment and compliance to health regimens.

Creating an educational climate and utilizing all appropriate opportunities to achieve educational goals becomes the responsibility of all health professionals. Only then can the meeting and maintaining of these goals be consistently measured.

Family-centered teaching requires that the family system, not an individual designated as a patient, be considered the patient. Family involvement must be routine. Society must become more aware of the power of the family system both to cripple lives and to expand their potential.

Family-centered teaching implies a multidisciplinary concept of education that embraces the family in its entirety during the total experience of wellness, illness, hospitalization, and recuperation. It suggests a many-faceted approach in meeting mutually established goals. It implies a systematic approach to the identification and resolution of family needs, and it demands an environment conducive to therapeutic relationships. Family-centered teaching demands a commitment to patients, their families, the community, and society at large to provide meaningful programming to promote, maintain, and restore health, to prevent illness, and to facilitate learning that has significance for health-promoting behavior.

REFERENCES

1. Anderson, R. E., and Carter, I. E. *Human Behavior in the Social Environment: A Social Systems Approach.* Chicago: Aldine, 1974. P. 6.
2. Bertalanffy, L., von. *General Systems Theory.* New York: Braziller, 1968.
3. Hall, J. E., and Weaver, B. R. *Distributive Nursing Practice: A Systems Approach to Community Health.* Philadelphia: Lippincott, 1977. P. 20.
4. King, I. M. *Toward a Theory for Nursing.* New York: Wiley, 1971. P. 12.
5. Murray, R., and Zentner, J. *Nursing Concepts for Health Promotion.* Englewood Cliffs, N.J.: Prentice Hall, 1972. P. 348.
6. Pratt, L. *Family Structure and Effective Behavior: The Energized Family.* Boston: Houghton Mifflin, 1976. P. 78.
7. Reinhart, A. M., and Quinn, M. D. (Eds.). *Family-Centered Community Nursing: A Sociocultural Framework.* St. Louis: Mosby, 1973. Pp. 88–91.

Resource Materials

SUGGESTED READINGS

Crawford, C. O. *Heath and the Family: A Medical-Sociological Analysis.* New York: MacMillan, 1971.
Downs, F. S. Technological advances and the nurse-family relationship. *Nursing Digest,* 2 : 22–24, 1975.
Hall, J. E., and Weaver, B. *Nursing Families in Crisis.* Philadelphia: Lippincott, 1974.
Haller, L. L. Families systems theory in psychiatric intervention. *American Journal of Nursing,* 3 : 462–463, 1974.
Hazzard, M. E. An overview of systems theory. *Nursing Clinics of North America,* 3 : 385–393, 1971.
Hymovich, D. P., and Barnard, B. U. *Family Health Care.* New York: McGraw-Hill, 1973.
Kantor, D., and Lehr, W. *Inside the Family: Toward a Theory of Family Process.* San Francisco: Jossey-Bass, 1975.
MacVicar, M. J., and Archibald, P. A framework for family assessment in chronic illness. *Nursing Forum,* 2 : 181–194, 1976.
Murray, R., and Zentner, J. *Nursing Assessment and Health Promotion Through the Life Span.* Englewood Cliffs, N.J.: Prentice-Hall, 1975.
Napier, A. Y., and Whitaker, C. A. *The Family Crucible.* New York: Harper & Row, 1978.
Orem, D. E. *Nursing: Concepts of Practice.* New York: McGraw-Hill, 1971.
Redman, B. K. *The Process of Patient Teaching in Nursing* (2nd ed.). St. Louis: Mosby, 1972.
Rogers, C. *On Becoming a Person.* Boston: Houghton Mifflin, 1961.
Smoyak, S. A. Toward understanding nursing situation: A transactional paradigm. *Nursing Research,* 5 : 405, 1969.
Sobol, E., and Tobischon, P. *Family Nursing: A Study Guide.* St. Louis: Mosby, 1970.
Thompson, L., Miller, M., and Bigler, H. *Sociology: Nurses and Their Patients in a Modern Society.* St. Louis: Mosby, 1975.

Sample Diabetic Teaching Assessment Record

Check teaching aids utilized
____ 1. "Getting Started" tape
____ 2. "Living with Diabetes" filmstrip
____ 3. "So You've Got Diabetes" movie
____ 4. Teaching tapes
    ____ Future of Diabetes
    ____ Diet Tips
    ____ Urine Testing Tips
    ____ Different Types of Insulin
    ____ Long Term Complications
    ____ Hyper-Hypoglycemia
    ____ Oral Hypoglycemic Drugs
    ____ Other _____

____ 5. Meal planning game
____ 6. Other _____

Check classes attended
____ 1. Introduction
____ 2. Dietary
____ 3. Medications
____ 4. Urine testing
____ 5. General care

Diabetic history
1. Age at onset of diabetes _____
2. Type of diet: home _____ hospital _____
3. Medication: home _____ hospital _____
4. Urine testing method _____
5. Family history of diabetes _____

Possible barriers to learning
____ 1. Decreased vision
____ 2. Hearing loss
____ 3. Speaks foreign language _____
____ 4. Decreased memory
____ 5. Other _____

Diabetes Teaching Guide and Checklist

	Yes	No	Date	Initials	Comments
1. Received and read teaching material					
2. Patient describes what diabetes is					
3. Patient is able to test urine using:					
a. Clinitest					
b. Tes Tape					
c. Acetest or Ketostix					
d. Keto-Diastix					
e. Diastix					
4. Patient					
a. Can keep an accurate record of urine testing					
b. Knows what a second voided urine is					
5. Answer the following:					
a. What will happen to the blood sugar if you eat too much or forget to take your medication?					
b. When your body cannot get enough sugar into the cells for energy, what will your body use for fuel?					
c. When too much fat is broken down what is the result?					
d. What urine test will tell you if your body is using fat for fuel and producing acetone?					
e. The name of the condition resulting from moderate to large amounts of acetone in the blood is?					

107

Diabetes Teaching Guide (Continued)

	Yes	No	Date	Initials	Comments
f. What would you do if you test your urine and find acetone in it?					
6. Patient can explain what an oral antidiabetic medication does					
7. Patient can explain what insulin is and how it works					
8. Insulin preparation and injection:					
a. Patient can describe when the insulin works					
b. Patient can demonstrate the ability to accurately withdraw the correct amount					
c. Patient demonstrates the ability to administer insulin					
d. Patient demonstrates the ability to keep a site rotation chart					
e. Patient is able to discuss the plans for care and storing of equipment and supplies					
9. Patient has had dietary consult:					
a. First					
b. Second					
10. Patient can accurately complete a selective food menu for his particular calorie level					
11. Patient can tell which foods are included in each broad category					
12. Patient is able to explain why diet is important in regulating diabetes:					
a. Kinds of food eaten					

108

b. Amounts of food eaten			
c. Time food is eaten			
13. Patient can explain the effect of physical activity on the balance of sugar and insulin:			
a. Normal activity			
b. Increased activity			
c. Decreased activity			
14. Patient can tell whether the blood sugar goes up or down with the following:			
a. Sore throat			
b. Infected cut			
c. Emotional upset			
d. A boil			
e. Skipping a meal			
f. Unusual exercise or exertion on rare occasions			
15. Patient can explain why it is important for him to do the following:			
a. Avoid skin lacerations and learn to care for a cut or skin irritation should one occur			
b. Keep skin dry, warm and unchafed			
c. Bathe regularly with warm water and mild soap			
d. Wear shoes outdoors			
e. Visit dentist every six months			

Diabetes Teaching Guide (Continued)

	Yes	No	Date	Initials	Comments
f. Visit an ophthalmologist every 6–12 months					
g. Visit physician regularly					
h. Consult a podiatrist when necessary					
16. Complications of diabetes					
a. Insulin reactions:					
1. Patient is able to explain the signs and symptoms of too much insulin					
2. Patient is able to list four things that might cause an insulin reaction					
3. Patient can explain the immediate treatment for insulin reaction					
4. Patient can explain why artificially sweetened food will not stop an insulin reaction					
5. Patient can tell what kind of food to carry at all times					
b. Diabetic acidosis:					
1. Patient is able to tell the signs of too much acetone in the blood					
2. Patient is able to tell some of the reasons why diabetic acidosis might occur					
3. Patient is able to state what he should do when he notices signs of diabetic acidosis					
17. Is Public Health Department of Visiting Nurses' Assoc. referral needed?					
18. Family members taught?					

II

Patient Teaching Activities

Discharge Planning and Patient Teaching

How can I help the patient continue to learn after he leaves the hospital? How can the discharge planner assure continuity of care and of teaching between the hospital and the community?

Patient education programming, to be most efficient and effective, requires many more activities than just the interactions of the teacher and the learner. Barriers to the patients' learning (see Chapter 6) exist, in part, because patients have such a short length of stay in the hospital and because they have not yet identified what problems will be faced upon return to the home environment. Thus, a means needs to be provided for patients to continue their learning as well as their care after they have returned to the community. Discharge planning, an essential component of continuity of care, is one means to insure continued teaching; the solution of identified care problems must continue after the patient leaves the hospital. The linkage between patient teaching and discharge planning is integral to continued learning as well as to continued identification and solution of patients' problems once they leave the protective environment of the hospital. The following chapter describes the activities of the discharge planner, why those activities are necessary, how they can be carried out, how they interface with patient teaching, and how to determine if they are effective. A sample of a nurse's patient discharge notes is provided to assist readers in devising or updating discharge planning activities in their own agency.

The information in this chapter should help the reader to

1. *List at least five factors that point to a need for discharge planning*
2. *Describe administrative supports necessary to ensure success of discharge planning*

3. *Describe the process of discharge planning*
4. *Describe the linkages between hospitals and home health or long-term care agencies*
5. *State the importance of patient transfer information*
6. *Devise a means of measuring the effectiveness of the discharge planning process*

Discharge planning and patient teaching are obviously related. To discuss one without discussing the other is quite inappropriate.

Let us consider Mrs. J., a 68-year-old woman admitted to the hospital with an established diagnosis of a fractured left femoral neck; she had a secondary diagnosis of diabetes mellitus. On the fifth postoperative day after insertion of an Austin Moore prosthesis, Mrs. J.'s blood sugar, which had previously been controlled on orinase, remained elevated, necessitating the initiation of lente insulin. Plans with the patient and family were completed for transfer to the skilled nursing facility as a stepping stone before going home. However, on the day before transfer, Mrs. J. recorded a temperature of 103°F. A diagnosis of cholelithiasis was made, and a cholecystectomy was performed. Postoperatively a chronic problem of urinary retention resulted in overflow incontinence. A neurogenic bladder secondary to the diabetes was diagnosed, and self-catheterization was deemed necessary for maintenance care. When discharge from the hospital appeared imminent once again, Mrs. J. was extremely eager to return to her own home. Assessment determined this choice as an appropriate one; after a 58-day hospital stay, the patient was discharged to her own home. The problems identified in this actual case study should stimulate thinking about the link between patient teaching and discharge planning. In this particular case, as well as in the largest number of cases, patient teaching addresses the task of preparing hospitalized patients for safely maintaining their personal care when they return home.

This chapter will focus on discharge planning and its relationship to patient teaching. The significance of a structured, identifiable approach to this issue will be discussed.

Continuity of care is a concept increasingly gaining recognition as an integral part of the health delivery system. To provide uninterrupted, progressive, comprehensive care to patients is a goal of modern health-care systems and is implicit in continuity of care. To have the patient in the right place, at the right time, at the right cost is part of the concept. Continuity of care can be expressed as a catalyst that will hasten the patient from sickness to health by the results of a planned activity for this progressive, comprehensive care. The vehicle by which this concept is activated is discharge planning.

Health-care providers have long passed the time when they can just think about what will happen to Mrs. J. when she leaves the hospital; a plan for posthospital needs must be developed during her hospitalization to ensure that when medical care is no longer warranted, she will be ready for discharge. Wensley most clearly points out that the walls of the hospitals must not become barriers for patients. Patients come from the community setting; hopefully, they will return to the community setting [11]. It is the responsibility of the health-care professional at the hospital level to prepare them for the other side of the walls. If the continuity of care concept is fulfilled, a program of specialized and supportive care for Mrs. J will have been developed so that her discharge will be timely, and her continued care will be facilitated; she will regain the optimum degree of health and rehabilitation.

Supporting factors that contribute to the rationale of discharge planning include the following:

1. The basic premise is that every patient shall be afforded the benefit of the highest quality care at any point of his or her health-care needs.
2. Patients should receive the benefits of the services of appropriate community resources.
3. The patient in the institutional setting can be overwhelmed by the complexities of technology and by the strange environment. No matter what and how the patient is taught, he or she may not comprehend everything. Follow-up teaching and evaluation are essential.
4. Regulatory mandates have spurred the development of quality assurance programs that demand discharge planning as well as patient education.
5. The more appropriate utilization of the acute-care bed is a mandate. Utilization review without the counterpart of a viable discharge planning program is a traumatic, problematic process in which the patient can be lost.

THE ROLE OF THE NURSE IN DISCHARGE PLANNING

Nursing has for years academically accepted the philosophy of continuity of care. But has nursing clinically fulfilled the obligations of the philosophy? Discharge planning is an integral part of nursing care. Every patient-care plan should have a discharge plan that results from the overall assessment of the patient's needs, beginning on admission (and continually updated). Each and every patient occupying a hospital bed has discharge planning needs. From these needs patient teaching evolves. The simple tonsillectomy or adenoidectomy patient, the herniorrhaphy patient, and the appendectomy patient demand attention for their posthospital care. Does the patient understand his or her activity limitations? Does he or she have prescriptions for necessary medications? Does he or she understand the use and purpose of the medications? Are there any diet restrictions? Each nurse providing patient care has a responsibility to see that these needs are addressed. Two out of every three patients will require more in-depth instruction, equipment, or other care [3]. Fifteen to twenty percent will require even more sophisticated care. Indeed, preparing the patient for discharge, including the assurance that the patient has gained sufficient knowlege to maintain safe care, is integral to nursing.

Realistically, does the staff nurse (in addition to the vast number of other duties he or she must assume) have the time and background preparation necessary to meet the sophisticated discharge planning needs of the 15 to 20 percent of the patients who require such? The acute needs of the patient must rightfully come first, and prioritization may place discharge planning lower on the scale when left to be incorporated in overall nursing care on the unit. But discharge planning is too important to receive such treatment.

EXTERNAL PRESSURES INFLUENCING DISCHARGE PLANNING

External pressures, though viewed negatively by some, can be a positive force in encouraging organized discharge planning programs. The Joint Commission of Hospital Accreditation requires the following [5]:

Discharge planning shall be initiated as early as a determination of the need for such activity can be made, in order to facilitate discharge at that point in time when an acute level of care is no longer required. Criteria for initiating discharge planning may be developed to identify those patients whose diagnosis, problems, or psychosocial or health-related circumstances usually require discharge planning. The utilization review plan may specify the situations in which nonphysician health care professionals are permitted to initiate discharge planning activity. The hospital's discharge planning activity shall not be limited to placement in long term care facilities, but also shall include provision for, or referral to, whatever services the patient may require in order to improve or maintain the patient's health status.

Various regulatory mandates have increased emphasis on discharge planning. Awareness has increased especially with the federally funded insurance programs like Medicare and the advent of utilization review. The interrelationship of discharge planning, inclusive of patient teaching, with utilization review is manifest.

The Professional Standards Review Organization (PSRO) Program Manual states "Where problems in post-discharge care or discharge placement are anticipated, discharge planning should be initiated as soon as possible after admission to the short-stay hospital. Discharge planning should include both preparation of the patient for the next level of care and arrangement for placement in the appropriate care setting" [12].

Further, the American Hospital Association's "A Patient's Bill of Rights" (see Appendix I) denotes that the patient has the right to expect information regarding his or her medical treatment plan as well as reasonable continuity of care [1].

Significant pressure is being exerted by patients and families themselves. As the average length of stay in the hospital is consistently shortened, the demands of the patient for a higher caliber of posthospital medical nursing care are greater than ever.

RATIONALE FOR A STRUCTURED APPROACH

If, indeed, we are to be successful in accomplishing the goals so described, it is clear that the practice of discharge planning must be formalized. It has been indicated that if discharge planning is left to everyone it will likely be lost in the vastness of the hospital. Someone should be designated as the person to coordinate discharge planning activities of the hospital. Whether a formal department or an individual, the discharge planner must work for flexibility consistent with the size and needs of the facility. The nurse who is designated as the "discharge planner," "continuity of care coordinator," or "home health coordinator," should have appropriate background; public health nursing or community nursing experience is important. If a nurse is taken from the hospital setting and placed directly in this new role, she should be afforded the opportunity to gain experience in home care and to research the community agencies. The nurse in the role of the discharge planner must also possess the skills of assessment, communication, diplomacy, initiative, and resourcefulness. This designated nurse can make or break the program [2].

A formal discharge planning program includes the development of written guidelines and procedures as well as job descriptions. The job description of this discharge planner should focus on four main functions: casefinding, assessment, planning, and referral (see Job Description for Continuity-of-Care Nurse in the section entitled Resource Materials). These functions will be discussed shortly.

SUPPORTS NECESSARY FOR A VIABLE PROGRAM

The awareness and support of the hospital administration is crucial to the success of a discharge planning program. If the administration has failed to recognize the impact of discharge planning on the overall quality of care at the facility, the program will not develop. Perhaps the administration has designated someone as discharge planner or has established a formal department in the institution but has done so only in response to the pressures mentioned above. Perhaps the administration feels the nursing staff alone can absorb the needs of discharge planning entirely within the framework of their day-to-day rendering of care; the administration may hold that another department is not necessary. In that case, discharge planning will founder and, as explained, will be prioritized out of existence. Until the administration of the hospital fully recognizes the requirements of implementation and the significance of the outcome of discharge planning, the chances of a viable program are minimal [6].

Paralleling administrative support as a vital factor in the effectiveness of discharge planning is medical staff support. The primary physician is the head of the health-care team. No discharge planner should interfere with the relationship between the patient and the attending physician. Therefore, it is extremely important that rapport and cooperation exist among the medical staff of the hospital. There are still physicians who resent the role of both the discharge planner and the patient educator. These physicians think that they can handle all the patient education and discharge planning tasks themselves. Nurses must remember that the basic preparation of physicians is disease oriented. They realistically have scant time either during their training or in their clinical practice to devote to posthospital planning. It is worth all of the time and effort necessary on the part of the discharge planner to gain respect of the physician. Initiative in the education of the physician may be necessary. Slowly, even the most conservative physician will begin to accept the assistance necessary to help his or her patient. Soon physicians will be asking for this assistance. The discharge planner working with the physician to effect the actual discharge plan is most acceptable to all concerned.

The understanding and support of nursing service administration is imperative. No matter where the discharge planning program finds itself on the organizational chart of a hospital, interrelationship with all of the nursing staff is the fact of life. The discharge planning nurse will have constant interaction with all staff of each nursing unit. No territorial boundaries are necessary; indeed they will prove disconcerting to the quality of care strived for if they do exist.

The Utilization Review Committee of the hospital is yet another group that must support an organized discharge planning program. As mentioned before, in this day of third-party payor pressure to assure that the patient remains in the acute-care bed only as long as medically necessary, discharge planning is gaining in importance. Utilization review committees are often comprised of physicians who are concerned about the continuity of care. They should be among the first to recognize the value of the discharge planner.

DYNAMICS OF IMPLEMENTATION

Casefinding

Casefinding, the identification of patients requiring an in-depth discharge plan, is accomplished in several ways. Surveillance of daily admission slips for various factors (diagnosis, age, address); surveillance of the nursing care plans; reliance on unit personnel; referrals from the patients or families themselves; referrals from the attending physicians; referrals from the utilization review nurses; referrals from the various ancillary department team members—all of these offer a source for the identification of patients needing a discharge plan. Continuity of care cannot await a physician's initiative. Casefinding must occur on the part of the discharge planner.

Assessment

Thorough assessment of the patient's posthospital needs is a necessity and draws upon the expertise of the nurse as well as other team members. The interplay of patient teaching with discharge planning will be evident during this process. The first study of discharge planning appears to have been conducted by Smith [10]. A prime goal of the study was to insure proper utilization of the hospital bed for acute care and to enhance referral to public health nurses. As a result of this research, Wensley [11] went further and urged development of criteria for the selection of patients for home care and in the process encouraged the assessment procedure. This assessment guide for the selection of patients for home care is still extremely useful today. The guide points out the following areas of consideration:

1. The complexity of a procedure, such as administration of a medicine or a treatment, that requires professional assistance in the home

2. An indication that a patient or his family is unable to give care or does not understand direction for follow-up care
3. Signs that patient or his family is unable to accept or is disturbed by some aspect of his condition or care
4. Evidence of need for reinforcement and clarification of instruction started in the hospital
5. The expressed needs of patients for follow-up nursing service, when professional personnel have corroborated the appropriateness of public health nursing to meet the needs
6. Some aspect of the physical or social environment at home and outside the hospital that may interfere with a patient's satisfactory self-care, for instance, a patient living alone or with family members in poor health
7. Following long-term hospital care
8. Evidence of need for anticipatory guidance (This is a commonsense presentation of facts to the family to help with their understanding of problems. Their frame of reference, life experiences, preconceptions, and motivations must be understood.)

Regardless of age or medical diagnosis, each patient can be evaluated in terms of the following: (1) present and future clinical course and potential, (2) attitude towards illness, (3) home environment, and (4) nursing needs, and whether they can be totally provided by the patient for himself or by his family [11].

The assessment of any patient preparing for discharge should be inclusive of these basic dimensions: mental status, activity, elimination, medications, nutrition, special procedures, equipment, special instructions, reaction to teaching, and need for further teaching. The form entitled Nurse's Patient Discharge Notes, in the section entitled Resource Materials, is an example of a tool used to promote this assessment process.

The social worker, the physical therapist, the dietitian, and every other team member will each have information to share with the nursing staff in order to make this evaluation complete. The social and emotional needs of the patient, as well as the physical needs, must be assessed if an appropriate plan for posthospital care is to be effective.

Let us return to Mrs. J., whose case study was introduced at the beginning of this chapter. The assessment near discharge revealed the following key factors:

1. Ambulation: Unsteady, bearing full weight on the left leg, using walker hesitantly. Her physical therapist felt further ambulation training necessary
2. Transfer: From bed to chair and to toilet with assistance of one aide and walker. Riser for toilet seat indicated
3. Elimination: Prone to constipation. Self-catheterization demonstration understood and returned only fairly well
4. Diet: The dietitian stated Mrs. J. appeared to understand her diabetic diet quite well. The husband and daughter would be preparing meals at first
5. Wound, skin, and nail care: Both the postop hip fracture and cholecystectomy sites were clean and healing. General diabetic management relative to skin and nail care appeared to be understood

6. Other specific diabetic management: Instruction for self-administration of insulin regarding dosage, technique, and site rotation appeared to be comprehended. Return demonstrations were fair and hesitant. The staff nurse felt Mrs. J. needed reinforcement of instructions
7. Clinitest: Understood and returned demonstration without difficulty. Signs and symptoms of hypo- and hyperglycemia repeated to nurse with some uncertainty
8. Equipment and supplies: Required walker and riser for toilet seat; supplies for insulin administration; supplies for self-catheterization (with instructions for resupply)
9. Prescriptions: Required prescription for insulin syringes and other medication
10. Appointments for physcian visits: Internist, orthopedic surgeon, and surgeon
11. Social-emotional: Conference with patient, husband, and daughter revealed a well-motivated, independent patient, eager to return to her own home, somewhat overwhelmed with the magnitude of self-care. Family concerned, husband able to be of assistance, daughter will assist to the extent necessary (The home is a two-story country farmhouse, bathroom on first floor. Arrangements were made to move Mrs. J.'s bedroom to the first floor temporarily.)
12. Mode of transportation: Ambulance was deemed the safest mode of transport due to distance involved, steps at home, and general condition of patient

Planning

Now that the assessment has taken place, the plan for posthospital care will be developed. The patient should be included in the planning process whenever possible. Family conferences are a necessity. The family interview during assessment will vividly depict that there are two sides to every story. Along with the need for the enlightenment of the discharge planner, the family or persons caring for the patient after discharge need to be involved and instructed as to the eventual care plan. The enthusiastic discharge planner has to be reminded that the continued care plan should be made with the patient and family, not for the patient and family. The discharge planner must be as resourceful as possible to formulate a plan that is most appropriate as well as most acceptable for the patient's continued care needs.

During this planning stage, input from all participating team members should be coordinated by the discharge planner. The current as well as the anticipated medical nursing needs should be communicated to the home-care nurse, the nursing home director of nurses, the rehabilitation hospital personnel, or the family member. The attending physician should oversee and approve the completed plan.

Plans made with Mrs. J. and her family included the following.

1. The county health department home nursing program inclusive of physical therapy was indicated. The nurse who was to care for Mrs. J. at home visited her in the hospital, scanned her hospital record with the discharge planning nurse, and was instructed by the physical therapist on ambulation exercises at home. The plans for the home-care program were begun.

2. The walker for home was ordered predischarge to assure proper fitting to the patient by physical therapy. The family was instructed on the purchase of a riser for the toilet seat. The daughter was instructed on supplies to purchase at the pharmacy for insulin administration and self-catheterization.

3. The husband and daughter were involved in diet instruction as well as overall diabetic techniques and management instructions with Mrs. J. Instructions included dietary and activity principles relative to constipation as well.

4. Self-catheterization instructions were reinforced to Mrs. J. with ample time for return demonstrations.

5. Prescriptions were written by the attending physician for insulin and syringes, with the recommendation of a laxative prn.

6. The appropriate physicians instructed Mrs. J. regarding activity, return visits, and expectations.

7. Copies of all teaching aids were prepared for taking home.

8. The home-care nurse was apprised of all teaching methods employed in the hospital for Mrs. J. and of the anticipated date of discharge.

9. Instructions were given Mrs. J. and family regarding home furniture, carpeting, stairs, and other such details.

10. The hospital unit was apprised of the referral to home care in order to initiate completion of transfer information, as well as the mode and time of transfer.

Interaction and coordination between the discharge planning nurse and the nursing unit occurred constantly.

Referral

Now that the plan has evolved, a referral to the appropriate resource must be completed. It is during the referral process that the need of a trained discharge planner is of further significance. Comprehensive knowledge of the community resources is indispensable if continuity of care is to be achieved. Assuring that the patient receives the benefits of services to meet his needs is important. It is not enough to provide the patient with a directory and telephone numbers. Comprehensive knowledge and personal contacts will result in a smooth and meaningful referral. What is important is that the resources be explored. The patient should then be linked with the one most appropriate.

Back to Mrs. J. On the day of discharge, a telephone call was made to the county health department's home nursing service to verify the discharge. The orders of the attending physician were given to this nursing service. The transfer form was completed in this instance by the discharge planning nurse who was knowledgeable in the type of orders indicated for home care. The unit clerk provided copies of appropriate reports to accompany the transfer form. Arrangements were made with the ambulance service to transport Mrs. J. home. The nursing unit was apprised of time and carrier.

All hospital patients, of all age groups, and of all service areas have a right to the benefits of a structured discharge planning program. The newborn and the new mother, the newly diagnosed diabetic child in pediatrics, the 20-year-old spinal cord injury patient, the 55-year-old amputee, the 70-year-old cerebrovascular accident patient, the 90-year-old Parkinson's disease patient, and the congestive heart failure patient are only a few. The importance of patient teaching in preparing these patients for discharge will manifest itself clearly.

Ideally, discharge planning begins with admission. In actuality, it will begin at the most appropriate time, based on continual assessment. Casefinding and monitoring of cases should begin upon admission. The critical point of consideration is that ample time be allowed for the entire process. The patient and family should not have to be pressured into approaching a move with one day's notice.

THE HOME HEALTH AGENCY AS A RESOURCE

The primary objective of any discharge planning program should be to return the patient to his or her own home and familiar environment. This can be accomplished at times only through the auspices of organized home-care programs. A home health agency is an organization established to provide health-related services in the home of the patient. Intermittent nursing care, skilled and rehabilitative, is administered by or supervised by a registered nurse working under the specific orders of a physician. Other services complementing the nursing services of the home health agency include physical therapy, social services, occupational therapy, speech therapy, nutrition, and home health aides. A home health agency may be an official agency such as a county health department or a voluntary agency such as a visiting nurses association. Although home health agencies exist in a high percentage of areas of the United States, there are areas that still lack the services. With the advent of Medicare in 1966, more agencies were established in response to the provision of funding for home health under this law.

Referrals to home health care from the hospital fortifies the rationale for a nurse to be involved as the coordinator. This nurse requires experience in the home-care setting. The referral to home care necessitates many times that the discharge planning nurse convince the attending physician and overall nursing staff that discharge under these conditions is advantageous. A trained discharge planner realizes there are but few patients who cannot be cared for at home if the conditions can be made safe and appropriate. At times a predischarge visit to the home is required in order to assure proper assessment and planning. Wensley's guidelines for the selection of patients for home care is a valuable tool in this process [11].

Patient teaching is again found closely aligned to this discharge plan. The diabetic, the ostomy patient, and the cardiac patient all require predischarge instructions; many will require postdischarge follow-through instructions. It is important to remember that no matter how much the patient seems to have comprehended during instructional activities in the confines of the secure hospital setting, with the nurse present to answer all questions, once the door is shut on those white uniforms, it is an entirely different situation at home. The most self-confident, intelligent patient in the hospital can become unraveled at home. Reinforcement is necessary if quality of care is to be maintained. In many instances the home health nurse should be called upon to perform this task. A liaison nurse from the local home health agency should be a member of the hospital's health-care team.

Home health care is underutilized in the United States and, therefore, there are patients lacking such services. In structured programs the nurse is emerging as an important figure in hospital discharge planning; the nurse's clinical experience enables him or her to assist the physician in selecting and developing a home-care program for the patient. This is an effective manner in which to enhance home care. For if left to the physician alone to initiate, home care will occur only seldom [7]. It can be concluded that the discharge planning program of any hospital will be most effective only with a viable link to the home-care program.

THE LONG-TERM CARE FACILITY AS A RESOURCE

Even though the primary objective of any discharge planning program is to return patients to their own homes, to do so is not always possible or appropriate. An alternative level of care posthospital is the long-term care facility. Again, proper assessment of the patient's medical nursing needs is imperative. Primarily three levels of care are available in long-term care facilities: skilled, intermediate, and sheltered. As the patient prepares to leave the hospital and it has been determined that transfer to a long-term facility is indicated, the appropriate level of care necessary to coincide with the patient's needs must be defined. Transfer of a heavy-care patient with skilled needs to an intermediate facility can be quite traumatic and necessitate another move for the patient.

To execute the physician's order to transfer a person to a nursing home can be no easy task. The nursing home transfer process is one of the most complex to implement. Not only must the medical nursing assessment be thorough to assure referral to an appropriate level of care, but the necessary knowledge of skilled care versus custodial care comes into the scene once more due to funding constraints, primarily Medicare. Interlaced with these clinical skills, the nurse must draw on her interview and counseling skills. The patient's and family's anxieties, fears, and guilt feelings surface readily during this process. Financing for long-term care is yet another issue of paramount concern.

Knowledge of the local facilities and personal contacts are crucial aids. There should be assurance that the patient will receive the benefits of optimum nursing care and rehabilitation. A discharge nurse is in the position to serve as facilitator and coordinator of the transfer with the final selection of the facility left to the patient or family. The medical nursing assessment of the patient, with specific needs identified, must be communicated to the appropriate nursing personnel of the facility. The social and emotional needs must be conveyed as well.

Patient teaching in the hospital nursing unit should not be halted because transfer to a nursing home is indicated. Many times, it must be remembered that the transfer is a stepping stone before returning home. A newly diagnosed diabetic in the hospital should have his or her insulin instructions initiated, as any other patient would, if at all possible. The same applies for the ostomy patient regarding self-care of the ostomy. The transfer activity process (from bed to chair, chair to bathroom) should not be forgotten. Transfer to nursing home does not negate the nursing responsibility of patient teaching; if it is at all feasible, teaching must continue.

The transfer to long-term care should not be made hastily. The patient and family require time for this process. Discharge planning must occur if this process is to be implemented in as untraumatic a manner and as appropriate a manner as possible.

TRANSFER INFORMATION

Brief comments on transfer information are needed in any discussion of continuity of care. As discussed above, no discharge plan indicating a referral to another health care facility or home health agency, is complete without appropriate, adequate transfer information being prepared to accompany the patient. This includes medical, nursing, and social and emotional information. A Patient Transfer Form is a standard form of any hospital. It should be considered an integral and important part of the medical record.

The various problems encountered and the approaches to meeting these problems must be conveyed to the receiving agency along with signed physician orders for continuity of care. The transfer form should be completed by the nurse rendering most direct, consistent care to the patient. Accompanying this transfer form should be copies of certain hospital records such as the current chest x-ray, complete blood count (cbc), urinalysis, and any other reports that may be helpful in rendering continued care at the receiving agency or facility. The ancillary departments involved with the patient should transmit reports as well.

Lack of comprehensive transfer information will disrupt the provision of continued and safe care for the patient and should be regarded as a vital deficiency.

TEAMWORK

The collaborative efforts between the nurse and the social worker is of prime concern if continuity of care is to come about. Each has expertise to contribute. Murdaugh, who after 13 years as a social worker became a consultant to a visiting nurse association, reveals there is a point beyond the human relationship skills of the nurse where the skills of the social worker are necessary [8]. Hirshon, a social worker and a registered nurse, thinks both professions have much to learn from each other. She points out that both roles have common characteristics: both deal with human conditions, both must interview and assess, both must teach, both may act as coordinators [4].

Some hospitals are fortunate to have had organized social service departments for years. The role of the nurse as a discharge planner has only recently come upon the scene. The need for referral to home-care programs is what has particularly prompted the nurse to be added to this team. Nursing is needed to round out the sphere of posthospital needs. Certainly the nurse and the social worker can learn from each other, share experiences, and effect a more realistic and total patient care plan.

Other members of the health team interacting in the discharge planning process include all of the ancillary services. Dietary, pharmacy, physical therapy, respiratory therapy, infection control, and pastoral care—all have contributions to make to individual patients. A prime responsibility of a discharge planner is to involve the appropriate team members and coordinate a final discharge plan. Without such coordination, the patient can be pulled in many different directions.

EVALUATION OF THE PROGRAM

Objective measures of the discharge planning process of any hospital are necessary. The audit, whether the nursing audit or the more desirable combined medical-nursing audit, is a concrete tool in identifying the deficiencies of both patient teaching and discharge planning. Due to lack of documentation or lack of actual implementation of the processes, a high percentage of audits will show the need for much improvement.

Other methods of evaluation include feedback information, on a planned basis, from the agency to which the patient is referred. The home health agency, for instance,can provide a written progress report of the patient several weeks after discharge to home. In the case of our patient Mrs. J., the home health nurse returned a feedback form to the continuity of care nurse two weeks post-discharge. A copy was sent to the nursing unit, physical therapy, dietary, and the patient education coordinator.

Constant interaction between the long-term care facilities and the discharge planner should occur, to provide at least verbal reports of referred patients' progress. Written or verbal feedback should be requested on a routine basis from all resources involved. Patient and family questionnaires may also be beneficial in assessing appropriateness and satisfaction of the referral.

The utilization review program is a means of measuring the effectiveness of discharge planning in a hospital. Denied days of patients' stays, unusual increase in the average length of stay, and a high number of termination-of-benefits letters, are among the indicators of problems in discharge planning.

Discharge planning as a process, whether or not structured, should have a built-in mechanism of evaluation of effectiveness. Otherwise, progress will not be made and the issue will be lost; most important, the patient will lack fulfillment of his complete needs.*

Summary

The purpose of this chapter is to call attention to discharge planning as an integral component of health care and to point to its obvious relationship with patient teaching. It is impossible to discuss the outcomes of one without involving the other. If patients are to be afforded the benefits of a planned, systematic process of providing for their vital, uninterrupted care, then the question each facility must address is, "How best can we meet this obligation?" Whether the discharge planner is the nurse assigned to the unit rendering total nursing care or a designated individual with specialized background and training, in modern health care systems a proven expanded role for the nurse has surfaced. The role of this nurse is to ascertain that the discharge-planning vehicle of continuity of care is not dismissed by other priorities, and that the right of planned, progressive, comprehensive care of the patient will be realized.

Coordination of all health team members, assurance that patient teaching is effected, knowledge of levels of care, knowledge of skilled care versus custodial care, ascertaining equipment for home use, assessment and determination of home health care versus institutional care, knowledge of funding sources and Medicare guidelines, interviewing and counseling skills, knowledge of community resources, personal communication of the patient needs with the receiving facility, coordination of transportation at transfer time—all have been identified as crucial to the discharge plan. Each nurse on the nursing unit does not have the time and the expertise to complete this important facet of total patient care.

Easily recognizable are the characteristics mutual to both patient teaching and discharge planning. Throughout this chapter *patient teaching* could be inserted for the words *discharge planning* in numerous instances. This is demonstrated in such areas as in the need for a structured approach, the need for a designated individual to coordinate casefinding and assessment, the need for evaluation, the supports necessary, and on and on. These two functions are clearly compatible with each other both in problems and approaches.

Until patient education and discharge planning are regarded as significant, especially by the hospital administrators, continuity of care will diminish to verbiage. The quality of care demands of our society are too important to allow

*A research project completed recently most aptly points out that a systematic assessment of patients' posthospital needs is not provided for the majority of patients being discharged. In the study, 14 hospitals were surveyed in the city of Chicago. Four were small hospitals (200 beds or less); ten were large hospitals (more than 200 beds). One half were teaching hospitals and the other half were community hospitals (no major teaching role). Four of the fourteen hospitals have a position that is primarily concerned with the function of discharge planning. Of these four positions, three are filled by nurses and one by a social worker. These positions have all been in existence a minimum of six years. Though various model types were reflected, it was obvious that these four hospitals saw the need for a formal program. Where a formal program does not exist, where discharge planning is everybody's job and no one is delegated the specific responsibility, it becomes in effect nobody's job [9].

this to happen. It is a human mandate, but more important, the teamwork that evolves to make this process work results in a rewarding and pleasurable mandate.

REFERENCES

1. American Hospital Association. *A Patient's Bill of Rights.* Chicago: The Association, 1972.
2. Bristow, O., Stickney, S., and Thompson, S. *Discharge Planning for Continuity of Care.* New York: National League of Nursing, 1976.
3. David, J., Hanser, J., Madden, B., and Pratt, M. *Guidelines for Discharge Planning* (rev. ed.). Downey, Calif.: Rancho Los Amigos Hospital, 1973.
4. Hirshon, R. Nurses and social workers—We can learn from each other. *American Journal of Nursing,* December, 1976.
5. Joint Commission for Accreditation of Hospitals. *Accreditation Manual for Hospitals.* Chicago: The Commission, 1979.
6. Jones-Bey, G., Klis, M. A., Sibley, H., and Quillinan, V. *Implications of Discharge Planning for the Hospital Administrator.* Chicago: Health Care Service Corp., 1978.
7. Lee, A. A fond farewell to patients shouldn't mean goodbye to care (Report of remarks by J. Byrne). *RN,* June, 1977.
8. Murdaugh, J. There is a difference. *Nursing Outlook,* 16 : 45, 1968.
9. Newcomb, B. J., Reichelt, Paul A., and Werley, H. Nursing Role in Post Hospital Referral for Home Care. *Journal of Nursing Administration,* In Press.
10. Smith, L. C. *Factors Influencing Continuity of Nursing Service.* New York: Institute of Research and Service in Nursing Education and the National League for Nursing, 1961.
11. Wensley, E. *Nursing Service Without Walls.* New York: National League for Nursing, 1963.
12. U.S. Department of Health, Education, and Welfare. Professional Standards Review Organizations Program Manual, 1974, ch. 8, p. 13.

Resource Materials

JOB DESCRIPTION FOR CONTINUITY-OF-CARE NURSE

Function

The Continuity-of-Care nurse is part of the nurse-social worker team effort to effect the concept of progressive, comprehensive care.

The Continuity-of-Care Nurse will focus on the area of the medical nursing needs of the patient with specific involvement in the transfer process to home health agencies, nursing homes, rehabilitation centers, and other acute health care facilities; the counterpart of the team shall be a social worker who will concentrate on the socioemotional, economic needs of the patient.

Duties

1. Function as a liaison between the hospitalized patient and the appropriate health care agencies/facilities that will provide continued care; will work in alliance with, and coordinate efforts of, the physician, the family, and all team members.
2. Casefind. Establish a routine mechanism of early identification of patients requiring specialized posthospital services.
3. Assess. Evaluate patient care needs, including level of care and requirements for posthospitalization.

4. Plan. Work in alliance with the patient, family, and all health team members.
5. Refer to appropriate resource. Must be knowledgeable of the scope of services of community resources.
6. Enhance home care program.
   a. Weekly conferences with home care nurse liaison, more often as indicated.
   b. Develop posthospital plans concurrently with home care nurse.
   c. Implement feedback information to nursing unit from the home health agency.
7. Maintain personal contacts with appropriate area nursing home personnel.
8. Assure that complete transfer information accompanies patient.
   a. Provide resource to nursing unit personnel for completion of transfer information for nursing homes and other health facilities.
   b. Continuity of Care Nurse will complete transfer form for home care program.
9. Verify that patient/family teaching methods are utilized as indicated.
10. Initiate family conferences.
11. Assist with obtaining necessary equipment and/or supplies for home care.
12. Facilitate appropriate mode of transfer and arrangements.
13. Serve as a resource for all nursing staff to ensure the meeting of patient discharge needs; participate in inservices to personnel relative to continuity of care.
14. Serve on Utilization Review Committee and other appropriate medical and nursing committees; work in cooperation with utilization review nurses.
15. Maintain contemporary knowledge base of acute patient care as well as all aspects of discharge planning.
16. Maintain case record of patients; contribute to monthly and annual reports.

Requirements

Registered nurse with minimum of two years clinical experience; hospital and community nursing experience preferred.

Worker Traits

1. Leadership and organizational ability
2. Attributes of teaching
3. Communication skills
4. Emotional stability
5. Self-confidence and initiative

NURSE'S PATIENT DISCHARGE NOTES*

Date _____ Time _____ a.m. _____ p.m.

(If transfer form accompanies patient, disregard this sheet.)

	Assessment (√ if applicable)	Teaching (√ if implemented)
Activity		
Locomotion		
Walks unaided	_____	_____
Walks with assistance	_____	_____

*Courtesy of Copley Memorial Hospital, Aurora, Illinois.

Uses: cane   _____   _____
     walker   _____   _____
     crutches   _____   _____
Unable to walk   _____   _____
Wheelchair   _____   _____
Stairs   _____   _____

Transfer
Sitting   _____   _____
Standing   _____   _____
Tub   _____   _____
Toilet   _____   _____

Bed
Up, ad lib   _____   _____
Complete bed rest   _____   _____
Limited schedule   _____   _____

Elimination
Voiding:
     Strain urine   _____   _____
     Incontinent   _____   _____
     Foley catheter   _____   _____
     Intake and output   _____   _____
Bowels: _____   _____
     Special instructions   _____   _____
     Involuntary   _____   _____

Medications
Prescription to patient   _____   _____
Return of medications   _____   _____
     brought to hospital

Doctor's Appointment   _____

Diet
Copy of diet to patient   _____   _____
Instructions to family   _____   _____
Fluids: Force   _____   _____
     Restrict   _____   _____

Appliances or Equipment
Walker   _____   _____
Crutches   _____   _____
Foley catheter   _____   _____
Dressings   _____   _____
Other: _____   _____   _____

Observations
Mental Status: ____ alert   ____ confused   ____ depressed
     ____ apathetic
Patient queried at discharge re: ($\checkmark$ if applicable and is positive)
____ pain   ____ vertigo
____ nausea   ____ visual impairment
____ dyspnea   ____ voiding
____ hearing

Nurses' Patient Discharge Notes (Continued)

Treatments/Procedures/Special Instructions

Specify _____

_____

Outpatient follow-up: i.e., P.T., R.T., Lab—Specify

_____

Continuity-of-Care Department involved

_____

Prosthesis taken home: ☐ Full dentures   ☐ Partial dentures
                              ☐ Hearing aid   ☐ Contact lenses
                              ☐ Glasses
                              ☐ Other _____
                                              (specify)

Valuables Release: ☐ Given to patient   ☐ Family

Mode of transportation: ☐ Car   ☐ Ambulance
Mode of discharge:
☐ Wheelchair   ☐ Stretcher   ☐ Walking

Accompanied by: _____

Discharge Summary

(Include condition, response to hospitalization, special instructions, reaction to teaching, socioemotional significance.)

_____

_____

_____

_____

_____

_____

_____

_____

_____

_____

_____

_____

_____

_____

_____

_____

_____

Nurse's signature _____

William L. Holzemer

10

Evaluation of Patient Education Programs

How do I know my patient has learned?
How can I determine the effectiveness of the overall patient education program?

A great deal of time, and therefore money, is spent in patient education activities. Health care organizations, faced with cost containment mandates, may have to prove that expenditures for patient teaching activities have been effective in producing learning outcomes. In order to do this, some type of evaluation will have to be conducted. The following chapter describes various reasons for conducting evaluation studies. A description of the many decisions (such as which variables to measure, how to measure them, and what to do with the information) is provided. Examples and illustrations are presented that will help the reader set up and conduct evaluation of patient education program activities.

The information in this chapter should help the reader to

1. *State several reasons for evaluating patient education programs*
2. *Develop a variable matrix for evaluating patient education*
3. *Select an evaluation design appropriate to the patient education situation*
4. *Select or construct instruments to collect evaluation data*
5. *Conduct data collection and analysis for evaluation of patient education*
6. *Write a report of the outcomes of the teaching-learning process*

DEVELOPING A PROTOCOL FOR EVALUATING
A PATIENT EDUCATION PROGRAM

Herein is presented a series of steps that may be followed to design an evaluation plan to examine patients' learning. The series of steps presented here were reported earlier [20].

The first step in designing an evaluation plan is to think about the *rationale* for the evaluation. Why evaluate a patient education program? Usually the prime reason for evaluating a patient education program is to determine if the program has been effective. A program can be determined to be effective, however, from many points of view. Usually an effective patient education program is defined as one that provides evidence of changes in patients' behavior in the desired direction. Dorothy J. del Bueno writes "Lack of evidence supporting any meaningful impact on patient education outcomes can be discouraging and demotivating to staff. A visible patient education program may be pleasing to the ego, but unless it is also effective, valuable resources have been wasted" [12].

Among the reasons patient education programs are evaluated are these: to document changes in patients' behavior, to increase staff morale, to justify expenditures, and to improve the program. Thinking about why a patient education program should be evaluated provides a greater understanding of the kinds of information that will be needed for the evaluation. The first task, therefore, is to write a rationale for the evaluation. The following are examples of rationales for conducting an evaluation of a patient education program.

What effect do our patient education programs have on our patients after they leave the hospital? I want to know if we have any carry-over effect into the home. Should we hire someone to visit the homes of our discharged patients to provide support for their ongoing adjustments?

Can we lower the readmission rate of certain types of patients due to our patient education program? I believe this data would be very important for our staff morale and budget support if it could be obtained.

I wonder if we should teach patients about self-administered medications individually or in groups? Has anyone evaluated this instructional option? Teaching patients in groups might provide psychological supports and lower teaching costs. On the other hand, participating in a group may be embarrassing to a particular patient.

I must justify my budget request for hiring a patient educator on the hospital staff. In order to accomplish this, I want to demonstrate the effectiveness and potential of various patient education programs that we have developed and might develop. Hopefully this data will provide me with the "ammunition" I need when time comes for budget hearings.

Sharing the rationale for the evaluation with those individuals interested in its results may help them to understand exactly why the evaluation is being conducted.

The next step in the evaluation process is to outline the *audience* for the evaluation. Who wants the information that will be collected? Does the supervisor want to justify costs? Does a grant officer require evaluation of the project? The task is to outline the audiences for the evaluation.

The reason for audience identification is that different audiences may require different kinds of information. For example, the teacher of the program may wish to focus attention on documented changes in patients' behaviors. Staff nurses may be interested in the effect of one particular program on other programs. A program director may want to monitor patient outcomes in an informal way. The kind of information that is acceptable and desired by one audience may not be acceptable or desirable to another.

A sample list of audiences might include the program developer, patients or consumers, family members of patients, teachers, staff nurses, medical staff, contract or grant officer, journal editor, and others. After the audiences for the evaluation have been outlined, the next step in the evaluation is to consider interviewing each audience member. Interviewing the audiences is discussed later in this chapter in the section on evaluation questions.

The established recognition of patients' rights suggests that a significant audience of the evaluation may be current and future patients. Perhaps the evaluation data can be used to demonstrate to patients the effectiveness of the particular program and thereby increase their motivation and interest in participating in the program. A patient has the right to expect a clear explanation of the benefits and risks associated with participating in any health-related activity, and certainly patient education is no exception.

Now the task is to build a *description* of the patient education program from a systems perspective. The systems perspective means writing a description of the program listing the inputs, processes, and outcomes. These are described below. This descriptive activity helps develop an understanding of the various components of the program in a logical, sequential fashion. The description is designed to inform the evaluation activity, not to be a complete, detailed account of the entire program. The description should be thorough, yet require only a few hours to complete. A sample program description based upon a systems model is presented in Table 2.

The first part of the description activity is to list the inputs to the program. What items or parts allow the program to occur? For example, inputs might include the following: patient's readiness to learn, patient's language status, curriculum objectives, space or setting available, machinery required to be assembled in order to allow the program to happen.

The next step is to outline the processes or those activities that occur during the program itself. Processes might include the following: teaching strategies, time spent with patient, kinds of nurse-patient interactions, patient's ongoing responses such as pain level or interest level.

The last step is to outline the outcomes of the patient education program. What are the outcomes expected for the patient? Patient outcomes are usually the most important aspect of the description. What effect is the program supposed to have on the patient's behavior? For example, diabetic patients should be able to test their urine and give insulin based on those results, or a colostomy patient should be able to change his bag and provide skin care to his stoma.

Table 2. Sample Program Description Based on a Systems Model

Inputs	Processes	Outcomes
Preoperative teaching program	Teaching activity Teacher attitude Eye contact Instructional format	Patient Percent of preoperative vital capacity remaining after surgery at 10–18 hr and 24–36 hr
AV delivery		
Nurse/teacher	Patient's status Anxiety level Pain level	Number of postsurgical hospital days
Patients Age, sex, preop status		
Setting/facilities	Time spent with patient	Incidence of postoperative respiratory complications Staff attitudes Patient's family attitudes Cost of program per patient

What outcomes are expected from the program other than patient outcomes? For example, perhaps an outcome of a patient education program in diabetes might be to improve staff morale or demonstrate staff competencies in this area. These outcomes are important, although not part of the category of patient outcomes.

One interesting aspect of evaluation is developing the expertise to become sensitive to unintended outcomes that result from an educational program [39]. For example, teaching a patient deep breathing exercises prior to surgery in order to decrease the postsurgical recovery time may be the intended outcome. However, a significant unintended outcome might be a lowering of the perceived stress of the anticipated surgery. This unintended outcome might never be detected if the length of hospital stay postsurgery was the only measure taken. It is a challenge to attempt to conceptualize what unintended outcomes may result from a patient education program.

The rationale, audience, and description of the program have now been written. The next step is to write the *evaluation questions*. What needs to be known about the program? The obvious questions will focus on patient outcomes. Have any changes in the patient's behavior occurred? Was this change what was expected? The task is to write the questions viewed as most important for the evaluation. After the list has been created, the list of evaluation questions should be organized into the inputs, processes, and outcomes model. Notice that most of the evaluation questions written probably focus upon outcomes and that insufficient attention may have been given to input and process questions. It may be the case that the type of patient admitted to a program has a greater effect on outcomes than the teaching method itself. Or it may be the case that failure to monitor the teaching behavior will result in a lack of understanding of what actually happened between patient and teacher. Table 3 presents a few evaluation questions organized into the systems model.

Table 3. *Variable Matrix for an Evaluation of a Patient Education Program on Diabetes*

Questions	Variable List	Data Source	Instrumentation
Input			
What is patient's knowledge of diabetes?	Knowledge of diabetes	Patients	Multiple-choice examination
Are there enough teachers for patients?	Staff availability	Supervisor	Interview
Process			
Are teachers effective in creating a climate conducive to learning?	Learning climate	Patients and setting	Interview/ observation
Was there sufficient time alloted to each content area?	Time availability	Patient and teacher	Interview/ interview
Outcome			
Has patient's knowledge of diabetes reached an acceptable level?	Knowledge of diabetes	Patients	Multiple-choice examination
What is the readmission rate for those patients who complete program?	Readmission rates	Records	Record review

Once the evaluation questions have been organized into the systems model, the list of evaluation questions should be compared with the description written earlier. Do the evaluation questions cover every significant area of the program? It may be important to add additional evaluation questions so that each descriptive area (input, processes, and outcomes) will have at least one evaluation question.

After the evaluation questions have been organized into the systems model and compared to the description of the program, the next step in designing the evaluation is to interview the audiences that have been identified. The purpose of interviewing the audiences is to determine what evaluation questions they believe are the most important to ask. What do they want to know about the program? For example, staff nurses may wish to know about the effectiveness of the program defined as changes in patients' behavior. Supervisory staff may be most interested in the cost of the patient education program or time spent by the nurses who teach it. There is an assumption here that there are not sufficient resources, time, or energy to answer all the possible evaluation questions. The questions must be prioritized or placed in some order of importance. Through the process of interviewing the respective audiences of the evaluation, it may be possible to prioritize the questions in a meaningful manner. Also, the list of evaluation questions already organized in the systems model can be shared with the audiences for their reactions. This process will hopefully ensure that no significant question is overlooked in the evaluation plan.

CONSTRUCTING A VARIABLE MATRIX

Once the evaluation questions have been listed and prioritized, the next step in the process is to translate the evaluation questions to a measurable format. This process is referred to as creating a *variable matrix*. A variable is defined as a characteristic or trait that can take on a value, for example, weight, height, knowledge, or attitude. First the evaluation question is written in a measurable format. For example, in designing a patient education program in diabetes, one may wish to ask, What do patients know about the disease? This question may be changed into a measurable question, What is the patient's knowledge of diabetes? The variable to be measured in this example is knowledge of diabetes. Second, the data source for the variable is located. In our example, the patient would be the source of the data on patient's knowledge of diabetes. Third, an instrument must be chosen appropriate for the identified data source to gather the desired information. In this case, the instrument might be a multiple-choice examination written by the program designer to assess patients' knowledge of diabetes. Table 3 presents an example of an abbreviated variable matrix.

The variable matrix presents clearly what variables are planned to be measured, what instruments must be either located or developed, and who must complete the instruments. The variable matrix helps to avoid duplication in data collection. For example, if it is decided to measure a number of characteristics about the patient that are felt to be important in determining the success of the program, the completion of the variable matrix would make it possible to tell how many times it will be necessary to request information from the patient. It may be possible to gather all the requested information at one time rather than returning at a later date for more information. The task of selecting an evaluation instrument is discussed after a brief examination is made in this chapter of selecting an evaluation design.

SELECTING AN EVALUATION DESIGN

While an evaluator is creating a variable matrix, the type of evaluation design to be adopted for the study will be considered. It is an interactive process in which helping to define the variables and their data source helps one to understand what type of evaluation design is feasible. Green discusses some of these interactions [18]. Although this section follows the section on variable matrix, it may be considered to be a simultaneous process of creating a variable matrix and selecting an evaluation design.

Four types of evaluation designs are briefly examined. They are the case study, survey research, experimental design, and clinical trials. This list is not meant to be an exhaustive list of the design; however, it is inclusive of the major designs available.

Case Study

The purpose of the case study design is "to study intensively the background, current status, and environmental interactions of a given social unit: an individual, group, institution, or community" [22]. Some examples of possible case studies in patient education programs include:

1. An in-depth study of a patient's behavioral patterns on a patient unit to examine the relationship between hospital-induced stress and smoking
2. An intensive study of the "culture" of a patient unit in a hospital and its effect on a patient's length of stay
3. A longitudinal study of a patient as admission, testing, patient education, surgery, recovery, and discharge are experienced

The major characteristics of a case study include the following. First, a case study provides a sufficient description of the person, patient, or unit. Sufficient description is defined by examining the rationale for conducting the study. The description should be relevant to the purpose of the investigation. Consequently, a case study may be very narrowly focused upon one specific aspect of a patient's case or very general and include all aspects of a patient's case. In general, the case study tends to examine a large number of variables for a few or single subject.

Survey Designs

A survey design is usually a questionnaire. The purpose of a survey design is to measure a number of variables for a large group of subjects. This is in contrast to the case study design that attempts to measure a large number of variables for a few subjects. Survey designs include a mailed questionnaire or a questionnaire that is completed in the presence of the investigator. Some examples of survey designs include:

1. A questionnaire mailed to patients at their homes to determine some aspect of compliance
2. A survey completed by patients at time of discharge concerning their anxiety level upon being admitted to the hospital
3. A questionnaire administered to newly diagnosed diabetics who have just completed a one-hour session on diet and diabetes

Two types of information tend to be gathered most often from a survey design using a questionnaire. These are demographic data about the patient such as age, weight, and years of schooling, and attitudinal information such as feelings about expected surgery, attitudes toward instructor of patient education class, and beliefs about health-care system.

The principal characteristic of a survey design is its ability to measure variables for a large sample of subjects economically. The variables, items, or events being measured have already occurred or are occurring, and the survey design is just a method of recording the results of these happenings. The investigator is not conducting an experiment in therapy in the traditional sense. Rather, the investigator is collecting data on events that have happened. The evaluator must then examine the results and attempt to hypothesize relationships between and among the variables that have been measured—for example, the relationship that may exist between perceptions of previous nursing care and recent nursing care at the time of discharge. Because the events are in the past when recorded by a survey design, a survey design is also referred to as post-hoc (after the fact) design.

In a survey design it is not possible to manipulate a variable and then to determine the effects of that manipulation. The evaluator therefore measures what is available to be measured.

Experimental Design

Three experimental designs are examined in this section. The literature on experimental designs is extensive, and the reader is urged to consult a reference text in this area for further understanding of this topic [8, 22, 34]. This section is labeled *experimental* because the investigator is causing an event or therapy to occur rather than just monitoring some phenomenon as in the case study or survey design. In patient education, the therapy or treatment is usually the instructional program designed to change patients' behavior. Three types of experimental designs are explored here. They are the case study design, the posttest-only design, and the pretest-posttest control group design.

The first experimental design is called the *case study design*, and it is unfortunate that the name is the same as the case study design previously discussed. Although both case studies have similar characteristics, there are important differences. In an experimental case study design, the investigator is manipulating a therapy and studying the effects of that treatment on a particular subject or subjects. Usually in an experimental case study, the investigator is able to gather pretherapy measures of the subjects, and he usually then follows the therapy with posttests or postmeasures.

For example, in a case study experimental design, a patient's recovery pulse rate is measured prior to participating in a 10-week exercise program. After the end of the 10 weeks, the recovery pulse rate is measured again and compared with the pretreatment pulse rate. Comparing the therapy scores with the post-therapy scores will provide the investigator with an indication of the success of the 10-week program for each particular patient. Note, however, that the investigator has no assurance that any observed change in the recovery pulse rate is due directly to the 10-week exercise course. Perhaps the patient lost weight during this time and that accounts for the increased recovery pulse rate. Or perhaps the patient experienced strong work-related stress during this 10-week period and that might account for the lowering of the recovery pulse rate. The experimental case study design is usually not considered a good design because no control group is available for comparison purposes.

In summary, an experimental pretest and posttest design conceptualized as a case study is not a good research design because it lacks a comparison or control group. Sometimes an evaluator must adopt this design because it is impossible to locate or select a comparison group. In those cases, gathering pretherapy measures to compare with posttherapy measures is a compromise that although not desired is better than no pretherapy information whatsoever. The second design is a posttest-only design. In this experimental design, a group of patients is randomly assigned to one of two groups. One group receives a treatment or therapy and then both groups receive a posttest or measure. A comparison is then made between the posttest scores for the two groups. For example, patients on a unit are randomly assigned to one of two groups. One group, called the experimental group, receives an instructional unit of self-care of IVs. The other group, called the control group, receives no instruction or treatment. The rate of infection for both groups postsurgery is monitored and compared. If the experimental group has a lower incidence of infection, then we may say that the instructional unit was effective. If a significant difference occurs, then the difference is assumed to be due to the treatment or therapy effect. By randomly dividing the group of patients into two groups an attempt is made to assure that no important differences exist between the two groups that might account for the difference in infection rate. Of course, it may be necessary to examine some variables that may be important in our study to determine that the groups are not different prior to receiving the instruction. Such variables might include age, sex, preoperative status, and prior number of hospitalizations.

A posttest-only design is a valuable design for evaluating patient education programs because it solves one of the ethical problems in this kind of evaluation. How can you have a group that does not get any treatment? In a posttest-only design, it may be possible to divide the group into two and provide the treatment for one group, test both groups on a posttest measure, and then provide the treatment for the control group. For example, 30 patients are randomly divided into two groups of 15 each. One group is given a 3-hour teaching program on self-administered insulin injections. Both groups are then given an examination to determine their extent of knowledge in the area. Following the administration of the examination, the control group can then be given the 3-hour treatment. Or in the IV instruction example, patients normally would not have received the instruction, so the second group was not missing an important part of their therapy.

The final design is the pretest-posttest design with control group. In this design, a group of subjects is randomly divided into two groups and all are pretested on the variables of interest to the study. One group then receives the treatment and then both groups are given a posttest.

Cosper, Hayslip, and Foree report on using an experimental and control group to study the effects of nutrition education of fifth graders [10]. They were able to demonstrate significant increase in knowledge of the experimental group over the control group but no significance between the groups on a 24-hour dietary recall. Other examples of research studies in patient education which included a control group are Lindeman [29], Downs and Fernback [14], and Nunnally and Aquias [32].

Pretesting both the experimental and control groups allows the investigator to be confident that the two groups are equivalent at the beginning of the treatment. Posttesting the groups then allows for a comparison of results to determine the effects of the treatment. Readers are urged to consult a text like Campbell and Stanley [8] for a more complete introduction to experimental designs.

Clinical Trials

Bradford Hill writes [19]:

The clinical trial is a carefully, and ethically, designed experiment with the aim of answering some precisely framed question. In its most rigorous form it demands equivalent groups of patients concurrently treated in different ways. These groups are constructed by the random allocation of patients to one or other treatment . . . . In some instances patients may form their own controls, different treatments being applied to them in random order and the effects compared. In principle the method is applicable with any disease and any treatment.

The clinical trial is conceptually similar to the pretest-posttest with control group design that we have already discussed. One characteristic that is generally different is that during a clinical trial it is not unusual to take multiple pretest measures and multiple posttest measures. For example, in a study of hypertension it may be desirable to gather multiple pre- and posttest measures of blood pressure due to the instability of the measure at any one particular moment.

Dershewitz and Williamson report the results of a controlled clinical trial designed to evaluate the implementation of a health education program intended to reduce the risk of childhood household injuries [13]. They found no difference between their experimental and control groups when they visited to see if the respective homes had been childproofed, although they did demonstrate a knowledge difference between the two groups. (See Witts for further discussion of clinical trials [43].

SELECTING AN INSTRUMENT

Now that the variables have been identified, the source of data specified, and a design selected, it is time to select or construct the instruments. Instruments can be examinations, survey questionnaires, interview guides, chart audits, etc.

Evaluating an Instrument

In order to judge the adequacy of an instrument, three kinds of information should be available. This information has been labeled validity, reliability, and utility by test constructors. Each type of information is briefly discussed.

The first step in evaluating an instrument is to understand the *validity* of the instrument. The validity of an instrument may be determined by answering the question, Does this instrument measure what it is supposed to measure? For example, if one is trying to measure patients' attitudes toward hospitalization and questions are asked only about their attitudes toward physicians and nurses, the instrument would not have validity. Other items on hospitalization should have been included. Information that demonstrates that the instrument measures what it is supposed to measure is an indication of instrument validity. There are three major kinds of instrument validity.

The first type of validity is *content validity*. If one is designing a multiple-choice examination in order to measure patients' learning, the test must cover the content of the teaching or the course objectives [24]. The comparison between content of teaching and the test itself is a measure of the content validity of the instrument. Content validity is usually determined by having an expert in the field examine the test against the course objectives and make a judgment that the appropriate material has in fact been covered on the examination or instrument.

The second kind of validity is *construct validity*. Construct validity generally refers to a psychological trait that an instrument is supposed to measure such as anxiety or perception of pain. These constructs do not exist in a physical sense, but they can still be measured by some instruments. Generally, one is urged to locate an instrument that has already demonstrated the construct validity of the trait because it is extremely difficult and expensive to conduct such a study oneself.

The final type of validity is *predictive validity*. This type of validity refers to the ability of the scores to predict some future, related behavior. An example of predictive validity would be an instrument that measured patient's knowlege of compliance prior to discharge that highly correlated with a measure of compliance six months later in the patient's home. Many difficulties are inherent in a study designed to measure predictive validity. The most glaring problem is the difficulty of measuring the desired behavior six months later, as in our example. Some commercially available instruments have reported predictive validity. If these instruments measure what one is interested in measuring, then careful consideration should be given to adopting them. However, most instruments do not have reported predictive validity. Predictive validity is usually reported as a correlation coefficient and is the strongest measure of validity.

At a minimum, an instrument should possess the characteristic of content validity. If appropriate, construct validity may be substituted for content validity. Predictive validity is the most powerful measure of instrument validity, yet rarely is it available. For a more thorough discussion in this area, see Cronbach [11].

The next issue to be considered in evaluating an instrument is the *reliability of the data*. Can you trust the data? If you were to repeat the administration of the instrument, would you get approximately the same results? Reliability of the data refers to how trustworthy the data are or how stable the scores would be over time. Usually, reliability is reported as a correlation coefficient between two sets of data. Commercially available instruments should report their reliability coefficients. Any instrument reporting less than .80 reliability should be carefully examined before it is adopted. See Juul for a discussion of correlation coefficients [23].

The reliability of a locally constructed instrument should be determined before using the instrument in the study. This is usually done during a pilot study or dry run of the project. Low reliability is interpreted to mean there is an error in the data and that the results do not reflect the actual score or ability of the person completing the instrument. Error in the data may be due to poorly written questions, confusion in directions, conditions under which the instrument was administered (for example, when anxiety is very high just prior to surgery), or problems with the scale of possible answers. For a more complete discussion of reliability, see Stanley [41] or Juul [23].

The final consideration in selecting a test is to gather information on the *utility of the instrument.* Utility of the instrument is a catch-all phrase that includes such items as cost, time to complete, type of directions, scoring mechanisms, and types of reports available. The description of a commercially available instrument should provide sufficient information for using the instrument. The American Psychological Association has published *Standards for Educational and Psychological Tests,* which may be helpful if more information is desired on utility. The kind of information that should be available on an instrument and documented in test manuals is clearly outlined [3].

Locating an Existing Instrument

The first possible source for an instrument for a study on evaluating a patient's learning is the literature in the area. What studies have reported instruments that might be similar to the study under design? It is often worthwhile to write the author of a study to see if the instrument from that study is available for further research. Usually there is no charge for such a use. Utilization of an instrument from the existing literature is one strong rationale for conducting a thorough literature search before beginning any project.

The next step in selecting an instrument is to explore the compendiums that are available; they list hundreds of instruments constructed by researchers to measure every type of behavior and product imaginable. Many of these instruments do not have acceptable validity or reliability information, so the reader must evaluate the instrument himself based upon the reported data. A good source to begin your exploration is with *The Seventh Mental Measurements Yearbook, Volumes I and II,* edited by Burros [6]. Approximately 1,100 instruments are reviewed in that text. Other compendia are available as well [5, 7, 9, 27]. If one is unable to locate an acceptable instrument from these sources or the literature, then an instrument must be constructed.

Constructing an Instrument

It is beyond the scope of this chapter to instruct the reader on how to construct various kinds of measurement instruments. Rather, this section will briefly review the various kinds of instruments available, provide examples of those instruments, and point out references for the reader to consult. If one is located or associated with a university or college, there will be individuals trained in instrument construction available. These people are usually located in departments of psychology, education, and sociology. It perhaps would be wise to seek their assistance in the project of creating an instrument for an evaluation study.

Five types of instruments will be briefly examined here. *Questionnaires* are usually developed to gather two kinds of information. This information includes demographic data, such as age and years of schooling, and attitudinal information, such as trust in doctor or nurse and perception of pain. The first step in the construction of a questionnaire is to outline the kinds of information that one wishes to gather. If one plans to gather data on attitudes or perceptions, it is strongly recommended that an expert in the area of test construction be consulted. Once the kinds of information desired are listed, the process of constructing a questionnaire is simply one of stating the questions in a clear and concise fashion so that the answers will be the kind of information desired. Usually one can locate an existing questionnaire—we all are constantly being asked to complete questionnaires of various kinds—and questions can be copied and modified. The challenge of writing a good questionnaire is that the questions will be so clear that the subjects will answer honestly and will take the time to complete the instrument. Instrument clarity will be of great assistance in gathering honest and complete information.

Various resources are available for improving skills at construction of questionnaires. Rezler presents an excellent overview on construction of attitudinal instruments [36]. Redman also presents an excellent review of various types of questionnaires, along with other instruments, that may be important in evaluating patient education programs [35].

An example of a questionnaire constructed for evaluation purposes, a Sample Page of a Demographic Survey, is presented in the section entitled Resource Materials. Another sample questionnaire is reported by Axford and Cutchen on staffs' attitudes toward patient education [4]. Kleinman and Olsen report on using the mail survey technique to study followup effects of 16 work shops on drug education [25].

The second kind of instrument to be discussed falls into the general category of *examinations*. Examinations refer to any type of instrument designed to measure either knowledge or skills of patients. Most of the literature on how to construct examinations is from the classroom. However, the procedures are the same whether constructing an examination to measure patients' knowledge of diabetes or nursing students' knowledge of diabetes.

First, examinations designed to measure learning or knowledge of the patient, which are referred to as *cognitive examinations* are discussed. A few items from a sample cognitive examination are presented in the section entitled Resource Materials: Sample Multiple Choice Items From Examination. The first step in developing an examination is to decide if the answer format will be open or free, such as fill-in the blanks or essay questions, or if the answer format will be closed or fixed, as in true or false or multiple-choice examinations. Both types of examinations, fixed or free format, require an equivalent amount of time to construct and score. Free format questions are easier to write but more difficult to score; fixed format questions are more difficult to write but easier to score.

The next step in the process is to outline the content to be covered on the examination. What are the content areas that need to be covered? Finally, individual items must be written that correspond to each content area outlined on the blueprint. For detailed information on the construction of examinations, the reader is directed to Adkins [1] and Passos [33] for additional information. Solleder outlined some of the considerations for taxonomy of cognitive level in evaluation, which may be helpful during the stage of constructing a blueprint [40]. There are different levels of cognitive questions. The simplest form is referred to as recall questions, and the most complex type of questions is referred to as synthesis.

The second kind of examination is referred to as *clinical evaluation*. Generally, the literature on clinical evaluation refers to evaluating students' clinical performance. However, in patient education we are often teaching patients a clinical skill. For example, the self-administration of insulin or irrigating a colostomy are clearly clinical skills. Therefore, much of the literature on evaluation of clinical skills of students' performance is appropriate for this discussion of evaluation of patients' clinical skills. The reader is directed to two references in this area. First, McGuire discusses the construction of simulated evaluations both oral and written which can be used for purposes of evaluation [31]. Second, Dyer discusses the evaluation of clinical performance by reviewing the construction of checklists and rating scales [15].

Usually clinical performance is evaluated by directly observing the patient completing the clinical skill. The evaluator completes either a checklist or rating scale while observing the patient. The checklist is a form which simply requires the evaluator to decide if the patient completed or did not complete a skill and the response is either Yes, No, or Not Appropriate. In a rating scale, the evaluator must judge the quality of the performance rather than simply stating that the performance was completed as in the use of a checklist. The rating scale requires a judgment on the degree of satisfactorily completing the task. The section entitled Resource Materials also presents sample items for checklists and rating scales. The reader is urged to explore the references provided to learn more about constructing instruments for evaluating clinical skills.

A face-to-face *interview* with a patient is a rich source of information. However, preparation for conducting an interview requires time and thought. It may be helpful to conceptualize an interview as an oral examination if your goal is to determine patients' knowledge about a topic. Or an interview may be conceptualized as an oral survey if your goal is to determine patients' attitudes or demographic information. Consequently, one must be prepared with a questionnaire or an examination to present to the patient. Redman discusses the role of interviewing in assessing patients' readiness to learn as a followup mechanism to explore issues such as compliance and as a teaching technique [35]. Interviews should be prepared for very carefully or personnel time and patients' time will be wasted.

Although a highly structured interview guide is a useful tool, training as a professional nurse is necessary to guide the interview in a nonthreatening, relaxed fashion. It will enable one to follow through with probes and questions of clarification as well as answering patients' direct questions. The ability to conduct an interview well is a highly valuable skill that requires preparation and practice. The trained, professional nurse learns to be observant about the patient and the environment every day of practice. The skill of *observation* is one that can provide another rich source of data to evaluate a patient's learning. There are generally two kinds of observations: structured and unstructured. A structured observation is similar to conducting a visual survey or questionnaire. The observer spends a great deal of time planning what is to be observed and how the responses will be recorded. In essence, a questionnaire is developed which is used as a checklist or rating scale while the observation is taking place.

An unstructured observation is one in which the observer may have hunches and ideas about what is important to observe but not enough information to focus the observation. Therefore, time is spent observing all those things in the patient's environment and behavior that the nurse is able to observe. Usually such an observer takes field notes about the observations. These notes may be taken while the observation is underway or written up after the observer leaves the patient. Unstructured observations usually are precursors to more formal, structured interviews once particular variables have been identified. It is a common methodology of the case study. McCall and Simmons outline many of the procedures for conducting structured and unstructured observations under the discussion of participant observation [30].

Another type of instrument that may be utilized to evaluate the effectiveness of a patient education program is a *written record*. Such records may be anecdotal notes, progress notes, or they may already exist as the patient's chart. These records are a rich source of data about the effectiveness of a particular program.

Planning to keep written records requires one to select those behaviors that will be recorded. It is recommended that behaviors be recorded that are characteristic of the patient ("wakes every morning around 6AM") and those that are specifically unusual for a patient ("slept until 10 AM this morning"). Not only must one decide what observations to record, but an attempt should be made to distinguish between factual information ("patient cried for 15 minutes") versus interpretation of observations ("patient is blue and upset and cried for 15 minutes"). Both factual and interpretive data are important, but the author of such comments should attempt to distinguish between the two types while recording behavior. See Redman for examples of forms used to record anecdotal nursing records [35].

A very important source of information about a patient is the patient's chart. Using chart audit as a means to collect data on the effectiveness of patient education programs is a promising yet difficult area. Tribble and Hollenberg reported on the use of quality assurance to develop, implement, and evaluate a diabetic teaching protocol [42]. They used the audit format of the Joint Commission on Accreditation of Hospitals.

A significant problem regarding the use of charts to audit performance is the inconclusive nature of the evidence that charting actually reflects regarding the care provided let alone any changes in patients' behavior. Various types of errors in charts have been noted. Rosenfeld differentiated between two categories of errors in recording to be those that reflect inaccuracies in record-keeping and those representing omissions of diagnostic or therapeutic decisions [38]. He found that physicians who made one type of error usually made the other, which led him to believe that charts may be in fact a valid assessment of clinical performance. Kroeger reported that in a study of practicing internists, only two-thirds of them kept records complete enough to make it feasible for nonphysicians to abstract data [26]. Gonnella compared chart data to actual interview data and found the chart data to be lacking [17]. Because of the reported inaccuracies in chart-audit procedures, it is not recommended that a chart audit be adopted as the sole method of data collection in an evaluation study. Rather, chart audit should be combined with the other types of data gathering techniques discussed in this chapter.

CONDUCTING DATA COLLECTION AND ANALYSIS

The first step in data collection is to standardize the methods under which the data are to be collected. For example, if patients are to be interviewed in bed, all patients should be interviewed in bed. The reason for standardization of data collection is that a large source of error in data collection can result from varying the way in which data are collected. When unusual situations are encountered in data collection, the investigator should note those conditions carefully so that the information will be available later to judge if the data must be discarded for a particular case. Controlling for the consistency in the administration of the instruments is one way to ensure the reliability of the data.

After the data have been collected, the next step is to analyze the data. There are many excellent sources for understanding how to report data. Juul [23] and Fox [16] review various statistical procedures including the following: descriptive statistics (means, graphic presentations, or standard deviations); inferential statistics (tests of significance like t-tests); nonparametiric statistics appropriate when assumptions of normality cannot be assumed (chi-square); and content analysis or a method of analyzing written interview comments, tape recordings, transcripts, and anecdotal records. Holzemer discusses reporting and interpreting evaluation data and presents concepts such as standard scores, correlation matrices, expectancy tables, item analysis for examination data, and an examination of the differences between norm and criterion referenced grading [21].

WRITING FINAL REPORTS

Once the data have been collected and analyzed, a report must be written to present the data in a meaningful yet concise way. Below are presented three outlines that could be followed in order to organize a report. The key words in writing an evaluation report are clarity and brevity. The reader of an evaluation report should be able to locate quickly the information that is of most interest to him without having to spend a great deal of effort searching through tables of data.

Three Samples of Report Organizations

1	2	3
Overview	Title page	Abstract
History and description	Abstract	Rationale
Program participants	Executive summary	Audience
Quality of program	Overview and introduction	Program description
Program cost	The problem	Evaluation questions
Program termination	Design and methodology	(Variable Matrix)
Program summary	Sample	Instruments
Appendices	Instruments	Results
	Analysis of data	Discussions and
	Summary and	summary
	conclusions	
	Appendix A: Technical	
	material	
	Appendix B:	
	Participants	

Often it is advisable to present an abstract of the report that may be less than one page. The abstract may be followed by a three to five page summary. This summary is then followed by the evaluation report itself. Even in the situation where an abstract and summary are written, it is often helpful to place many of the technical tables in an appendix so that the reader may consult the data if he so desires but does not have to confront it in the text of the report.

It is also recommended that once an evaluation report has been written, significant members of the audience be allowed to read the draft of the document before it is published. Depending upon the nature of the evaluation, it may be crucial to validate quotations and judgments prior to printing. As judgments in evaluation are value statements and people differ in their values, it is only fair to expect differences of opinion. Data can be presented in many different ways to expose or to hide particular points. The evaluator must make the final decision as to how the information will be presented; however, unless the evaluator is very wise, it is advisable to check with the significant audiences prior to publishing an evaluation report. Embarrassing errors may have to be withdrawn if one is not careful. Lee and Garvey recommend that "staff patient education performance must be evaluated and rewarded if management expects patient education to be accomplished" [28]. This chapter outlines a series of steps to take in order to design an evaluation of a patient education program. This information collected in the evaluation can be presented to management to demonstrate the effectiveness of the program, illuminate problem areas, and create an objective database for making judgments about financial support for staff and programs. Evaluating a patient education program is a challenging task that requires as much attention, creativity, and funding as does the designing of a patient education program itself.

REFERENCES

1. Adkins, D. C.   *Test Construction: Development and Interpretations of Achievement Tests* (2nd ed.). Columbus, Ohio: Merrill Publishing Company, 1974.
2. American Hospital Association.   *Hospital Inpatient Education, Survey Findings and Analyses, 1975.* Atlanta, Georgia: Center for Disease Control, 1977.
3. American Psychological Association.   *Standards for Educational and Psychological Tests.* Washington, D.C.: The Association, 1974.
4. Axford, R., and Cutchen, L.   Using nursing research to improve preoperative care. *Journal of Nursing Administration,* December, 1977. Pp. 16–20.
5. Burros, O.K. (Ed.).   *Personality Tests and Reviews.* Highland Park, N.J.: Gryphon 1974.
6. Burros, O. K. (Ed.).   *The Seventh Mental Measurements Yearbook, Volumes I and II.* Highland Park, N.J.: Gryphon, 1972.
7. Burros, O. K. (Ed.).   *Tests in Print II.* Highland Park, N.J.: Gryphon, 1974.
8. Campbell, D. T., and Stanley, J. C.   *Experimental and Quasi-Experimental Designs for Research.* Chicago: Rand McNally, 1963.
9. Chun, K-T., Cobb, S., and French, J. R.   *Measures for Psychological Assessment: A Guide to 3,000 Original Sources and Their Applications.* Ann Arbor, Mich.: Institute for Social Research, The University of Michigan, 1975.
10. Cosper, B. A., Hayslip, D. E., and Foree, S. B.   The effect of nutrition education on dietary habits of fifth-graders. *The Journal of School Health.* 47 : 475, 1977.
11. Cronbach, L. J.   Test Validation. In R. L. Throndike (Ed.), *Educational Measurement, Second Edition.* Washington, D.C.: American Council on Education, 1971. Pp. 443–507.
12. del Bueno, D. J.   Patient education: Planning for success. *Journal of Nursing Administration,* June, 1978. Pp. 3–7.
13. Dershewitz, R. A., and Williamson, J. W.   Prevention of childhood household injuries: A controlled clinical trial. *American Journal of Public Health.* 67 : 1148, 1977.
14. Downs, F. S., and Frenbach, V.   Experimental evaluation of a prenatal leaflet series. *Nursing Research,* 22 : 498–506, 1973.
15. Dyer, E.D.   Evaluation of Clinical Performance: Rating Scales and Checklists. In A. G. Rezler and B. J. Stevens (Eds.), *The Nurse Evaluator in Education and Service.* New York: McGraw-Hill, 1978. Pp. 125–141.
16. Fox, D. J.   *Fundamentals of Research in Nursing* (2nd ed.). New York: Appleton-Century-Crofts, 1970.
17. Gonnella, J., Goran, M., Williamson, J., and Cotsonas, N.   Evaluation of patient care: An approach. *Journal of the American Medical Association,* 214 : 2040–2043, 1970.
18. Green, L. W.   Evaluation and measurement: Some dilemmas for health education. *American Journal of Public Health,* 67 : 155, 1977.
19. Hill, B.   *Principles of Medical Statistics.* New York: Oxford University Press, 1966.
20. Holzemer, W. L.   A protocol for program evaluation. *Journal of Medical Education,* 51 : 101, 1976.
21. Holzemer, W. L.   Reporting and Interpreting Evaluation Data. In A. G. Rezler and B. J. Stevens (Eds.), *The Nurse Evaluator in Education and Service.* New York: McGraw-Hill, 1978. Pp. 297–322.
22. Isaac, S., and Michael, W. B.   *Handbook in Research and Evaluation.* San Diego, Calif.: Robert R. Knapp, 1971.
23. Juul, D.   Description and Analysis of Test Data. In A. G. Rezler and B. J. Stevens (Eds.), *The Nurse Evaluator in Education and Service.* New York: McGraw-Hill, 1978. Pp. 279–283.
24. King, E. C.   Constructing classroom achievement tests. *Nurse Educator,* 3 : 30, 1978.
25. Kleinman, S. P., and Olsen, L. K.   An evaluation of the long-range effects of drug

education workshops. *The Journal of School Health,* 43 : 578–583, 1973.
26. Kroeger, H., Altman, I., Clark, D. A., Johnson, A. C., and Shelps, C. B.   The office practice of internists 1: The feasibility of evaluating quality of care. *Journal of the American Medical Association,* 193 : 371–376, 1965.
27. Lake, D. G., Miles, M. B., and Earle, R. B., Jr. (Eds.). *Measuring Human Behavior.* New York: Columbia University, 1973.
28. Lee, E. A., and Garvey, J. L.   How is inpatient education being managed? *Hospitals,* 51 : 75–76, 1977.
29. Lindeman, C. A.   Nursing intervention with the presurgical patient. *Nursing Research,* 21 : 196–209, 1972.
30. McCall, G. J., and Simmons, J. L.   *Issues in Participant Observation: A Text and Reader.* Reading, Mass.: Addison-Wesley, 1969.
31. McGuire, C. H.   Evaluation of Clinical Performance: Written and Oral Simulation. In A. G. Rezler and B. J. Stevens (Eds.), *The Nurse Evaluator in Education and Service.* New York: McGraw-Hill, 1978. Pp. 101–124.
32. Nunnally, D. M., and Aquias, M. B.   Patients' evaluation of their prenatal and delivery care. *Nursing Research,* 23 : 469–474, 1974.
33. Passos, J. Y.   Evaluation of Classroom Performance. In A. G. Rezler and B. J. Stevens (Eds.), *The Nurse Evaluator in Education and Service.* New York: McGraw-Hill, 1978. Pp. 83–100.
34. Popham, W. J.   *Educational Evaluation.* Englewood Cliffs, N.J.: Prentice-Hall, 1975.
35. Redman, B. K.   *The Process of Patient Teaching in Nursing* (3rd ed.). St. Louis: Mosby, 1976.
36. Rezler, A., and Stevens, B. (Eds.).   *Evaluation in Nursing Service and Education.* New York: McGraw-Hill, 1978.
37. Riordan, N. M.   An analysis of variables affecting maternal knowledge of growth and development. Master's thesis, College of Nursing, University of Illinois at the Medical Center, Chicago, 1978.
38. Rosenfeld, L.   Quality of medical care in hospitals. *American Journal of Public Health,* 47 : 856–865, 1957.
39. Scriven, M.   The Methodology of Evaluation. In R. E. Stake (Ed.), *Perspectives of Curriculum Evaluation.* American Educational Research Association Monograph Series on Evaluation, No. 1. Chicago: Rand McNally, 1967.
40. Solleder, M. K.   Evaluation in the cognitive domain. *The Journal of School Health.* 42 : 16, 1972.
41. Stanley, J. C.   Reliability. In *Educational Measurement* (2nd ed.). Washington, D.C.: American Council on Education, 1971. Pp. 356–442.
42. Tribble, N. M., and Hollenberg, E.   The impact of a quality assurance program on diabetes education. *The Nursing Clinics of North America,* 12 : 365–373, 1977.
43. Witts, L. J.   *Medical Surveys and Clinical Trials: Some Methods and Applications of Group Research in Medicine.* London: Oxford University Press, 1964.

Resource Materials

SAMPLE PAGE OF A DEMOGRAPHIC SURVEY*

Thank you for agreeing to complete this survey. This study will be very helpful to those of us concerned with planning education for parenthood. It is very

---

*From N. M. Riordan, "An Analysis of Variables Affecting Maternal Knowledge of Growth and Development." Master's Thesis, University of Illinois at the Medical Center, College of Nursing, 1978. Used with permission.

important that you answer every question. It is not necessary to identify yourself by name. All of your answers will be strictly confidential.

General Information

1. Your age: _____
2. Race: a. Black   b. White   c. Oriental   d. Other
3. Employment status:
   a. Full-time mother
   b. Working full-time
   c. Working part-time
   d. Other: _____
4. Highest year of school completed (circle):
   Grade school   1 2 3 4 5 6 7 8
   High school   1 2 3 4
   College   1 2 3 4
   Graduate school 1 2 3 4 5
5. How many children do you have? _____
   List their ages: _____
6. What is your family's yearly income?
   a. less than $3000
   b. $3001–$6000
   c. $6001–$9000
   d. $9001–$12,000
   e. $12,001–$15,000
   f. more than $15,000

SAMPLE MULTIPLE CHOICE ITEMS FROM EXAMINATION*

Survey
Circle the one best answer. All questions refer to the average or typical child.
1. Most babies walk on their own by what age?
   a. 4–7 months
   b. 8–11 months
   c. 12–15 months
   d. 16–19 months
2. A baby usually doubles his birth weight at what age?
   a. 3 months
   b. 5 months
   c. 7 months
   d. 9 months
3. Which of the following statements is true about play in the preschool child (3–5 years)?

*From N. M. Riordan, "An Analysis of Variables Affecting Maternal Knowledge of Growth and Development." Master's Thesis, University of Illinois at the Medical Center, College of Nursing, 1978. Used with permission.

a. He is very concerned with rules and fairness.
b. He plays most often alone, although often doing the same things as other children are doing.
c. He plays cooperative games with other children, at least for short periods of time.

SAMPLE DIABETIC TEST

Please circle ◯ the correct answers to the following questions.

1. Diabetes will "go away" when the blood sugar and urine are kept normal.
   True   False
2. The pancreas plays an important role in diabetes.
   True   False
3. Diabetes occurs only in the 30–60 age group.
   True   False
4. Calories are made up of carbohydrate, protein, and fat.
   True   False

SAMPLE CHECKLIST AND RATING SCALE ITEMS

Checklist*   Yes   No

1. Scrubbed top of vial with disinfectant sponge   _____   _____
2. Punctured rubber vial with needle, without contaminating _____   _____
3. Withdrew all of fluid from vial   _____   _____
4. Expelled excess air from syringe without losing fluid   _____   _____
5. Measured fluid to within 0.1 ml of the correct dose   _____   _____

Rating Scale

1. The atmosphere in the patient education classroom seemed (circle one):

   1   :   2   :   3   :   4   :   5
   (relaxed   (tense &
   & friendly)   unfriendly)

2. Did this patient education class give you enough opportunity to share and discuss your concerns with other patients?

   a. Yes
   b. Not sure
   c. No (but did not want this opportunity)
   d. No

*From B. K. Redman, *The Process of Patient Teaching in Nursing* (3rd ed.). St. Louis: Mosby, 1976. P. 187. Used with permission.

Barbara J. Mohr

11

Quality Assurance and Patient Education

How do quality assurance activities relate to patient education programming? How can I integrate patient education activities into the newest quality assurance standards from the Joint Commission on Accreditation of Hospitals (JCAH)?

Evaluation of patient teaching programs includes more than just how well the patient has learned. Evaluation activities must also address overall institutional effectiveness in meeting all standards of care including teaching. The newest standards for quality assurance recommend a coordinated effort that crosses departmental lines in an institution. This coordinated effort may help not only to reduce overall patient care costs but may also help to solve patient care problems that have more than one cause. The following chapter explores the relationship between quality assurance and patient education. The newest concepts of quality assurance programming are presented, and examples are provided of how the newest standards of quality assurance can be applied to patient education activities. Patient-care evaluation is described with an institution-wide focus.

Information in this chapter should help the reader to

1. *Derive operational definitions of quality of care and quality of teaching*
2. *List the components of a comprehensive quality assurance program*
3. *Measure the impact of patient education on overall quality patient care*
4. *Describe the relationship between utilization review and patient teaching activities*
5. *Relate clinical monitoring activities to the patient educator*
6. *Establish a system of accountability for teaching patients*
7. *Describe the relationship between education activities and quality assurance*
8. *Mobilize institutional resources to establish a viable quality assurance program*

This chapter is designed to acquaint the reader with current quality assurance concepts and the manner in which many of them relate to patient education. Several reasons exist for carefully examining the relationship between an institution's quality assurance program and its patient education program. First, patient education as an integral component of quality patient care is a premise enjoying increasingly widespread acceptance [13, 20, 25]. Second, cost containment concerns mandate that the health care system build on, improve, and integrate existing mechanisms rather than create separate and uncoordinated functions. Third, a thorough understanding of the institution's evaluative mechanisms will allow the patient educator to use quality assurance data to assess the needs for specific patient education programs and to evaluate the impact of patient education programs. Before the relationship between quality assurance and patient education can be explored, it will be necessary to assure some familiarity with the newer concepts in quality assurance.

TRADITIONAL QUALITY ASSURANCE CONCEPTS

With few exceptions, prior to the 1970s quality care was assumed if competent health-care professionals practiced in a setting where the organizational structure and physical environment were considered sound. Quality meant attention to such measures as education, licensure, and speciality certification. Surveys by local health departments and accrediting agencies concentrated on features such as the physical facility, the safety of equipment, and the completeness of internal policies and procedures.

However, in the early 1970s a number of related activities led health-care professionals to question the assumption that quality care was synonymous with a safe physical environment. The federal government and third party payers, faced with rapidly rising health-care expenditures, called for demonstration that their dollars were being spent appropriately. The courts increasingly were asked, after the fact, to determine whether quality care had been given. Consumers of health care sought to know why personal expectations, already at a high level and spurred higher with each public announcement of new medical cures, were not being fulfilled.

Responding to these pressures, the Joint Commission on Accreditation of Hospitals (JCAH), the voluntary accreditation body formed in 1951 by several major groups within the private health sector, added new standards requiring the governing boards of health-care institutions to develop formal procedures to monitor and assure the quality of professional services. At about the same time the federal government also responded by establishing Professional Standards Review Organizations (PSROs), regional physician groups, to monitor the cost and the quality of medical care.

One particular procedure, the "medical audit," has received a great deal of attention by both the JCAH and the PSRO. Today, almost all hospitals conduct a small number of medical audits for the purpose of systematically reviewing patient care [2]. These audit studies generally focus on groups of patients with similar medical diagnoses or surgical procedures and rely on documentation in the patient's medical record to confirm compliance with predetermined criteria. Any unacceptable variations from the criteria (as determined by practitioners) are singled out for remedial action.

Although this method of evaluating patient care is widespread, critics have argued that the procedure is too expensive, does not result in lasting behavior change, and does not improve the health status of patients [14, 18, 29]. Reasons cited by those who contend the failure of these studies include inappropriate topic selection [32], invalid or indiscriminate criteria [9], too much emphasis on continuing education as the sole corrective action [4, 9], and simple resistance to change [18]. Thompson states that "rigid requirements emphasizing identification of deficiencies against which 'corrective action' is necessary has caused us to be defensive and to overlook many potential uses of patient care audit findings" [28]. Others believe that too much is expected of the audit; while it can be an effective study method, the audit must not be taken as the only method and should be integrated with other quality assurance functions [27, 31].

NEW DIRECTIONS

Quality assurance today has been influenced by many of these past criticisms and is undergoing some major conceptual changes. Two of the most significant changes are the encouragement of methodological flexibility in contrast to the early emphasis on one strict procedure, and the realization that the audit is just one component of a truly comprehensive quality and accountability system.

Methods

The first substantive change in the quality assurance field is reflected in the April 1979 revisions of the JCAH quality assurance standard. This new standard urges innovative and flexible study procedures that may vary depending on the nature of the study. The shift in emphasis away from one study method (audit) with specified protocols allows experimentation in the use of a variety of means to identify and resolve patient-care problems. Thus, the quality assurance field is "experiencing a time of introspection, redefinition and increased options—a time to go back to the drawing boards" [10].

The advantage of such introspection is the luxury it affords to rethink some very basic questions such as the definition of quality. One of the frustrations of the current status of quality assurance may be that the health-care field has been struggling to measure something that has not been defined. Although the effort to define quality must be made before it can be measured, the task is not an easy one. Consider, for example, the different perspectives of those persons who might define it. Health-care professionals might define quality in terms of the technical skills needed to perform certain tasks. If third party payers were to determine quality, they might respond in a manner that emphasizes the most cost-effective methods of delivering care. A health-care administrator might use occupancy or utilization statistics or the number of board-certified physicians or baccalaureate-prepared RNs on staff as a measure of quality. And finally, the patient might define quality very differently and talk in terms of access, efficiency, and fulfillment of personal expectations.

Even taking into account all of these diverse perspectives, one can derive an operational definition of quality. Richard E. Thompson proposes that the following six elements be included in the definition [28]:

1. Optimal achievable patient results
2. *Primum non nochere*—first do no harm
3. Patient and family understanding
4. Cost effectiveness
5. Reasonable documentation
6. Appropriate utilization of resources

This operational definition of quality is particularly attractive because of the flexbility it allows in determining methods for implementing various quality review activities. Rather than being placed in the position of having to defend one method of review against another, the assessor can determine methods with an eye toward more than a single aspect of quality. For example, in order to determine achievement of optimal patient results, one would need a retrospective review (after the patient is discharged) since patient results such as normal blood pressure or knowledge of postdischarge instructions may not be evident until some time very close to discharge. However, quality also includes adherence to the directive *primum non nochere,* which implies preventive monitoring concurrently (while the patient is still in the hospital) so that complications are avoided. An ideal quality review system would take advantage of both retrospective and concurrent review methods.

Similarly, the debate concerning the efficacy of studying professional activity (process) or patient results (outcome) will most likely continue for some time [3, 15, 19, 22]. However, an ideal study method would include attempts to relate professional activity to patient outcomes for at least two reasons: first, to see if optimal results are being obtained in the absence of some activity considered by the providers to be crucial, and second, to confirm that certain processes are causally linked to favorable outcomes.

Finally, the operational definition of quality allows the inclusion of cost concerns in the same study in which quality is being evaluated. For example, suppose an institution discovers that garamycin or carbencillin is the most expensive drug in use. An arbitrary directive restricting the purchase or use of these drugs would be inappropriate without first determining whether these drugs are ordered only when indicated and avoided when less toxic alternatives could be substituted. If subsequently the pharmacy records show a decrease in the utilization of these drugs, has quality been improved or has cost been reduced? Surely, both goals have been accomplished.

Regardless of the methods chosen for quality review, there are five elements common to most strategies [30]:

1. Identification of problems in the delivery of quality care
2. Selection of appropriate objective assessment strategies
3. Assessment of the problem against established criteria to determine the extent of the problem and identify probable causes
4. Interpretation of appropriate methods aimed at solving the problem; and
5. Reassessment of the problem to ascertain resolution or reduction to an acceptable level

Audit Does Not Stand Alone

The second major change in quality assurance efforts is one that seeks to place the audit within the broader context of a comprehensive quality assurance program. Quality assurance is no longer equated just with the audit. Instead the audit is being viewed as one of many activities necessary to maintain and document high quality care.

PATIENT-CARE EVALUATION AND PATIENT EDUCATION

Of the quality assurance components, patient-care evaluation (formerly called audit) is perhaps of most significance to the patient educator, for it is through patient-care evaluation studies that the impact of patient education is measured. Because it is generally acknowledged that the bulk of actual patient teaching should be done by clinicians involved in the patient's care [17], evaluating the impact of patient education presents some special problems. The most reasonable way to avoid any misunderstanding when the patient educator criticizes the performance of others is to incorporate the evaluation of patient education into currently existing patient-care evaluation studies. For those who may not be familiar with patient-care evaluation methods, the section entitled Resource Materials presents a sample set of criteria developed to evaluate retrospectively the care of patients with diabetes mellitus. As can be seen from this list, criteria 9 through 15 are intended to determine from documentation in patient records if hospitalized patients can demonstrate or verbalize desired behavior prior to discharge. The advantages to the patient educator of being aware of and involved in this type of activity are many. Data from this type of study will help the patient educator to make needed modifications in specific patient education programs. For instance, suppose the patient educator has been involved in conducting group classes for the diabetic patient population. As part of the evaluation of a particular class, a pre- and posttest of the patients' knowledge of diabetes is given. It is possible that the same patient who did well on a posttest of cognitive skills necessary to correctly administer insulin would be unable to follow through on the actual self-administration demonstration prior to discharge. The implication for the patient educator is in altering the class methods to allow for participant demonstration and practice of the desired behavior.

Patient-care evaluation studies can also be useful in identifying where the services of the patient educator as a consultant to other staff members might be most productive. Depending on patterns of compliance with patient education criteria by service, unit, discipline, or practitioner, it is possible to identify those persons who are doing the best job and to identify where the consultation of the education specialist might produce the most results.

The necessity for the input of patient educators into the evaluation process is asserted by Jencks and Green who claim that clinicians' ideas for conducting health education are often wrong [17]. Without a patient educator to help analyze data from patient-care evaluation studies, inappropriate actions may be recommended to deal with identified deficiencies in patient education. For instance, clinicians might recommend the use of expensive visual aids whereas enlisting family support might be a more effective method of increasing patients' knowledge or desired behavior.

Patient educators should be involved not only in the analysis of data from patient-care evaluation studies but also in the design of such studies. They might suggest the addition of criteria that would yield valuable information. For instance, the patient educator with knowledge of learning curves and the tendency for quick deterioration of desired behavior changes might suggest the value of including criteria to review all readmissions of patients with diabetes within a specified time. Because of the probable relationship between failure to comply with the therapeutic regimen and readmission, this data can be valuable in assessing the impact of patient education. In fact, if readmission rates are lower for patients who have participated in a specific patient education program than for a similar group of patients who had not participated, a step toward demonstrating cost benefits has been made.

One final advantage to increasing the collaboration between patient educator and the patient-care evaluation activity is that the patient education evaluations that document impact on physiologic or functional patient outcomes like reduction of blood pressure increase relevance to clinical practice [16]. Thus the acceptance by clinicians of patient education as a significant therapeutic measure is enhanced.

It is definitely to the advantage of the patient educator to become thoroughly familiar with and involved in patient-care evaluation activity. For those who may be new to the job of coordinating patient education activities or who may be unfamiliar with their institution's evaluation activity, it would be useful to review the last ten patient-care studies conducted inhouse. In addition, audit committee chairmen or department heads should be interviewed to see if individual studies include criteria to evaluate patient education. Are the criteria appropriate? Where are the problems? Has any action been taken to improve patient education? What educational program needs have been identified? It might also be useful to become familiar with some of the recent advances in patient care evaluation study methods, some of which are summarized in Table 4.

UTILIZATION REVIEW AND PATIENT EDUCATION

An institution's utilization review program is charged with the awesome responsibility of monitoring and assuring appropriate allocation of scarce health-care

Table 4. The Changing Face of Audit/Patient-Care Evaluation

Change	From	To
Name	Audit	Patient-care evaluation
Evaluator	Medical staff committee	Multidisciplinary committee involvement
Topic	Most frequent diagnosis procedure or surgical procedure	Suspected problem of clinical concern
Source of Information	Only the patient's medical record	Additional sources such as departmental logs, patient's bill, discharge abstracts, practitioner profiles, etc.
Criteria	Developed only by providers	Developed by providers with input from patients
Reason for Evaluation	Compliance only	Collect needed information in order to make better decisions about patient care
Object	Whip nonconformers into line	Improve quality, utilization, and documentation of patient-care services

resources without adversely affecting the quality of patient care. Components of such a program include concurrent review for the necessity of admission, surgery, or diagnostic and therapeutic procedures. Appropriate utilization of operating rooms, intensive care units, emergency room services, ancillary services, and even drugs are examples of areas that are monitored regularly as part of an effective program. Patient educators can play a major role in efficient utilization of these resources. For example, inadequate patient instruction and preparation may be the reason for cancelled or repeated diagnostic procedures such as certain x-ray series, radiation therapy, or telemetric monitoring. Clearly such inefficiencies are irritating and costly for both the patient and the institution.

On the other hand, adequate patient instruction may reduce patient post-operative reliance on sleeping medications, analgesics, or the need for intermittent positive pressure breathing treatments. In such cases, utilization review data may be extremely valuable in demonstrating the effectiveness of patient education programs. There are many questions that will be answered by utilization review data. Does the preoperative teaching program reduce the length of stay? Do patient education programs reduce readmission rates or result in shorter hospital stays for those patients who must be readmitted? Changes in utilization patterns such as shorter lengths of stay and reduction of readmission rates or outpatient visits as a result of patient education can be transferred into substantial cost savings. In fact, the Blue Cross Association cites a study at Tufts-New England Medical Center in which patient education effected a 45 percent reduction in total cost per patient with a specific diagnosis [33]. These kinds of cost-benefit studies are absolutely essential to patient educators if adequate third party reimbursement and administrative support for patient education programs are to be realized.

Because of the obvious relationship between discharge planning (preparing the patient for a less acute level of care) and effective use of inpatient facilities, no utilization review program is complete without a major emphasis on discharge planning. Discharge planning not-only is a major component in utilization review but also essential to quality and continuity of care. Discharge planning data can also be another valuable source of information for the patient educator. The liaisons with community agencies established by the discharge planning department may provide a partial answer to the dilemma posed by being able to evaluate health education outcomes only on a short term basis, that is, at discharge from the hospital. Since health-education induced behavior changes are time dependent [12], it would be useful to have feedback from the home health program, for instance, concerning observed behavior change following a hospital education program. An effective relationship between the persons responsible for an institution's patient education program and those responsible for the utilization review program is to the advantage of both parties.

CLINICAL MONITORING

Clinical monitoring refers to ongoing activities designed to maintain high professional standards of care. Such activities include review of antibiotics and other drugs, review of the use of blood and blood products, surgical case review to determine appropriate indications for surgery, mortality review, medical records review, and infection control. The two most important clinical monitoring activities from the standpoint of the patient educator are antibiotic review and infection control.

Antibiotic and Other Drug Reviews

The need to include antibiotic review as part of an institution's quality assurance program is well documented by Simmons and Stolley who estimate that as many as 33 percent of medical/surgical patients receive at least one antibiotic during hospitalization [24]. Some of these patients will develop life-threatening adverse reactions. The purpose of antibiotic or any other drug review is to determine appropriate utilization of the drug including administration, specific dosage, and monitoring of patient response including possible side effects or adverse reactions.

The patient education implications in drug review are well known because failure to comply with prescribed drug therapy very often accounts for nonachievement of optimal patient results. The patient educator will be responsible for helping hospital staff teach patients proper information about drug therapy. Then specific patient education criteria should be included in studies of specific drugs.

Infection Control

An institution's infection control program is designed to identify, control, and ultimately prevent hospital-acquired (nosocomial) infections or those infections brought to the hospital by the community. The importance of this function to quality patient care is illustrated by the fact that nearly 1.5 million persons annually are subjected to infections while hospitalized [26]. Responsibilities of the infection control program include the development of surveillance mechanisms that identify patterns of infection by unit, service, practitioner, procedure, and pathogen. In addition, an active plan that can respond quickly to outbreaks of infectious diseases, by discovering their source, route of transmission, and population susceptibility, should be well established. Finally, specific protocols for the management of patients needing such measures as isolation, Foley catheters, and IV therapy are the responsibility of the infection control program.

Patient education is a major concern of a preventive infection control program and the expertise of the patient educator may be called upon to assist with that function. Any patient discharged with a communicable disease will require extensive patient instruction to prevent the spread of the disease. It is very possible that the expertise of the patient educator will be called upon for input into either design of clinical monitoring studies or interpretation of data from these activities.

SAFETY AND RISK MANAGEMENT

Prompted by increasing malpractice claims, rising insurance premiums, cost containment pressures, and the resulting trend to self-insure, many health-care institutions have developed risk management programs [5, 11]. These programs aim to control institutional liability and focus on the analysis of incident reports, and the development of safety procedures (for example, protocols for sponge counts, obtaining of informed consent, and labeling of patient specimens and personal belongings). Some institutions have hired patient representatives or ombudsmen to intervene on behalf of patients with complaints.

The relationship of risk management activities with patient education activities is largely unexplored. However, the potential of patient education for increasing patient satisfaction [13], and consequently decreasing the number of litigations against the institution or physician [21, 23, 29] is enormous, and the patient educator may play a vital role in this emerging quality assurance activity. A portion of an effective risk management program will be reactive in nature, beginning with the filing of an incident report or feedback from the patient representative noting a dissatisfied patient. Any potential claims judged on the basis of patient harm or injury are forwarded to the hospital administrator, the hospital's attorney, and the patient's physician so that a plan to handle the situation can be prepared.

Although reaction should be part of a risk management program, Fifer labels the majority of these measures incomplete because they deal with issues of custodial liability (that is, responsibility for the patient's safety while in the hospital) rather than with professional negligence or deficiency of medical care [11]. In a California medical insurance feasibility study that reviewed over 20,000 patient records, it was estimated that "nearly one in every 20 experienced a provider-caused patient disability or potentially compensable event

(PCE)" [7]. The screening criteria used in this study were subsequently adapted for institutional use on a concurrent basis [9]. Those institutions that have adopted this system screen every patient record to provide early identification and warning of hospital-induced PCEs. Examples of some of the criteria used to screen patient records include those related to cancelled or repeated diagnostic or therapeutic procedures, drug or transfusion reactions, unscheduled return to the operating room, and unscheduled transfer to special care units [9].

If patient educators are aware that an institution has implemented such a concurrent program in risk management, it is possible that the identification of the most common patient complaints may result in a request for the patient educator to develop a video tape explaining reasons for extended waiting time and usual procedures in the emergency room. Similarly, analysis of incident reports for patterns by location, type, severity, practitioner, and any other relative factors may call attention to the fact that inadequate patient education is sometimes the major reason cited in accidental falls [21]. Other risk management activities such as the monitoring of PCEs, review of claims, allocations, or modifications of policy or procedures all have potential patient education implications. For example, it is entirely possible that the help of the patient educator would be sought if an institution elected to revise its consent forms in order to ensure better patient understanding or to adopt a Patient's Bill of Rights to be distributed to every patient upon admission.

CREDENTIALING AND PERFORMANCE APPRAISALS

Credentialing is the process whereby an institution identifies those patient-care functions that may be safely performed by an individual practitioner. The decisions about who may do what are based on the individual's experience, education, references, and current competence. In the past, credentialing was instituted only for physicians seeking membership on the hospital medical staff. Currently the term is used to describe the mechanisms for assuring the competence of many health-care professionals. Whether an individual's performance is evaluated through a formal credentialing mechanism or a yearly performance appraisal, quality assurance data on patterns of individual clinical performance should be a determining factor.

One way of increasing individual accountability for patient education activities is to include responsibility for the function in job descriptions and subsequent performance appraisals. A patient educator may wish to investigate how many disciplines or departments think that patient education is an important enough function to be included in the performance appraisals.

EDUCATION

Although the function of education is more of a response to the findings from patient-care evaluation, utilization review, clinical monitoring, and risk management activity, the intrinsic relationship between these activities and education warrants its placement among the quality assurance functions. Brown's

"Bi-Cycle theory" first acknowledged this relationship [6]. Brown states that the quality assurance activity assesses the need for certain educational activities. The effectiveness of the education program is then evaluated through restudies to see if desired behavior change has occurred. Quality assurance personnel are well acquainted with this concept since many patient-care studies end with the recommendation for patient education, staff education, or even community education.

The relationship of education to the other quality assurance functions has been pictorially described as a circle. The circle begins with identification of a problem, and, if the analysis of the problem reveals the need for certain educational activities, these are carried out. The effectiveness of the education program is evaluated through restudies to see if the desired behavior change has been effected. Although the circle theory was first used to discuss the relationships between quality assurance activities and continuing education of health professionals, it also describes the relationship between patient education and quality assurance activities. Data from the quality assurance studies identify the need for certain patient education programs that are then evaluated through restudies to see if patients' behavior has changed.

INTEGRATION: FITTING THE PIECES TOGETHER

As is evident from the discussion of the six components of a quality assurance program, many of these activities overlap, and the placement of them in separate categories is difficult. That is why many institutions with a well-planned quality assurance program will centralize the responsibility for coordinating all quality assurance activities in one individual, department, or committee. This coordination will include an emphasis on assuring appropriate feedback to and from those persons performing the various quality assurance functions. Such integration reduces duplication, increases communication, and maximizes the potential usefulness of data generated by each of the separate activities. Figure 4 may be useful in visualizing how these components are conceptually related. There are, however, as many organizational structures for achieving this integration as there are health-care institutions. Many institutions, for example, will determine that antibiotic review could best be achieved through the infection control program. Other institutions will incorporate portions of surgical case review, transfusion review, and medical records review into the patient-care evaluation program. Still others will combine patient education and discharge planning in an independent department. The expertise of the patient educator may be called upon almost daily by those persons responsible for an institution's quality assurance program. The help of the patient educator may be needed with the selection of patient study topics or for input into decisions about how the information should be used. The advantage to the patient educator is that this kind of involvement will help the patient educator with the very difficult tasks of identifying specific patient education needs and evaluating the impact of patient education.

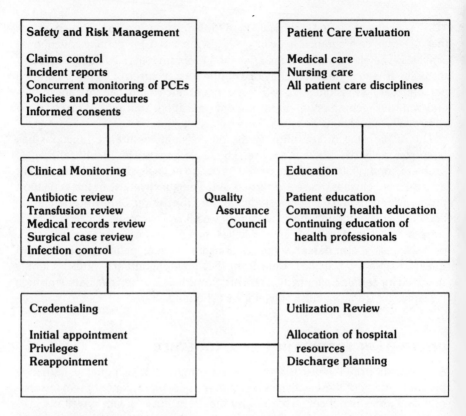

Figure 4. *Conceptual model for integrating quality assurance functions. The model illustrates the relationship among individual organizational functions and the various quality assurance components.*

REFERENCES

1. Batalden, P. B., McClain, M. P., O'Connor, J. P., and Hanson, A. S.   Quality assurance in the ambulatory setting: An operating program. *The Journal of Ambulatory Care Management,* 1(4) : 1–13, 1978.
2. Brook, R. H.   Quality, can we measure it? *New England Journal of Medicine,* 296 : 170, 1977.
3. Brook, R. H., et al.   Assessing the quality of medical care using outcome measures: An overview of the method. *Medical Care,* [Suppl.] 15 : 1–164, 1977.
4. Brook, R. H., et al.   Quality assurance today and tomorrow: Forecast for the future. *Annals of Internal Medicine,* 85 : 809, 1976.
5. Brook, R. H., and Williams, K. N.   Malpractice and the quality of care. *Annals of Internal Medicine,* 88 : 836, 1978.
6. Brown, C., and McConkey, R.   The Quality Assurance System. In *Medical Peer Review Theory and Practice.* Saint Louis: Mosby, 1977.
7. California Medical Association.   *Report on the Medical Insurance Feasibility Study.* San Francisco: The Association, 1977.

8. Craddick, J. W.   The medical management analysis system: A professional liability warning mechanism. *Quality Review Bulletin,* 5(9) : 2–8, 1979.
9. Fifer, W. R.   Explaining the ineffectiveness of medical audit (letter to editor). *Quality Review Bulletin,* 4 : 5, 1978.
10. Fifer, W. R.   Quality assurance: Debate persists on goals, impact, and methods of evaluating care. *Hospitals* 53(7) : 163–7, 1979.
11. Fifer, W. R.   Risk management and medical malpractice: An overview of the issues. *Quality Review Bulletin,* 5(9) : 9–13, 1979.
12. Green, L. W.   Evaluation and measurement: Some dilemmas for health education. *Nursing Digest,* 6 : 69, 1978.
13. Green, L. W.   The potential of health education includes cost effectiveness. *Hospitals,* 50 : 57, 1976.
14. Haggerty, R. J., and Demlo, L. K.   Study urges redirection of quality assurance programs. *Hospital Progress,* 58 : 76, 1977.
15. Hejyvary, S. T., and Haussmann, R. K.   *Monitoring Nursing Care Quality: Quality Control and Performance Appraisal.* Wakefield, Mass.: Contemporary Publishing, 1976.
16. Inui, T. S.   A common bond: Exploring the interface between health education and quality assurance. *Quality Review Bulletin,* 4 : 6, 1978.
17. Jencks, S. F., and Green, L. W.   Establishing a hospital-based patient education program. *Quality Review Bulletin,* 4 : 8, 1978.
18. Jessee, W. F.   Quality assurance systems: Why aren't there any? *Quality Review Bulletin,* 3 : 16, 1977.
19. Kane, R. L., et al.   Relationship between process and outcome in ambulatory care. *Medical Care,* 15 : 961, 1977.
20. Lee, E. A., and Garvey, J. L.   How is inpatient education being managed? *Nursing Digest,* 6 : 12, 1978.
21. Meyer, N. H., and Wendorf, B. H.   Analysis of incident reports and malpractice claims from a group of health care institutions. *Quality Review Bulletin,* 5 : 29, 1979.
22. Nobrega, F. T., et al.   Quality assessment in hypertension: Analysis of process and outcome methods. *New England Journal of Medicine,* 296 : 145, 1977.
23. Sax, A. B.   Patient relations in risk management. *Quality Review Bulletin,* 5 : 14, 1979.
24. Simmons, H. E., and Stolley, P. D.   This is medical progress? Trends and consequences of antibiotic use in the United States. *Journal of the American Medical Association,* 227 : 1023, 1974.
25. Somers, A. R.   Promoting health, consumer education and national policy: Part III, Summary and recommendations. *Nursing Digest,* 6 : 1, 1978.
26. Stamm, W. E.   Nosocomial infections due to medical devices. *Quality Review Bulletin,* 5 : 23, 1979.
27. Stearns, G., Imbiorski, W., and Fox, L. A.   *Solutions,* Chicago: Care Communications, 1979.
28. Thompson, R. E.   Evaluating quality isn't worth the cost . . . unless. *The Hospital Medical Staff,* 7 : 1, 1978.
29. Vaccarino, J. M.   Malpractice: The problem in perspective. *Journal of the American Medical Association,* 238 : 861, 1978.
30. Vanagunas, A.   Quality assessment: Alternate approaches. *Quality Review Bulletin,* 5 : 7, 1979.
31. Vanagunas, A., Egelston, E. M., Hopkins, J., and Walczak, R. M.   Principles of quality assurance. *Quality Review Bulletin,* 5 : 3, 1979.
32. Williamson, J. W.   Formulating priorities for quality assurance activity: Description of a method and its applications. *Journal of the American Medical Association,* 239 : 631, 1978.
33. White Paper: Patient Health Education. Blue Cross Association. August, 1974.

Resource Materials

CRITERIA TO SCREEN RECORDS OF PATIENTS WITH DIABETES MELLITUS

Validation of diagnosis:
1. At least one documented blood sugar greater than 200 milligrams percent

Admission—Justified by any of the following:
2. Poorly controlled diabetes requiring insulin or oral hypoglycemic agents
3. Diabetic acidosis
4. Insulin coma or shock
5. Severe or frequent hypoglycemic reactions
6. Hyperglycemia

Discharge status:
7. Blood sugar less than 180 milligrams percent
8. Urine acetone negative

Knowledge—Patient demonstrates ability to:
9. Correctly administer insulin or oral medication
10. Calculate diet (with proper distribution of carbohydrates, proteins, etc.)
11. Test urine for sugar and acetone
12. Care for feet and skin with specific attention to any open wound

Knowledge—Patient verbalizes knowledge of:
13. Diabetes, and how illness or change of activity can affect control
14. Signs and symptoms of hyperglycomia and hypoglycemia, and how to treat them
15. Appropriate follow-up as directed by physician

Complications—Return any patient records with evidence of:
16. Ketoacidosis
17. Hypoglycemic reactions
18. Urinary tract infection
19. Readmission within six weeks

12

Cost-Benefit and Cost-Effectiveness Analysis of Patient Education Programs

How much does patient education cost?
Is patient education worth the cost?

Cost containment is a great concern in health care today. Mention of the term causes hospital and nursing service administrators to shudder. Demands from regulatory agencies, as well as demands from a growing tide of health-care consumers, make it impossible to ignore analysis of the benefits and data on effectiveness of programs in light of their costs. Cost analyses are another form of evaluation that affect patient education programming. Intuitive guesses about cost and productivity will no longer suffice in justifying a program's existence. Accurate data will become more and more important in supporting both the benefit and economy of health care and patient teaching. The following chapter describes the overall concept of cost containment. Cost-benefit and cost-effectiveness analyses are compared and contrasted, and examples of conducting cost-analysis studies are presented.

Information in this chapter should help the reader to

1. *Describe the rationale for cost-containment requirements*
2. *List the steps for decision making when conducting cost-analysis studies*
3. *Define cost-benefit analysis*
4. *Define cost-effectiveness analysis*
5. *Describe approaches to use when evaluating alternatives in patient teaching*
6. *Apply cost-benefit and cost-effectiveness analyses to make decisions in patient teaching activities*

Patient education is recognized as an essential component of nursing practice. As early as the middle and late nineteenth century, nursing leaders in England saw the importance of teaching families about sanitation, cleanliness, and care of the sick [10]. More recently, the American Nurses' Association's statement of standards, functions, and qualifications includes teaching as a nursing function [1]. Today, the trend toward health maintenance and preventive care is making patient education even more important; however, other factors in the current national situation also make economy a prime consideration. This chapter presents a brief explanation of the need for cost containment, the theory of cost-benefit and cost-effectiveness analysis, and the use of these techniques in the evaluation of patient education programs.

NEED FOR COST CONTAINMENT

The high cost of health care has become a focus of public and political concern. Hospital costs have risen 400 percent in the last 20 years. Although all costs have been steadily rising, hospital costs have averaged greater increases than the increases in the consumer price index [5]. The cost of nursing care contributes to the cost of hospitalization, and there is evidence that nursing expenses have been increasing in both absolute and relative terms [11]. In other words, at the same time that the expenses of nursing services have been increasing in absolute dollar terms, nursing services have been growing as a component of total hospital expense.

The rising cost of health care necessitates delivering nursing care not just effectively, but economically as well. Nursing care now ranks as the highest cost in the running of a hospital [6], and nursing leaders have recognized the importance of controlling the cost of nursing care. A recurring theme at the American Nurses' Association's 1976 convention was an awareness of the need for costs to be controlled at the same time that nursing care and health services are improved [2]. Thus, it is imperative that nurses begin to evaluate nursing care in terms of cost as well as quality.

COST-ANALYSIS TECHNIQUES

Nurses who must decide which type of patient education program to implement are faced with an alternative choice problem. Anthony suggests a series of steps to follow when approaching an alternative choice problem [3].

1. Define the problem
2. Define the most likely alternative solutions
3. Measure and weigh the consequences of each alternative in either quantitative or qualitative terms
4. Make a choice among the alternatives

Although this type of analysis is usually used in business to select the course of action providing the greatest profit, such techniques may also be applied in nonprofit organizations such as hospitals. Anthony states that many alternative choice problems involve a choice between two ways of reaching the same objective [3]. The action with the lower cost is usually the better alternative in a profit-seeking company because the lower-cost action leads to higher profits. The lower-cost alternative is also usually better in nonprofit organizations because it means that the objectives can be accomplished with fewer expended resources.

Both profit-seeking and nonprofit organizations can quantify the resources invested in solving a particular problem in monetary terms. When dealing with problems that involve both inputs and outputs, however, it is extremely difficult to quantify the outputs (benefits or effects) in a nonprofit organization. In profit-seeking companies, outputs are measured by revenue, and the best alternative is the one that produces the greatest differences between differential revenue and differential costs, that is, the one that leads to the greatest profit [3]. Outputs frequently cannot be measured in monetary terms in a nonprofit organization.

Thompson and Cannon also list the following reasons hospital administrators commonly give for their failure to use cost or managerial accounting techniques [12].:

1. Cost-accounting and engineering standards cannot be applied to hospitals the same way they are applied in industry where the product is homogeneous.
2. Hospitals are complex entities with no definite unit of production for the measurement of output.
3. Because each hospital is different, there is no one system applicable to all institutions; therefore, each facility must develop its own system.
4. Hospitals are usually too small to cost-justify sophisticated information systems.

Although all of these reasons are valid to a point, formal analytical techniques *can* be used with alternative choice problems in nonprofit organizations, and hospitals must strive to improve their performance and take advantage of all available management tools, if they are to survive [3, 12].

Cost-Benefit Analysis

Anthony describes two approaches for analyzing costs and benefits in nonprofit organizations [3]. The technique described here is a combination of Anthony's approaches that the author has used and found to be workable [4]. In this approach, a careful estimate of the cost of each alternative is made, and the outputs (benefits) anticipated under each alternative are expressed in some quantitative way. An alternative is selected or rejected by deciding whether its benefits are worth the cost. For example, suppose that a woman who liked the look of antique furniture was shopping for a new desk for her home. She found that she could buy an authentic antique desk that required refinishing for $500 or a new reproduction of the same style for $300. After careful thought, the woman decided to buy the reproduction because authenticity was not worth $200 extra to her, and she thought the reproduction was more attractive and usable.

Cost-Effectiveness Analysis

Analysis of cost-effectiveness is a special, more narrow form of the cost-benefit approach, and differs in several ways. Under cost-effectiveness analysis, the enumeration of benefits need not be so complete as under the cost-benefit approach [7]. Instead, certain results are specifically selected and all other results are regarded as held constant or of secondary importance. Under cost-effectiveness analysis, costs are calculated and compared for althernative ways of accomplishing a specific set of objectives. When an objective or output is specified, the aim is to minimize the cost of attaining it. For example, a businessman must attend a meeting in another city at 8 A.M. the following morning and finds that he can choose between the following modes of transportation:

Type of Transportation	Cost in Dollars	Arrival Time
Bus	10	8:15 A.M.
Rental car	15	7:30 A.M.
Plane	25	7:30 A.M.

Cost-effectiveness analysis would lead him to select the rental car because this alternative minimizes the cost of attaining his objective. In this example, the result selected for analysis was arrival time at a destination, and other results, such as length of travel time and passenger comfort were considered to be of secondary importance.

Klarman indicates that cost-effectiveness, rather than cost-benefit, is used when various benefits are difficult to measure or when they cannot be rendered commensurate [8]. The cost data necessary for cost-effectiveness analysis are, however, the same as for cost-benefit.

Basically, when using the cost-effectiveness approach, the decision-maker sets standards for a given objective or set of objectives, specifying the level of achievement required. Alternative actions are then investigated. The action with the lowest cost that meets the predetermined standard is selected as the best alternative.

When using cost-benefit analysis, the decision-maker does not start out with predetermined outcome standards. Instead, the costs and benefits of each alternative are determined and expressed as a ratio of costs to benefits. The cost-benefit ratios provide the decision-maker with information about the costs of obtaining different results. Thus, cost-benefit analysis does not identify the cheapest alternative. Instead, it provides the decision-maker with information about various results that can be obtained for different costs, and the decision-maker uses this information to select an alternative.

As indicated earlier, cost-effectiveness analysis requires the establishment of outcome standards. Nurses are currently developing outcome criteria for patients with different diagnoses for purposes of quality assurance. Cost-effectiveness analysis should become an increasingly useful technique for making decisions about nursing actions as patient outcomes are more clearly defined.

APPROACHES TO EVALUATING ALTERNATIVES IN PATIENT TEACHING

To use cost-benefit or cost-effectiveness analysis to evaluate and compare alternative approaches to patient education, the nurse must objectively measure both the costs and the results of each type of program being considered. The same methods for measuring costs and results are applicable to both types of analysis.

The first step in cost analysis is to identify all of the factors that contribute to the total cost per patient of the program. The following cost factors are frequently associated with patient teaching:

1. Personnel costs: The cost of paying hospital personnel for the time spent implementing a patient education program
2. Equipment costs: The cost of acquisition and depreciation of audiovisual or other equipment used to present a patient education program
3. Material costs: The cost of preparing printed material for a patient education program
4. Facility costs: The cost of using a classroom (heating, lighting, and housekeeping) for a patient education program

Each of these cost factors can be measured as follows.

1. Personnel costs: Monitor the amount of time needed to implement the program. For example, how long does it take a nurse to teach a patient to cough, turn, and deep breathe? How long does it take a patient escort to transport a patient to and from a class? An average time figure should be determined for each patient teaching activity. This figure is multiplied times the employee's hourly wage or the average hourly wage for that category of personnel. If the employee provides a service to a group of patients at the same time (for example, a nurse teaching a group of patients to perform deep breathing exercises), the cost of the employee's time is divided by the number of class members to obtain a cost-per-patient figure.
2. Equipment costs: Monitor the amount of machine time needed to present the program once. Obtain information concerning anticipated hours of performance from the manufacturer (how many hours can the machine be expected to run before it wears out). Divide the purchase cost of the machine by the number of hours of expected performance to obtain a cost-per-hour-of-use figure. Multiply this figure by the fraction of one hour needed to present the program once. Once again, this equipment depreciation figure

should be divided by the number of patients in a group teaching class to obtain a cost-per-patient figure. To calculate the depreciation cost for a slide program or a film, find out from the manufacturer how many times the program may be shown without serious loss of quality. Divide the purchase price of the program by this figure to determine the depreciation cost of each presentation. If the program was developed by the institution, rather than purchased, the cost of preparation time may be included. Divide by the number of class members if applicable. Machine depreciation can be combined as a total equipment depreciation cost figure per patient.

3. Material costs: Determine the cost of preparing one pamphlet by dividing the purchase or printing cost by the number of pamphlets purchased. As in the case of slides and films, preparation cost may be included if the pamphlet was developed by the institution.

4. Facility costs: If presentation of the program does not require additional heating, lighting, and housekeeping in the classroom, this cost factor is not applicable; however, if a special room is built or reserved for patient education, this cost should be considered, especially if space shortage is a problem within the facility. One way to determine this cost is to find out how much the facility charges parties who rent space in the building and use this figure to calculate the cost per patient of utilizing the classroom to present the program once.

These are only guidelines for calculating program costs. Each institutional program is unique, and individual situations differ widely. The important thing is to obtain an accurate total cost per patient by identifying each applicable cost factor, determining the actual cost per patient for each factor, and including all of the costs in the total.

Measurement of the results (benefits or effects) of patient teaching is directly related to the objectives of the program, that is, to desirable patient outcomes. It is very important to measure the results of the teaching in a way that will provide objective information, preferably numerical, rather than impressions and opinions. Although qualitative information such as how participants react to a program can be helpful and may lead to the development of new measurement systems, the use of cost-benefit and cost-effectiveness analysis requires quantitative, or numerical, measurement of results.

The following list of suggested approaches to evaluating patient teaching demonstrates how objective information about results can be obtained:

1. Patient visits: Observe patient's return demonstrations and listen to the patient verbalize knowledge of self-care. Develop a tool to rate the adequacy of the patient's response in numerical terms (for example, a score of 80 percent).

2. Paper and pencil tests: Develop and administer a written test to evaluate the patient's knowledge of self-care.

3. Nursing documentation: Review nursing documentation for indications that the patient can demonstrate self-care and verbalize pertinent information.

Score on the basis of the percentage of charts containing such documentation. Information obtained from a primary source such as the patient is preferable, however, to information obtained from the medical record, a secondary source.

4. Physical indicators: Measure patient's vital capacities, temperatures, and the like.
5. Length of stay: Monitor the length of patient's hospital stay.
6. Readmission: Monitor readmissions with related problems (for example, ketoacidosis or wound infection).

To summarize, a method must be developed to measure whatever effect the program is designed to produce. The information obtained should answer the question, "To what degree are the objectives of the program being met?"

The following hypothetical examples illustrate how cost-benefit and cost-effectiveness analysis could be used to make decisions about nursing actions. Let's say that a Director of Nursing is concerned because nursing audit has revealed a deficiency in the area of teaching ostomy patients self-care. The Director decides that there are two alternative approaches to correcting this deficiency: hire a nurse clinician to teach ostomy patients, or inform the nursing staff of the deficiency and enlist their help in correcting it. The Director believes that each nurse should teach his or her own patients, but she must correct the deficiency and thinks that hiring a clinician would ensure that the patients would be taught because accountability would be more clearly defined. The Director decides to use cost-benefit analysis to obtain the information needed to make the decision.

The Director selects one nurse who is interested in and knowledgeable about the care of patients who have ostomies. This nurse teaches half of the new ostomy patients self-care for the next three months while the remaining half are cared for by the nursing staff. The Director evaluates the results of each program in terms of direct measurement of patients' ability to perform self-care and verbalize pertinent knowledge, nursing documentation concerning teaching activities and patients' response, and staff nurse job satisfaction.

The only cost involved is the cost of the nurses' time. The nurse chosen to function as the clinician is at the midpoint of the staff nurse salary scale, which is $7 per hour, and the hospital has an equal distribution of short- and long-term employees. Thus, the average hourly wage figure is the same for both programs, and the pilot study revealed that both the staff nurses and the clinician spent a total of two hours teaching a new ostomy patient self-care.

The Director used the information she obtained from the pilot study to produce the cost-benefit ratios illustrated in Table 5. These results led the Director of Nursing to decide to make the staff nurses responsible for teaching their own ostomy patients for the next three months. At that time, the staff nurses' documentation would be reviewed again, and they could continue to do their own patient teaching if their documentation reached 90 percent. The Director chose this approach because the cost-benefit analysis revealed that for the same cost the two programs produced equally good patient outcomes, and

Table 5.

Type of Program	Cost	Benefits		
		Patients' ability to perform self-care	Documentation	Staff nurse job satisfaction
Nurse Clinician	$14	90%	100%	20%
Staff Nurse	$14	90%	50%	95%

the staff nurses derived more job satisfaction from doing their own teaching. In addition, the Director thought that the staff nurse program allowed for better utilization of personnel. Several times during the pilot study there were no new ostomy patients in the hospital. At these times the staff nurses were still productive because they had flexible job responsibilities, but the clinician was not. The Director plans to use the results of the analysis to motivate the staff nurses to improve their documentation.

The next example illustrates the application of cost-effectiveness analysis. A group of nurses is concerned by the discovery that 50 percent of their postoperative patients develop respiratory infections. They want to develop and implement a group preoperative teaching program, but they cannot decide whether they should present a live program, an audiovisual program, or a program combining both approaches. The nurses decide that they want to reduce the incidence of postoperative respiratory infections to 25 percent. An evaluation of the costs and effects of each program reveals the information illustrated in Table 6. The nurses select the live program because it meets their predetemined standard. If the nurses had utilized cost-benefit analysis, they might have chosen the combination program because it offers more "benefit" at little extra cost.

Although differences between costs and results of programs sometimes seem insignificant, the impact of small differences can be tremendous. It can be very enlightening to relate the findings of an analysis to the cost of providing patient teaching projected over several years. For example, it would cost the institution in the preceding example $10,750 to provide the combination preoperative teaching program for 1000 patients per year for five years, whereas the live or the audiovisual program could be presented to the same number of patients for $10,000 and $5000 respectively. An extension of the projection to results of the programs indicates that the institution, in choosing to provide the combination program to 5000 patients at a cost of $10,750, could expect 750 of these patients (15 percent) to develop postoperative respiratory complications. The institution, in choosing to provide the live program to the same number of patients at a cost of $10,000, could expect 1250 of the patients (25 percent) would develop postoperative respiratory complications. Finally, if the institution chose to present the audiovisual program to the same number of patients at a cost of $5000, it could expect 1500 of the patients (30 percent) to develop postoperative respiratory infections. The decision would depend upon the

Table 6.

Type of Program	Cost Per Patient	Infection Rate
Live	$2.00	25%
Audiovisual	$1.00	30%
Combination	$2.15	15%

institution's objectives and the resources available for attainment of these objectives.

It is desirable to compare differences among the results of alternative educational approaches for statistical significance using appropriate types of statistical analysis. Statistical significance indicates that the differences were due to the education programs, rather than to chance. It is not necessary, however, to analyze differences in cost for statistical significance. The significance of money is dictated by such factors as the availability of resources and the goals of an institution. Therefore, the importance of the differences in cost depends upon the supply of money, nurses, transporters, facilities, and equipment accessible to the decision-maker and upon what an organization wants to accomplish.

Nichols believes that a natural outcome of public dissatisfaction and nationwide demands for changes in health care is that each profession faces the need to establish values in terms of quality care, availability of care, and cost of care [9]. Thus, nursing is charged with the responsibility for controlling the cost of nursing care and, therefore, must develop methods of delivering nursing care that are both effective and economical. Intuitive estimates of the costs and effects of alternative methods of providing patient education are inadequate. The price of nursing care today mandates careful investigation of contributory costs and results that can be obtained, and cost-benefit and cost-effectiveness analysis are two techniques that can provide the information nurses need to arrive at and justify sound decisions about patient care.

REFERENCES

1. American Nurses' Association. *Functions, Standards, and Qualifications for Practice* (rev. ed.). New York: The Association, 1973.
2. *American Nurses' Association's Convention News.* 6, June 8, 1976.
3. Anthony, R. *Management Accounting Principles.* Homewood, Ill.: Richard D. Irvin, 1970.
4. Crabtree, M. A cost-benefit analysis of individual and group preoperative teaching. Master's thesis, University of Illinois, 1977.
5. Feldstein, M., Moore, F., and Warren, R. The high cost of hospital care—A seminar. *Archives of Surgery,* 105 : 962, 1972.
6. Gallagher, G. Let's have better nurse deployment. *Nursing '76,* 6 : 64D, 1976.
7. Klarman, H., Francis, J., and Rosenthal, G. Cost-effectiveness analysis applied to the treatment of chronic renal disease. *Medical Care,* 6 : 48, 1986.
8. Klarman, H. Application of Cost-benefit Analysis to Health Systems Technology. In M. Collen (Ed.), *Technology and Health Care Systems in the 1980s.* Washington, D.C.: Department of Health, Education, and Welfare (Publ. NSM 73 – 3016), 1972.

9. Nichols, M.   Quality control in patient care. *American Journal of Nursing,* 74 : 456, 1974.
10. Redman, B. K.   *Process of Patient Teaching in Nursing* (2nd ed.). St. Louis: Mosby, 1972, P. 1.
11. The Increase in Nursing Expenses. *Hospitals,* 43 : 28, 1969.
12. Thompson, G., and Cannon, W.   Hospitals, like industry, must apply cost-accounting techniques. *Hospitals,* 52 : 129, June 16, 1978.

Financing Patient Education
free? fee? funded?

How can we pay for patient teaching activities?
Will third party reimbursement cover the costs of patient teaching?

Patient education programming costs have traditionally been reimbursed through the daily room rate charges in hospitals. Thus, patients pay for services based on whether they are in a private or semiprivate room and not on the basis of the amount of service (including health-related teaching) they receive. Now a trend is developing in which fees for the actual amount of service delivered to the patient are being computed. Patient teaching does take time, and this time costs money in terms of wages, salaries, and benefits. Material costs (including handouts, media, and equipment) and overhead expenses (electricity, heat, and space) need to be recovered through some form of reimbursement. The following chapter describes several methods for paying the expenses of patient teaching. External funding sources are described, and some strategies that might be useful in receiving funding are described. Information is presented that may be useful in developing a proposal for external funding.
  Information in this chapter should help the reader to

1. *Compare and contrast three methods for financing formal patient education programs*
2. *Describe strategies for receiving external funding for patient education activities*
3. *Develop a proposal to seek funds to pay for formal patient education programs*

One of the important areas to be considered in a formal program of patient education is finance. Health professionals have been informally imparting necessary health information to those in their care for years. Much of this was and is carried out at the bedside, treatment area, or wherever the need arose. However, formal programs of patient education with objectives, content, materials, evaluation, and follow-up necessitate a person or persons to develop, coordinate, and evaluate this facet of health care for hospital consumers. This kind of program involves nonpatient contact and a commitment on the part of the institution to support patient education morally, verbally, and financially. This commitment is expressed through the administrative backing of a hospital-wide philosophy and policy on consumer health education and the financial backing of the department designated for this task [5].

FREE

One traditional way for hospitals to finance formal patient education programs is through the allowable room rate. In May 1974, the American Hospital Association issued a statement on health education roles and responsibilities for health-care institutions. "Financial responsibilities for health education that is integral to the treatment and care of the patient is a legitimate part of the cost of caring for the patient" [1]. The disadvantages of allocating health education as part of the room rate are as follows:

First, all the patients pay for the health education of a few. If there are 40 patients on a unit and five are diabetic and are receiving more involved patient education, all 40 may be paying for the education of a few. A financial base for health education should allocate the responsibility for the development and implementation for an in-hospital patient education program on a broader basis. Weinberger observed that "Health Education is everyone's concern and no one's responsibility" [14]. A financial base that includes a Department for Consumer Health Education attempts to take that responsibility.

Second, nurses and other health professionals do not usually become involved with the cost of health care. Administrators and business office decision-makers do not usually get involved in patient care. This lack of knowledge and communication makes it difficult for health professionals to improve and expand patient education by way of materials and personnel. Without a definite cost basis the import of patient education is lost on nonpatient-care hospital officials. Materials are not developed or ordered, evaluation of teaching is not carried out, and the general importance of health education is misunderstood. There are some health-care facilities that have made the decision to provide health education as a service to the patient and to the community. The American Hospital Association states, "Health Education that is designed to maintain the good health to the community at large and to prevent illness should be viewed as a service to the community" [1]. In many institutions, the staff providing the program planning or teaching is given released time or time back for hours spent beyond the general work shift. However, problems arise when the patient census picks up and the 'time back' becomes lost in the work load.

One health education director has developed a way of offering job enrichment opportunities to nurses in order to have a health education program [9]. After the program topic has been established by a multidisciplinary health education committee, a job description is written for the person teaching in that particular program. Then a short-term, part-time position is advertised designating the number of hours and the subject of the program. The person chosen for the short-term project develops the program content, materials, and evaluation procedure, and implements the program [8, 16].

The third and perhaps biggest disadvantages of hiding patient education in the room rate is that the patient does not see it. For years, industries that sell a product to the public have pursued high visibility tactics to present their product. Consumer health education programs need to present their product—a healthier lifestyle—in the most attractive and noticeable way possible. Just as commercial products advertise their price, so patient education programs should say, "This is what you get for what you pay, and it's worth it!" Most human beings today will adhere to a care regimen if they know they must pay for it.

FEE

There are advantages to a direct charge for health education of patients. First of all, when a direct fee is charged, the program tends to be very visable and is more apt to be planned formally and allocated to a responsible department. This allows for the collection of follow-up data that can demonstrate the effectiveness of education on increased health maintenance of the patient. Second, the patient realizes he is paying to receive information regarding his present level of health, the diagnostic and therapeutic interventions ordered, and the health information and habits needed to maintain his health at home. This dollar exchange tends to make the patient more attentive to the information provided. One hospital offers a five-day course for the diabetic and family, as well as for other health professionals. [7]. Sometimes the fee for the week is reimbursable and sometimes not. Consumers of the program fit that educational week into their life through vacation or time off work, juggling family, job, or school activities, because they realize the importance of this health education to their health. Another hospital offers consumer health classes in diabetes, hypertension, weight control, and smoking on a fee basis. The fee is based on the instructor's class time and materials with a number set for minimum and maximum group participation. The average consumer in these courses is usually more motivated and interested in changing unhealthy habits than the participants in a free monthly health series open to hospital patients, visitors, staff, and community at the same hospital. Still another hospital offers health education programs to the consumer and designates the content and corresponding fee. The patient has a choice of whether to accept the program. When the patient knows what is being offered and the benefits to him or her, few refuse the program even though it is explained that the insurance company may or may not reimburse the cost of the program. [8].

FUNDED

Throughout the 1970s much rhetoric expounded the need for consumer health education in order to increase and maintain a healthier lifestyle. In 1972 the President's Commission on Health Education recognized the need for third party reimbursement for health education as part of the basic service charge [12]. Today this direct patient charge may or may not be reimbursed by third party payers. The White Paper on Health Education developed by Blue Cross in 1974 has been used by some to indicate that company's support of health education. In fact, Blue Cross has not always provided direct reimbursement for patient education [2]. Reimbursement policy seems to be made as a state by state decision by the policy makers of the particular Blue Cross State Insurance headquarters. Welch reviews and explains the system of health care financing in our country and encourages nurses to become more active in influencing the development of a comprehensive health-care system[15]. Some guidelines for presenting such a proposal might include:

1. Put your institution's policy, philosophy, and plan in writing and know who is supporting the program.* [10].

2. Find out whom to talk to at the state headquarters of whatever insurance agency your institution deals with. (Your facility's business or patient accounts director should be able to tell you who this would be.) Nordberg and King have related their particular method for obtaining third party reimbursement for at least two formal patient education programs [6]. Some areas like Minnesota and Maryland have Blue Cross Associations that are reimbursing inhouse patient health education programs [6, 8]. Many state Blue Cross Associations are not, however, but will discuss the possibility.

3. Make an appointment with the insurance agency's state-level Special Project Director. Health-care facilities are very dependent upon third-party insurers and it is necessary for health education professionals to be cognizant of insurance terminology and language. Kirchner, in *Medical Economics,* endeavors to explain this complicated language to health professionals [4]. Brief your business office representative on your program if he or she is not familiar with it. A representative from the administration would be helpful, especially the Vice President of Nursing.

4. Present your program, including objectives, content, evaluation, and follow-up, to the insurance agency official. Show what your actual cost would be, what the charges will be, and how it will be coded. It should be coded one way if it is prescribed by a physician or is part of the patient's diagnostic treatment procedure, and in another way if it is patient or family requested. Some third-party reimbursement systems are mostly dependent upon the physician's order: no order, no reimbursement. The American Nurse's Associa-

*Ideas on planning for health education programs can be gleaned from other chapters in this book and from *A Model for Planning Patient Education: The Report of the Commission on Education Tasks and Chronic Illness,* Public Health Education series, American Public Health Association; The American Hospital Association, The Center for Health Promotion, Chicago; and S. Pritchett, *A Workbook on Patient and Family Community Health Education,* Atlanta: Pritchett-Hull Associates.

tion is working to change this, but currently most hospitals are still dependent upon the physician order for third-party reimbursement [13]. This does give the third-party insurer a responsible person for determining all reimbursable therapy. It also has a tendency to down-grade the consumer's part in making decisions for his or her own health care, and it *is*, after all, the consumer who pays the premiums and who makes the daily, at home, lifestyle decisions about his or her health.

5. Once you have met with one company, go on to the next. Some states have insurance companies that have patient education included in their coverage. If yours does not, write, call, or visit the person in charge of company policy, state your case, and ask him or her to consider reviewing the present policy.

6: Private, state, and federal grants can also provide funding possibilities. Investigate your local civic and community organizations that might be interested in promoting health education. Address your letter to the organization's president or project director, stating your goal and general terms. If they are interested, pursue this goal in a personal interview. Take to the interview a written statement of your institution's backing, the health program objectives, content, evaluation, follow-up, and expected cost. Be ready to bargain. Know what are your priorities: do you need funding for audiovisual materials, handouts, or instructors' time? Could you use volunteer help from the organization? If the organization sponsors your program, use *every* available means to publicize their involvement. The hospital auxiliary can be one great area of support for health education. It can provide funds, equipment, and volunteers for the health education program. The advantages of an auxiliary funded project are many. The people involved are from the local area and do much to aid in the marketing of health education to friends and relatives. They also represent many volunteer-hours that reduce health care costs.

Other sources for health education are just beginning to open up. The state university closest to you should have an area designated for the government publications and document holdings. Public Law 94-317 amends the Public Health Service Act to include health education and may be of benefit in the research of your particular project [3]. This area of the state university library should also hold copies of the Federal Register and Government Publication Listings which give possible funding sources. The Center for Health Promotion of the American Hospital Association may also provide you with resources in your particular area. The innovative program that came from the College of Medicine and Dentistry of New Jersey might serve as a model for consumer health education for your area [13].

No longer can we have patient education without accountability. Patient education that achieves certain behavior changes must show more effective use of health-care systems and a corresponding reduction in health-care cost. The literature shows that health education for consumers has reduced the cost of health care. However, we need more data on the cost of comprehensive hospital health education and third party participation in this effort. [11]. Health education for patients, family, and the community has always been a concern of nursing. However, if we truly believe the path to a healthy lifestyle includes consumer health education, we must develop and present valid programs that fall within a responsible cost for both the consumer and the provider.

REFERENCES

1. American Hospital Association. *Statement on Health Education, Role and Responsibility of Health Care Institutions.* Chicago: The Association, 1975.
2. Blue Cross Association.   White Paper: Patient Health Education. Chicago: The Association, 1974.
3. Health Information and Health Promotion Act. Public Law 94-317. 94th Congress, S. 1466, Washington, D.C.: Government Publications, 1976.
4. Kirchner, M.   The real world of hospital finance. *Medical Economics,* 55 : 219, 1978.
5. McNerney, W. J.   The missing link in health services. *Journal of Medical Education* 50 : 11, 1975.
6. Nordberg, B., and King, L.   Third party payment for patient education. *American Journal of Nursing,* 76 : 1269, 1976.
7. Personal communication with Diabetes Education Center, Minneapolis, May 1979.
8. Personal communication with Peggy Martinson, R.N., B.S.N., Core Patient Education Instructor, Methodist Hospital, Minneapolis, Jan. 1979.
9. Personal communication with Mary Woodrow, R.N., M.S.N. El Camino Hospital, Mountain View Calif., July 1979.
10. Public Health Association. *A Model for Planning Patient Education.* Washington, D.C.: Government Printing Office, 1972.
11. Simonds, S. K.   Hospital patient counseling: Problems, priorities and prospects. *Health Values,* 1 : 41, 1977.
12. Simonds, S. K.   President's commission on health education. *Hospitals,* 47 : 54, 1973.
13. Somers, A.   Consumer health education: To know or to die. *Hospitals,* 50 : 52, 1976.
14. Weinberger, C. W.   The role of the federal government in educating the public about health. *Journal of Medical Education,* 50 : 138, 1975.
15. Welch, C. A.   Health care distribution and third party payment for nurses' service. *American Journal of Nursing,* 75 : 1844, 1975.
16. Woodrow, M.   Cost-consciousness prompts three-phase education service. *Hospitals,* 53(9) : 98, 1979.

David J. Kinsey
Ronald K. Schaffner

14

Media in Patient Education

What is the role of educational media in patient teaching programs?
Can media replace the busy instructor in patient teaching?
What are the advantages and limitations of various media formats?

Television sets, as well as other mediated instruction formats, proliferate in educational settings today, enhancing educational outcomes, and at times replacing the live classroom instructor. Research has shown mediated instruction to be effective in achieving learning outcomes, but much of this research has been done on healthy subjects. A prior chapter has already pointed out that when the learner is a patient, learning ability may be altered. Therefore, media may not be as effective in producing patient learning outcomes if used without a live instructor to provide emotional support. The following chapter describes the reasons why media help to improve learning outcomes. A variety of media tools are described, and information is provided about how these tools are chosen, how they are applied, and how the outcomes of their use are evaluated.
   Information presented in this chapter should help the reader to

1. List five factors inherent in media that enhance patient education outcomes
2. Describe various media tools that can be used to meet patient educational needs
3. Describe how media fit in as part of the instructional design process
4. List various formats of instructional media that are used in conjunction with "live" patient education
5. Describe a means of indicating the level of instructional effectiveness of media in patient education

Patient education through media can be defined as the organized use of materials other than direct lecture to achieve predetermined patient learning goals. Within the framework of such a definition, which covers printed and classroom-oriented materials as well as audio or visual media, it may safely be asserted that no patient education program can be fully effective without a mediated instruction component.

RATIONALE

The remarkable effectiveness of media materials properly integrated into a patient education program results from the interaction of several factors.

Variety.   Repetition, a fundamental technique for reinforcing learning, becomes counterproductive when associated with boredom. By permitting the patient to receive the same message in more than one way, media permits reemphasis without demotivation.

Multisensory Appeal.   The old adage "a picture is worth a thousand words" has been shown by twentieth-century educational researchers to fall far short of the full truth, for it says nothing at all about the combined effect of picture *and* words presented simultaneously. Experiences that appeal to more than one of the five senses are not only more interesting to the patient but also produce several times the retention rate of materials that are simply read or heard. If images and words can be supplemented by touch (as with models and realia), sense of position (practicing skills), or response (asking and answering questions), both knowledge and attitude change are further enhanced.

Logistics.   Mediated instruction can accommodate a very large volume of instruction and do so with fewer scheduling concerns. Instructional materials can deliver experiences that would otherwise be impossible at a time and place that fit the individual patient's schedule and needs and do not disrupt staff schedules. By allowing patients and families to learn at the most opportune times, without requiring the presence of an expert lecturer or patient education coordinator, costs can be held far lower than for a comparable volume of one-to-one instruction.

Quality.   The quality of the instructional experience is enhanced in various ways besides the synergistic effect of multisensory reinforcement. A mediated instructional program does not suffer from migraine or forgetfulness, but always presents the same content in the same sequence. Mediated instruction can be prevalidated and does not depend on the varying teaching capabilities of the many health-care personnel who may be involved with teaching activities. In some cases where visualization of the information is an important factor, forms of mediated instruction that include a visual channel are obviously superior. Furthermore, one can usually assume that more thought, planning, and consultation have gone into the production of a mediated program than the preparation of a lecture or personal patient visit.

Relationship to Instructor. None of these advantages in any way devalues personal contact, interaction, and flexibility. We stated at the outset that fully effective patient education cannot be achieved without mediated instruction. Since personal instruction and the use of media reinforce each other, the corollary statement is that fully effective use of instructional media cannot be achieved without a personal contact component.

CHOOSING TOOLS

Patient education needs have been described elsewhere in this book, and a variety of media tools to meet these needs will be discussed in this chapter. How these tools are chosen, how they are applied, and how the outcomes of their use are evaluated is what this chapter is all about.

What should already be quite clear is that if the media are tools of a program of patient education, they cannot be the program itself. Education is a human activity and cannot be reduced to a conglomeration of indiscriminately dispensed, rigidly applied systems of audiovisual hardware and software. Mediated instructional units can convey information, but they cannot conduct assessments of patient need, cannot evaluate, cannot determine an appropriate teaching strategy, and have no sensitivity to differing emotional needs of patients and their families.

If this aspect of the use of the media in a program of patient education seems overemphasized, it is because the media are often put in place as a substitute for a more comprehensive program, and this is certainly not in the interest of the hospital or the patient. The use of instructional media is appropriate when it is applied as a part of the instructional design process but not in lieu of it.

Once overall program goals and more specific instructional objectives have been decided, the process of format selection can begin. For the purpose of this discussion, a media tool is defined as any aural or visual communication used as a part of an organized teaching activity with designated leaders and formalized goals and objectives. These tools range from the very simple to the very complex and include materials that are presented to the patient in a variety of forms or, to use a term most often used in reference to the form of nonprint materials, *formats.* In this discussion, all forms of instructional communication tools, with the exception of personal communication, whether print or nonprint, will be termed formats.

Instructional media in some formats are designed to be used by the live teacher as an adjunct to personal communication. These include drawings, graphs, overhead transparencies, flip charts, models, and real objects that are sometimes termed *realia.* Other instructional media are designed for more passive applications and include posters and displays. Perhaps the most important classification of instructional media is the group of materials that are designed for "stand-alone" utilization. That is, they do not need continuous instructor intervention. This classification includes audiocassette tapes, films, slide/audiotape programs, videotapes, and sometimes other media or media mixes.

A knowledge of the many available audiovisual formats and their suitability to various institutional settings is prerequisite. This information can be acquired in several ways. If the hospital is large enough to have a staff media specialist, he or she can offer assistance or arrange for some training sessions. Perhaps an opportunity to work alongside the media specialist until the needed skills are acquired can be arranged. There are numerous other opportunities, however, to learn media selection skills. Inquire at colleges, universities, and vocational schools about media courses. A surprising number of media-related courses are available even in many rural areas. Workshops are another source of information that are often professionally specific and transmit a great deal of information in a very short time. The American Hospital Association, The National Medical Audiovisual Center, and Knowledge Industry Publications are among several dozen organizations that offer workshops in a variety of media-related areas. Books and professional periodicals are another excellent source of information on media selection and utilization. University media professionals can provide information on currently available media publications suitable for the neophyte. The American Hospital Association's videocassette, *Selecting Media for Patient Education,* is a brief but useful treatment of the subject.

Once goals and objectives have been set, a search for appropriate formats can begin. The prospective user will discover an abundance of excellent patient education software, but he or she will also discover that there is very little format consistency. Some material is available on overhead transparencies, some on filmstrips with accompanying cassette tapes, some on videocassettes, some on reels of 16mm motion picture film, some on 8mm motion picture film cartridges (some of these have sound and some do not), some as slide sets, some on slide sets with an accompanying LP record or cassette tape, and some as hybrids that combine formats (such as the LaBelle Audiscan Cartridge which uses 16mm film as a still filmstrip and also carries a magnetic sound tape in the same plastic shell). Obviously the hospital media user must make some preliminary decisions about *hardware* before approaching the task of *software* selection.

Again, the advice of other media users, college or vocational school course-work, workshops, and books will be of value in making informed decisions about hardware purchases. There are several common-sense considerations, however, that can help you make a decision even if you cannot attend a class or a workshop. Is the hardware item easy to operate? Will it be used with a single patient or with a group of patients? Are there special environmental considerations such as darkening the room? Will the sound of the machine or the program soundtrack disturb others nearby? Will equipment maintenance be a problem? Is sufficient software available in that particular format? Can the hospital afford a sufficient number of the particular hardware item? Can the equipment accommodate software that can be made within the hospital? Do patient education goals and objectives require more than one format (for example, to accommodate both individual and large group instruction)? These are all important questions that must be answered before hardware purchases are made.

With all the foregoing considerations in mind, let us examine some popular formats and the hardware and software that pertain to each.

Personal Instruction Aids

A number of different types of media are useful as aids to personal instruction. Flip charts, diagrams, and illustrations are among the class of graphic materials that require no equipment for presentation. When these are professionally prepared and properly protected so that they do not become dog-eared in everyday use, they are often remarkably effective as clarifiers and reinforcers. Overhead transparencies are a slightly more sophisticated graphic presentational method that is particularly useful when layers of transparencies, *overlays*, can be used to describe a progression or a change. An overhead transparency projector is required for showing the transparency films, and the method is perhaps better suited to classroom use than to use in patient rooms, where lack of a proper screen and crowded conditions can provide some limitations.

Availability of prepared graphic instructional aids is very limited; most require local production. Although the materials used in production of these items are often inexpensive, labor costs for quality illustration can be quite high.

Also in this group are realia (real objects) and models. These often neglected materials can provide a realistic, three dimensional experience at relatively low cost.

The effectiveness of all of the media in this classification is highly dependent on teacher skill. None require complicated hardware to use and most require no hardware at all.

Audiotape

Audiotape is, of course, a sound-only format. Audiotape on reels is useful to the patient educator only as a means of recording originals, or as they are sometimes called, masters. It can be easily edited with a simple splicing block, single-edge razor blade and special splicing tape, to remove mistakes or unwanted material. Audiotape on reels is too cumbersome to use as a distribution medium in patient education, but audiotape packaged into cassettes is excellent. They are inexpensive, available in many lengths, easy to use, and universally familiar. The required hardware is likewise inexpensive and simple to operate.

There is little prepared audiocassette software available for patient education. Perhaps for this reason there is not much use of the audiocassette by itself in patient education applications. But the tapes are so easy to make and to use, and so inexpensive, that this medium should not be overlooked as the hospital builds its media arsenal. Combining the audiocassette with printed diagrams and illustrations is another possibility that is often overlooked. With a cassette duplicating machine that can be purchased in the $500 to $1500 range, good quality cassette copies are quickly and easily produced.

Audiocassettes are especially suitable for outpatient teaching because of their portability and low cost. Since almost everyone has a cassette player at home, or can borrow one, take-home instructions about aftercare are an obvious use for audiocassettes and are perhaps more likely to be used than printed materials.

35mm Slides

Although 35mm slides (also called 2-by-2 slides) are occasionally used by themselves as adjuncts to classroom lectures, a more frequent patient education application is the use of 35mm slides that are used in synchrony with an audiocassette soundtrack. Sometimes the slides must be changed manually in response to audible cues from the soundtrack. Commonly, the slide projector is connected to a special audiocassette player, which uses inaudible pulses recorded on one track of the cassette tape to automatically advance the slides. Today, most of these automatic slide/cassette tape systems conform to specifications of the American National Standards Institute (ANSI) and are compatible with one another.

The slide/cassette format offers several attractive advantages. There is considerable prepared software available in this format, the software is relatively inexpensive, equipment to play the programs is available both for individual and group applications, and the equipment is fairly easy to operate and not too expensive. Except for the lack of ability to display motion, the slide/cassette tape offers many advantages including simplicity, versatility, ease of editing and up-dating, and low cost. For many institutions, inhouse production capability is a very important advantage of this format. A basic slide/audiocassette production set-up consists of a single lens reflex camera with macro lens, copystand and lights, a reel-to-reel audio recorder and microphone, a cassette recorder and perhaps a cassette tape duplicator. Although the needed equipment can be acquired in the $3000 to $5000 range, the cost of artwork and script development must also be considered.

Filmstrips

Filmstrips with audiocassettes provide the same visual and audio effect as slide/audiocassette programs. Software availability is excellent. However, the need for manual threading, framing, synchronizing, and storing makes this format more difficult to use. Inhouse production and updating are also impractical.

These drawbacks may lead to the choice of a less complicated and more flexible format. Programs already owned, or available only in filmstrip, may be converted to slide/audiocassette format by mounting the frames separately and re-pulsing the audiocassette.

Motion Pictures

Motion picture films on reels, usually 16mm films, are perhaps best suited for group instructional applications. Although software availability is quite good, use in patient rooms is usually unsatisfactory. Projectors are often somewhat noisy, and unattended operation is probably not a good idea. For group instruction in a classroom, however, 16mm films offer a large picture, adequate sound, and the very important advantage of the capability to display movement.

Super-8mm films offer most of the advantages of the 16mm format, except that their smaller size permits packaging in easy-to-use cartridges. These are usually of the endless loop type, and the beginning of the film is found by playing the film clear through to the end, since no rewinding is possible with this arrangement. Since these cartridges are usually designed for use in table-top rear screen projectors, they are suited for individual and very small group instruction, but are not suitable for large groups. Software availability is limited, the cartridges vary from manufacturer to manufacturer, and the cartridges are not interchangeable. All software titles are not available in all packaging formats, so careful examination of software availability in the area of interest is recommended before any purchase is made.

Neither the 16mm or Super-8mm film formats lend themselves to local software production and consequently most users will be entirely dependent on the availability of prepared software.

Videotape

Several volumes would be required for a totally comprehensive examination of the potential uses of videotape in connection with patient education. Since videotape encompasses nearly all the capabilities of the other media and since it is such a versatile format for local production, this format deserves the special consideration of the patient education designer.

As a playback-only medium, videotape can be used in a variety of ways. A portable cart with videotape player and small monitor is easily used in a patient room. A videotape player with a large-screen monitor can easily accommodate groups of up to a dozen learners. When used with one of the newer large-screen television projectors, adequate visibility can be achieved in a small auditorium. For the hospital with a master antenna system to distribute local television channels to patient rooms, the addition of tape players, switching equipment, monitors, and modulating equipment can achieve the distribution of patient education programming throughout the hospital for reception on any patient room television set.

In the latter configuration, a number of hospitals are distributing two distinct varieties of programming on their inhouse systems. *General health education programming,* mainly prevention-oriented and viewable at the patient's option, is a currently popular activity of many hospital patient education programs. Frequently, this programming is also shown on television sets in hospital lobbies and other waiting areas for viewing by visitors to the hospital. A second programming mode is often referred to as *specific medical instruction* or *prescription television* and refers to programming ordered by a physician or another teaching health professional that relates directly to the treatment or aftercare plan. Both of these services are generally elaborate and costly, but are able to accomplish a much larger volume of instruction than would be possible using conventional instructional methodologies.

Although there are numerous videotape formats, including several developed especially for the home market, the current format of choice for patient education applications is the ¾" U-Matic cassette. Software availability is excellent in this format, and until some standardization of the ½" home-type videocassette format occurs, unlikely in the near future, patient education software will continue to be produced in the more universal ¾" tape size.

Inhouse production of videotape programming offers almost unlimited possibilities in patient education applications, but because it is such a complicated and expensive process, the achievements of small-scale users are often quite dismal. Unless the hospital can afford the continuing expense of media professionals to operate and maintain the equipment, inhouse production of videotape programming is perhaps best avoided altogether. Television production workshops for beginners, like those sponsored by the American Hospital Association, Eastern Airlines, Knowledge Industry Publications, and others, are helpful in acquainting prospective users with the benefits and the pitfalls of inhouse videotape production. Visiting other hospitals that have videotape production facilities and viewing their videotape products is another way to make a determination about your own hospital's potential for establishing such a service.

Computer-Assisted Instruction

Microprocessor technology is now reaching into all aspects of American life from spelling toys to medical libraries. Computer-assisted instruction, usually on an individual basis, is now available to health-care professionals. No doubt applications and formats suitable to patient education will appear shortly.

The patient educator should be aware of current developments in various media formats. Obsolescent formats and products must be avoided, and the temptation to acquire new and expensive gadgets of unproven practicality must also be resisted. The audiovisual marketplace contains a bewildering array of genuine advances and pretentious gimmickery. The antidote for the lure of flashing lights and dealers' pitches must always be the question, "Is this the simplest, cheapest way to accomplish the desired effect?"

Software Selection

Once basic format and hardware decisions have been established, the task of selecting software to implement instructional goals can begin.

Many software catalogs are available. Unfortunately, most of these are published by commercial producers or by university film libraries and are limited in their coverage. A universal AV catalog that would parallel the function of *Books in Print* has yet to be developed.

Of most use are directories that cover more than one producer or source. Some are found annually in professional periodicals, while others are published by clearinghouses or review organizations. A list of these directories is included at the end of this chapter. Professional journals in scientific and health-care fields often list or review new audiovisual programs.

Medical libraries that have a telephone link to the National Library of Medicine's MEDLINE article reference service can use the AVLINE portion of the memory bank to find programs on specific topics. Only programs that have been approved by a review board are included. As a result, the most recent programs are not listed. This severely limits the usefulness of AVLINE for patient education because patient-oriented programming is a relatively new field for many production houses.

Perhaps the most practical source of information about software *and* facilities is correspondence with or a visit to an institution with a well-established, large-scale patient education program.

Programs must be evaluated for such factors as content, audience level, technical quality, and relevance to intended use. Each program should be examined by at least one potential user, one content expert, and one media specialist.

Programs should be selected on the basis of their relationship to the goals and objectives of the patient-care plan. The selection can be made by the patient education coordinator, a nurse specialist on the particular unit, a physician, or by all three together. A sample preview and evaluation form is shown in the section entitled Resource Materials.

EVALUATION OF MEDIATED PATIENT EDUCATION

The individual nature of patient education, with its captive yet transient audience, makes objective evaluation difficult and expensive. The time, budget, and skills required to do a rigorous follow-up study of patient behavior after discharge are beyond the reach of most institutions.

Thus, most of the formal justification of mediated patient instruction still rests on studies of nonpatient media, and the assumption that what works for other audiences will work with patients.

The rapid growth of the mediated patient education field has increased the need for formal studies. Until this need is met, informal evaluation can be carried on through observation and tests. Pre- and posttests are now more frequently supplied by program producers and can also be devised by individual instructors. Such testing, even informal oral quizzes, can greatly reinforce learning and validate the program.

In almost every hospital setting, no matter how great the limitations, some measure of the effectiveness of whatever form of mediated instruction is employed can be obtained by merely talking to the patient about what he or she has learned. Even here, some skills will be needed to avoid putting answers in patients' mouths in order to fulfill our expectations of what has been accomplished. But carefully constructed questions, posed in a caring, helpful way, will provide at least some indication of instructional effectiveness.

We find ourselves in the midst of two apparently contradictory movements in the health-care field. A clamor for cost containment is heard from both govern-ment and consumer. At the same time there is a demand for new programs of education and prevention.

The only way to meet both these challenges is innovation. Since patients who are active participants in their recovery get well faster, leave the hospital sooner, and have a smaller hospital bill than those who assume a more passive role, and since media greatly facilitate the inclusion of the patient's family in this process, mediated patient education will be a large part of the solution, and it is available now.

Resource Materials

GENERAL BIBLIOGRAPHY

Biomedical Communications Decision Makers' Guide: Patient Education Systems and Hospital Television Systems. Los Angeles: Decision Publications, 1977.
Grover, P. L., and Miller, J. Guidelines for making health education work. *Public Health Reports* 91 : 249, 1976.
Journal of Biocommunications. See especially the patient education issue of March 1978, and the annual media directory issue.
Kinsey, D. J. *Patient Education Using Television.* Kettering, Ohio: Kettering Medical Center, 1979.
Prynne, T. A. *Handbook on Hospital Television.* Columbia, S. C.: Educational Re-sources Foundation, 1972.

PROGRAM SOURCES

Audio Visual Source Directory. (Sources for audiovisual services and products.) Tarrytown, N. Y.: Motion Picture Enterprises Publications, Spring/Summer 1978.
Hospital Training Health Care Media Profiles. (Descriptions and evaluations of au-diovisual materials.) New York: Olympic Media Information, 1976.
Results of survey conducted by American Hospital Association, 1979.
Videolog. (Programs for business and industry.) New York: Esselte Video, 1979.

EQUIPMENT

Bensinger, C. *The Video Guide.* Santa Barbara, Calif.: Video-Info Publications, 1977.
Kemp, J. E. *Planning and Producing Audiovisual Materials* (3rd ed.). New York: Crowell, 1975.
Marsh, K. *Independent Video.* San Francisco: Straight Arrow Books, 1974.
National Audio-Visual Association. *The Audio-Visual Equipment Directory.* Fairfax, Va.: The Association, 1978 – 1979.
Zettl, H. *Television Production Handbook* (3rd ed.). Belmont, Calif.: Wadsworth, 1976.

SOFTWARE EVALUATION FORM

Preview Procedure

Make appointment by calling Education and Training.
Bring the Notice of Software Received to the Resource Room of Education and Training.
PURCHASE will be initiated by Instructional Design if recommended by user, media specialist, and/or content specialist.

Evaluation

Proposed Use

1

Times Used/Year	Audience Size	Copyright Date	Length (Minutes)

	Unacceptable		Average			Outstanding	
Check one box in each line	1	2	3	4	5	6	7
Organization	[ ]	[ ]	[ ]	[ ]	[ ]	[ ]	[ ]
Authenticity of content	[ ]	[ ]	[ ]	[ ]	[ ]	[ ]	[ ]
Clarity	[ ]	[ ]	[ ]	[ ]	[ ]	[ ]	[ ]
2 Learning interest	[ ]	[ ]	[ ]	[ ]	[ ]	[ ]	[ ]
Audio quality	[ ]	[ ]	[ ]	[ ]	[ ]	[ ]	[ ]
Video quality'	[ ]	[ ]	[ ]	[ ]	[ ]	[ ]	[ ]
Overall quality	[ ]	[ ]	[ ]	[ ]	[ ]	[ ]	[ ]
Relevance to proposed use	[ ]	[ ]	[ ]	[ ]	[ ]	[ ]	[ ]

Program audience level (i.e., physician, nurse, student, layman, etc.)

3

4 Recommendation   [   ] Purchase   [   ] Rental   [   ] Return

Brief Description of Program

Comments

Evaluator signature	Department or section	Date

Hospital Information Systems
the computer comes to patient education

Are computers of any use in patient teaching?
What are computers being used for in hospitals?
How can computer use be increased for the benefit of the patient?

Computer-Assisted Instruction (CAI) has been a part of educational technology for many years. Computers are also being used to streamline a number of functions within the health-care setting. Computers are not, however, being used to the extent they could or should be used in patient education. The following chapter describes the usefulness of computers in various health-care related functions. The fact that computers are not being used as much as they could be for patient education is explained, and two avenues for action are described to increase the utilization of computers for effective patient education.

Information in this chapter should help the reader to

1. *Describe three different categories of hospital information systems*
2. *Describe areas of potential use of computer-generated data in patient education*
3. *List two avenues by which computers may be incorporated more fully into patient education*

"Skylab is falling." NASA Newsbulletin,
June, 1979.

The patient education movement has been continually gaining impetus and importance for the past decade. With the advent of Professional Standards Review Organizations (PSRO), outcome and process audits, and the Joint Commission for the Accreditation of Hospitals (JCAH) standards all discussing patient education as an important facet of the health-care delivery system, more and more health-care professionals have begun to recognize the importance of, and incorporate within their specific field, the practice of patient education. Goldiamond succinctly captures the importance of the professional's function in this role by stating that patient education "need not be of the kind or depth which produces a skilled professional [but] it might be one which simply supplies the individual [patient] with the tools for analysis and change in the problem areas of the treatment concerns" [7]. Thus, the patient education process assumes a professional-client interaction. Within this interaction, certain types of data are disseminated—information about diagnosis, prognosis, symptoms, and medication or preventive measures. The list is legion, but the time constraint to perform this function is finite.

Enter the computer. Within the same time frame during which patient education has been recognized, legitimatized, and incorporated as standard operating procedures within the health-care system, the use of computers in the health-care industries have been adapted for clinical and informational purposes. It is interesting to stop and ask how much of the health-care industry currently relies on the computer. When was the last time you were in a hospital laboratory that was not at least partially computerized? When did you last ask someone in medical records to locate a chart? When did you last try to locate a patient's whereabouts at an information desk? And these are mundane and pedestrian computer applications. Walk into an intensive care unit and investigate the type of patient monitoring performed there. Some types of intensive care monitoring devices not only monitor the patient's vital signs but normalize the data, perform trend analyses, and predict (statistically) future problems or complications. Enough? Think of the entire accounting-billing function. You would probably never receive a bill (or a paycheck) if it were not for the computer. The computer is now a colleague with most if not all of those involved in the delivery of health care.

HOSPITAL COMPUTER APPLICATIONS

Various authors and writers have defined the hospital computing functions according to the purposes and procedures of the computer application. Many classification schema of computer applications are arbitrary and situational with most authorities differentiating between clinical and administrative applications. Austin and Green's comprehensive work is definitive. They list three generic approaches to categorizing hospital information services [2]:

1. Clinical (or Medical) Information Systems (CIS)
2. Administrative Information Systems (AIS), and
3. Fully Integrated (Total) Hospital Information Systems (THIS)

Clinical Information Systems

The CIS encompasses those computer applications utilized to support patient-care activities. Under this categorization is subsumed the information processes that assist in diagnosis, treatment selection, laboratory and pharmacy applications, patient monitoring systems, quality review functions, and medical record indexing, retrieval, and abstracting. Typically, these systems are developed specifically to meet the needs of the given department with data elements specific to the given department. Often the data is entered in batch* with daily updates of information. A critical dimension of the CIS is that often the system and data are generated for the use of a particular department without attending to the interdepartmental needs of the hospital. Consequently, data and results of the system are rarely used in other departments.

The major advantages and disadvantages are obvious. A specific department's information processing needs can be met at a minute level with systems tailored to meet explicit demands and requests at the expense of duplicating and storing many of the generic functions required of any system (for example, patient demographic information, historic data, and treatment data).

The use of this type of informational services within the health-care industry is limited. A 1976 study conducted by the Hospital Finance Management Association of approximately 2000 hospitals indicated that, when the medical record function is excluded, not more than 20 percent of the hospitals surveyed utilized the computer for any other clinical applications [4].

It is important to note that increasingly specialized departmental requirements in the form of more sophisticated diagnostic procedures, reports to outside agencies, and creative attempts to improve the quality of care delivered have created an environment that proliferates highly specialized computer applications for specific functions and departments.

Administrative Information Systems

Administrative information systems refer to those computer applications utilized in nonmedical functions for a given department. Specifically, this includes scheduling, financial reporting, materials management, personnel functions, patient billing, and accounts receivable.

Again, the AIS is generally a batch system with daily, weekly, monthly, or even quarterly updates. More often than not, the AIS is concerned with hos-pitalwide information processing. The development of these systems is gener-

---

*In batch means that all data to be entered in the computer is collected and then entered at one time, in one batch, and not necessarily at the moment the information is generated or the moment the event occurs.

ally more sensitive to governmental, legal, and financial constraints in the establishing of data and reporting structure. The critical dimension of the AIS is that a major constraint is placed on the hospital as a whole (for example, FICA tax in payroll), and all departments are treated identically along this parameter. Also, the reporting function of the AIS is identical for all departments with only higher administrative levels receiving all the data.

In the 1976 Hospital Finance Management Association survey, a distinct minority of the hospitals surveyed utilized the computer for some type of clinical assistance. However, an overwhelming majority of the hospitals surveyed utilized the computer for some type of administrative function [4].

Again, the major advantages and disadvantages of the AIS are obvious. It is safe to assume that administrators would drown in a sea of requisitions, charge slips, and inventory control forms without administrative computer assistance.

Total Hospital Information Systems

The THIS refers to those computer applications in which the administrative information and clinical information are integrated in one complete, complex, and comprehensive unit. Typically, requests for data or information are initiated in a department (nursing station), electronically transmitted via cathode ray tube (CRT—a TV screen) to another department (for example, the hospital lab), where action is taken to produce the information requested (test performed), electronically reported via CRT simultaneously to the requesting department (nursing station) and appropriate administrative units (patient accounts). Given a successful CIS and AIS, it would seem logical that a THIS would be a simple outgrowth. However, the National Center for Health Services Research and Development listed approximately a dozen different commercial vendors offering a THIS in 1971 [8]. In 1979, only one of these vendors was still offering such a product.

Obviously, the potential benefits of a THIS are enormous. Equally obvious are the risks involved in the development and implementation of such a system. The critical dimensions of the THIS that differentiate it from the AIS or the CIS are generally:

1. On-line data entry and retrieval with real-time* data updates, especially in the results-reporting function
2. Transmission of information to all major departments of the hospital
3. The use of a common database by all departments in the hospital

PATIENT EDUCATION AND THE COMPUTER

By now you are probably beginning to ask yourself, "What is a chapter on hospital information systems doing in a book about patient education?" Unfortunately, the answer is "Not much!" Giebink and Hurst's review of 29 computer

---

*Real time means that data is fed into the computer at the moment the event occurs, thus causing the information to be as accurate and up-to-date as possible.

projects in the health-care industries documented 14 different areas in which the computer assisted health-care professionals. These 14 areas can be generally classified either as typical CIS or AIS functions. However, within the 29 computer projects, the medical records function was addressed approximately 90 percent of the time by the computer applications, while patient education was addressed approximately 6 percent of the time [6]. It is unfortunate that designers and implementers of such computer systems disregard or ignore the potential for patient education.

One can only imagine the multiple uses of the data generated by the computer when applied to patient education. Lab results can be used as one of a limitless set of examples. What if a hard copy of the lab results were generated for the patient? What if generalized complaints of illness or ailment could be concertized into something specific such as a low blood sugar? Discussions regarding the effects of medication and/or diet and the effects of maintaining such a regime can be demonstrated to the patient. Too often we ask or tell our patients to follow some prescribed course of action without demonstrating the effects of that action. No wonder patients stop taking what we give them or stop doing what we tell them as soon as they walk out the hospital door. But lab results given within the context of an educational program that relates the desired outcomes to the patient's involvement might ensure the patient's cooperation in taking an active part in regaining and maintaining health.

Another example where the computer could help is diet planning, especially for complicated diets such as required for hemodialysis patients. A chronic complaint of the dialysis patient (especially the person who must prepare the food for a dialysis patient) is the lack of knowledge regarding what kinds of nutrients or additives are in what kinds of foods. How much potassium is in a 16-ounce can of tomato sauce? A computer generated list of such food items would be invaluable. Or why not create a computer-generated daily menu that patients could use at home?

The computer can be of invaluable assistance in the planning, implementing, and documentation of patient teaching-learning interactions. The computer can generate a set of standardized guidelines that present disease-specific information useful to guide the teacher who is to present information to the patient. The computer can be used to keep records of the patient's progress through a teaching-care plan, and the nurse can easily enter the documentation of successful learning outcomes at the CRT located at the nursing station.

Obviously, the list of examples of computer use in patient education is infinite. It is only bound by the imagination (or lack of it) of the health-care provider.

The Bottom Line

The bottom line is simply the source of the analogy. Most computer applications in hospitals are *not* there for patient education. They are generally administrative or clinical applications for which the institution has specific goals, budgets, and technical and financial constraints. Patient education is currently, at best, a spin-off or by-product. There are, however, at least two avenues of action.

The first of these is that much of the data generated for clinical purposes could be utilized *as is* for supplementing patient education activities. Lab results are the obvious example. Of course this is a stop-gap measure and, of course, no significant strides will be realized in favorably impacting the design of such applications for patient education. But on a very pragmatic, idiographic level, it might just work!

Second, and more important, those advocates of patient education must become involved in the planning and implementation of computer applications within an institution. Patient education should be seen as an achievable, realistic benefit of the system as important as cost reduction. In this manner, both users of the system and planners of the system can at least voice the opinion, the request, the demand that patient education be addressed during the design and implementation of a system.

Oh yes, Skylab did fall. But it was people who put it up there with the help of the computer and the computer helped track its descent. It's a disgrace that our hospitalized patients know more about spaceships and celestial bodies than about achieving and maintaining health. We as a country drink too much, smoke too much, and eat too much, especially of the wrong foodstuff. Patient education is one means of reversing that trend, and computers are one of the tools available to the health care professional in achieving that goal.

REFERENCES

1. American Hospital Association. Statement on the Roles and Responsibilities of Hospitals and Other Health Care Institutions in Personal and Community Health Care Education. Chicago: The Association, 1974.
2. Austin, C. J., and Green, B. R. Hospital information systems. *Inquiry,* 15 : 95, 1978.
3. Bekey, G. A., and Schwartz, M. D. *Hospital Information Systems.* New York: Marcel Dekker, 1972.
4. Chervenak, L. EDP is up. *Hospital Financial Management,* 31 : 24, 1977.
5. Garret, R. D. *Hospitals: A Systems Approach.* Philadelphia: Auerbach, 1973.
6. Giebink, G. A., and Hurst, L. L. *Computer Projects in Health Care.* Ann Arbor: University of Michigan Health Administration Press, 1975.
7. Goldiamond, I. Protection of human subjects and patients: A social contingency analysis of distinctions between research and practice and its implications. *Behaviorism,* 4 : 1, 1976.
8. U.S. National Center for Health Services Research and Development. *Hospital Computer Applications Programs.* Vols. 1, 2, 4. U.S. Department of Commerce, 1974.
9. Virts, S. Introducing the hospital-wide information system to hospital and medical staffs. *Medical Informatics* 77 : 993, 1977.

III

Roles and Settings for Patient Teaching

The Role of the Patient Education Coordinator

How can a systematic approach to patient teaching be coordinated throughout an institution?
How can the Patient Education Coordinator facilitate patients' learning outcomes?
What organizational factors hinder smooth functioning of patient teaching?

A systematic approach to patient education necessitates many different kinds of activities including gathering resources, evaluating commercial materials and seeking approval of their use, and planning a comprehensive program. The health-care provider already complains that there is not time enough to do everything, and less effective teaching and learning is often the result. The role of the Patient Education Coordinator has evolved, then, out of the need to facilitate teaching done by busy personnel. The following chapter describes the role of the Patient Education Coordinator as it actually exists in a hospital. The various functions that are served by the Patient Education Coordinator are described. Sources of patient education goals are described. The formation of a steering committee is described as a helpful means to accomplish patient education. A means for dealing with barriers and frustration is described.
    Information in this chapter should help the reader to

1. *Describe the personal characteristics of an effective Patient Education Coordinator*
2. *Identify and answer three questions that help establish the goals of patient education*
3. *Describe the formation and functions of a patient education steering committee*

4. *Identify means to support and facilitate the bedside nurse's patient teaching activities*
5. *Describe strategies for dealing with trouble spots in patient education*

Patient education programs are just beginning to gain momentum, and the position of Patient Education Coordinator is a newly created one. This chapter will point out some of the effective mechanisms to help accomplish the goals and help define the role of the Patient Education Coordinator. Such things as organization, administrative expectations, committee structures, development of teaching programs, preparation and motivation of the nursing staff, and increasing the responsibility of the patient for self-care and health maintenance will be discussed.

It takes a special kind of person to coordinate patient education, to bring it all together and make it work. A BSN or MN, or classes in "Psychology of Learning," "Adult Learners' Needs," and "Behavioral Modification" are all helpful no doubt, but what are the personal characteristics needed for success at this new job? It is helpful if the Patient Education Coordinator (PEC) is assertive, confident, persuasive, and verbally fluent. Also advantageous are broad personal interests, social poise, enthusiasm, imagination, humor, and flexibility [3]. The PEC needs to strike a balance between social behavior and task-oriented behavior so that the nursing staff is not threatened. Establishment of friendly relationships should take a place of importance. To have credibility, the PEC must know how to take care of patients and know the functions and stresses involved in daily patient care. Not only are skills important but experience must also verify understanding of nurses themselves and the problems inherent in their role as educators. The Resource Materials section presents a representative job description for a Patient Education Coordinator.

As the need to contain hospital costs is very real, the trend seems to be toward using the staff nurse as teacher. In this case the PEC must look at the staffing pattern to determine how much time the nurse can usually be spared from the unit for committee work. Will staffing require LPNs to teach also? Are there student nurses who may supplement the teaching? Is it necessary to draw frequently from a "float pool"? All of these answers will influence the decisions the coordinator makes in doing his or her job.

The PEC has a major function in helping the staff identify the goals of patient education. These goals arise as three questions are asked. "Who should be taught?" *Every* patient has some learning needs. Even physicians and nurses who are patients have questions about procedures and findings. Almost every contact of the care provider with the patient furnishes an opportunity to teach, answer questions, or explain procedures. The problem seems to be in convincing the care-provider that he or she is indeed responsible and potentially capable of providing this teaching.

"What does the patient need to know?" First, he or she needs to know enough to be safe. Second, the patient needs to know enough to participate in the decision-making process. He has a right to know the alternatives of treatment, the risks associated with each, and the possible consequences of no treatment at all. To presume to make these choices for someone else is the ultimate in arrogance. "What does the patient need to know in order to attain a maximum degree of wellness?" The patient's decision about the necessary components of his life and his definition of "quality of life" determine the effort he will make to achieve maximum wellness. He decides the objectives of learning. Values, not needs, determine behavior. An increase in knowledge is no guarantee of a change in behavior.

These are the goals—to assure safety, informed consent, and maximum health potential for all patients. How does one begin to go about meeting these goals? First, the PEC should survey the assets available. There is probably already patient teaching going on in the hospital, for example, prenatal classes and diabetic teaching. Others may exist as well. The PEC must develop communication with other departments—the library, physical therapy, x-ray, laboratory, dietary, outpatient—to find out what kind of things those departments do in staff, student, and patient education. It will be helpful to maintain an exchange of information on a regular basis with these other departments. In addition, the hospital administration is likely to be much more receptive to the request for new equipment if it is to be used by several departments.

This initial assessment will take time, but it should be done thoroughly. As materials and equipment are being collected, staff members who are enthusiastic about patient teaching will identify themselves. Some of them will approach the PEC directly and ask to be involved. The coordinator should ascertain their particular interests and write their names in a notebook for future reference.

Some patient needs will be identified in this exploration, especially if the PEC makes an effort to overlap into shifts other than 7 to 3. Nurses on the 3 to 11 shift on a surgical ward may ask about Pre-op classes, on a medical ward about x-ray instruction sheets. It is important to remember these needs, but the decision about where to start is not made this way. It is made by the use of a committee.

The degree of freedom the PEC is allowed in committee selection will depend upon the organizational structure and the amount of control retained by the administrative officers. However, the committee chosen to select the patient education programs to be developed should include representation from all the specialty areas—Medical, Surgical, Ob/Gyn, Pediatrics, Orthopedics, and ICU. Members should be chosen carefully for their interest, vision, and ability to express themselves. This is not a time-consuming committee; it meets initially a few times to develop a philosophy and objectives and to determine the first one or two programs. Since it takes several months to develop most programs, it is possible the committee will meet only four or five times a year. Although there may or may not be a physician on this committee, it is prudent to involve physicians whenever they are willing to be involved. An effort should be made to choose a physician who has a broad range of interests or initial programs may be concentrated in one specialty area. The hospital situation and committee membership can best determine this question.

A good beginning point for the steering committee is a summary of admission diagnoses for the past two or three years. The medical records department can provide this information. From this information it is possible to determine the largest patient populations and to choose the first target groups.

The process for developing the specific program is much more time consuming. It also involves selection of a committee, and, by all means, a physician should be included. Search for one whose specialty is in the area and who seems comfortable working with nurses. Hopefully, he or she will have an open attitude toward nurses providing teaching for patients and be able to persuade his or her colleagues of the benefits of better informed clients. Representation from any other involved departments is also necessary (for example, dietary or physical therapy). Choose nurses who are interested and experienced in the specialty. Development of programs utilizing nurses experienced and working in the specialty areas naturally eases into the concept of having nurses skilled in teaching one or two areas of patient education and using each other as resources [1]. A workable size for the committee is from six to ten members.

The committee should participate in the work. Request that one or more of them review the literature and discuss with their colleagues during committee meetings the current concepts of diet, benefits of exercise, or the possible therapeutic effects of relaxation techniques. Encourage them to help develop teaching aids, instruction sheets, and diagrams. They are the experts, and they have the contributions to make. The job of the PEC is to bring it all together, to see that objectives and expected patient outcomes are written, to see that the content is manageable and adaptable to the different levels of understanding and education found in patients. The language is especially important: it must be realistic. The program should include necessary information, but not overload the patient. As Barbara Redman says, "It is better to give six pearls than a carload of information the patient can't incorporate" [4]. A list of "Questions To Ask the Doctor" is extremely helpful for the average patient [2]. The nurse can help the patient compile a question list to have ready for the physician's next visit.

The PEC must also seek suitable teaching aids and check catalogues for film strips and booklets. The committee makes the final choices. The PEC may inquire as to what people in other hospitals are using. The more methods by which the content is presented, the more understanding is likely to take place. Whether the patients are to be taught on a one-to-one basis, in a class setting, or a combination of both will influence the choice of methods and materials. It is not possible to do true in-depth teaching during the short time and under the stressful circumstances in the hospital. The plan should include follow-up classes or referrals to community agencies for their group programs where possible.

For those patients for whom compliance is essential, behavior modification has had success. The American Heart Association has classes in weight control and hypertension and the American Cancer Society has smoking clinics that may be valuable. The support of others who are coping with the same problems can be invaluable. A very impressive program for both adults and young people is supported by the American Diabetes Association. The Association sponsors summer camps for children in some states, and their monthly publication

"Forecast" is excellent. This organization also has a group for patient educators. There are many other support systems that the PEC should know about.

If a hospital has closed-circuit television, the PEC has a tremendous advantage. Much of the routine information can be provided by TV in the patient's room. This is especially true of information that must be given to large numbers of patients at frequent intervals.

The PEC should expect that the teaching program will require several revisions before it is presented to the appropriate medical group. Having an articulate, supportive physician as a member of the committee is an obvious advantage, but he or she may or may not be the one to present the program. The individual who is selected must be very comfortable with the entire content. It may be expedient to divide the program, with, for example, the dietitian explaining one portion and the physical therapist another. These people should be prepared to answer questions from the medical group and provide a rationale for decisions that were made. It will be a definite advantage to have "standing orders" for patient teaching approved where feasible.

Now comes the hard part—implementation. There will be some disappointments. Once-enthusiastic nurses will be unable to find the time to teach. Individual physicians will announce that they do not want their patients in the program, and patients themselves will exhibit an incredible amount of indifference and resistance. Now one remembers all the "people" factors. Dale Carnegie once said, "Let us remember we are not dealing with creatures of logic. We are dealing with creatures of emotion, creatures bustling with prejudices and motivated by pride and vanity."

The nurse may be uncomfortable with her teaching skills, the program content, or her lack of support from colleagues and supervisor. "Nurses need the support of other nurses in their teaching efforts" [1]. The PEC must make it as easy as possible for the nurse to teach. Primary or total-patient care would seem to facilitate patient teaching because of the depth of involvement with the patient and family. Team nursing does have some built-in problems, not the least of which is accountability.

Patient teaching is, in reality, a part of patient care. A written care plan that includes learning objectives and expected patient outcomes with dates and a complete patient history seems to be part of the answer. Nursing care plans are developed from standards of care. It is an advantage to have input into the Nursing Standards Committee. A good care plan developed from a comprehensive standard will outline the objectives for the bulk of patient teaching.

As a supplement to this, the PEC may develop a rather inclusive discharge plan as part of the nursing care plan. It should contain verbalized understanding by the patient or significant other of the disease process, activity, special cares (tubes, dressings, casts), medications, diet, and return appointments. It should also list the patient's limitations and whatever referrals have been made. This care plan, including the discharge summary, is written in ink and becomes part of the permanent record.

The PEC must try to provide ways to develop or reinforce the skills of the staff nurse to make her more comfortable in the teaching role. A concept of the way adults learn is a good place to begin. Once the process of learning is understood, teaching skills may be reinforced by teaching with another nurse who is more experienced and by the availability of several methods of providing the information. Often times a simple but complete checklist may be used to include significant content.

Many nurses seem to require support in mastering communication and helping skills. "To be minimally helpful, one must be functioning at a particular level of empathy, concreteness, genuineness, and self-disclosure, and communicate respect and immediacy in the relationship" [5].

The time to teach comes only from making it a priority, and this will happen only with administrative support. If the expectation is voiced in administrative goals, it will be reflected in division goals. If personnel are evaluated on performances that include more than completion of tasks, their priorities will shift. If coordinators emphasize their desire to meet the learning needs of the patients, staff will conform to expectations. There will, of course, be no more minutes in an eight-hour shift, but there will be time for what the nurse feels is important.

One of the methods some hospitals are exploring in order to find time to teach is a two-hour shift overlap by utilizing a 9 A.M. to 5:30 P.M. shift. This method serves two purposes—it provides two hours a day devoted solely to patient teaching as well as rewarding the nurse-teacher with choice hours.

There are physicians who appear to be threatened by a nurse's efforts to teach patients. It is best to go slowly, clear the material with the physician (if that is his concern), and attempt to determine the reasons for his or her lack of trust. Involvement of a physician in the planning of programs promotes acceptance. Part of the answer may be for the nurse to resume making rounds with the physician. In some areas this seems to be one of the casualties of nursing's effort to escape the "handmaiden" role. It is probably one of the most important factors, however, in communication of the physician's plan of care.

This may be a bit idealistic in some situations, so a "Request for Patient Teaching" has been developed. This is a simple checklist of the program's components, a question whether the physician would like to preview the handout materials, and a request for the physician to share with the nursing staff his expectations for the patient (see Two Requests for Patient Teaching in the section entitled Resource Materials). Patients themselves, especially in a small community, will ask for the services their friends and neighbors have received in a similar situation. So the important thing is to get started; increase patient satisfaction and the word will spread.

What does one do if one "hits the wall" when one finds that resources are spent, the idea bank is broke, and it seems impossible to move forward an inch? A marathon runner tries to "run through the wall." In patient education, one can usually afford to withdraw, regroup, and approach from another angle. Sometimes it is a good idea to take refuge in a smaller program in a receptive area for a few days. The Ob/Gyn area is pleasant for some PECs because there patient teaching has long been a way of life. After a week or so most PECs can usually go back to the original project with new ideas and a fresh perspective. They will have isolated some of the original problems and can usually determine another course of action.

One other important factor is that of a role model. An obese instructor of weight reduction, a no-smoking advocate who reeks of tobacco smoke, or the exercise "pusher" who drives her car to the corner grocery all lack credibility. Some time might be well spent examining one's own life style. Do you *really* believe what you are teaching? The things that the PEC tries to influence others to do must be incorporated into his or her own value system to be convincing.

This chapter makes an admittedly pragmatic attempt to answer some questions concerning role development and staff retationships for the Patient Education Coordinator. It discusses some of the things that have worked and some of the trouble spots. Obviously, these will vary from institution to institution. However, the basic premise of the consumer's right to pertinent information will remain; as hospitals continue to make the transition from crisis care to prevention, the informative portion of health care will consume an increasingly large percentage of the dollars spent. The increased life-span of the population, the availability of communication media, and the awareness of individual responsibility will contribute to improved health and well-being. The gains we are making now are helping to form the foundation for better health for all of us.

REFERENCES

1. del Bueno, D. Patient education, planning for success. *Journal of Nursing Administration,* 8 : 4, 1978.
2. Green, L. W. What evaluation of recent patient education efforts is telling us. 2nd Annual Symposium of Patient Education, 1978.
3. Motivational Dynamics. *Modern Management Techniques.* Minneapolis: Control Data Corporation, 1975.
4. Redman, B. K. Curriculum in patient education. *American Journal of Nursing,* p. 1365, Aug., 1978.
5. Redman, B. K. *The Process of Patient Teaching in Nursing* (3rd ed.). St. Louis: Mosby, 1976.

Resource Materials

PATIENT EDUCATION COORDINATOR'S JOB DESCRIPTION*

Position Summary

A Registered Professional Nurse who functions under the Director of Inservice and is responsible for coordination of Patient Education for all Nursing Units. It is expected that the majority of Patient Teaching will be done by the staff nurse during the course of patient care.

Typical Duties

1. Coordination of teaching of inhospital and ministay patients and their families in order to prepare them for the transition from an acute level of

*Courtesy St. Mark's Hospital, Salt Lake City, Utah.

care to other levels of care, or to the home setting, with improved capability for health maintenance.

2. Promotion of consistency in program content and teaching concepts to be utilized by the staff nurse for patient teaching:

   a. With committees consisting of persons skilled in the area, identifies learning needs, develops teaching plans, and acquires appropriate teaching materials to meet these needs
   b. Evaluates programs and makes recommendations to Inservice Staff of programs for staff development
   c. Confers with nursing personnel
   d. Orients new personnel to patient education programs
   e. Consults with and gives guidance to nursing staff in unique situations
   f. Teaches one-to-one with patients who require such service

3. Works in conjunction with the Director of Social Services to develop, evaluate, and determine the most appropriate patient education and discharge planning program.
4. Coordination with other Health Care Professionals such as Medicine, Dietary, Pharmacy, Physical Therapy, and Occupational Therapy to develop patient education programs and meet specific patient needs that will enhance patient responsibility and independence.
5. Promotion of continuity of patient care through written instruction sheets, booklets, prescription inserts, and referral to community services such as Public Health, Community Nursing, Visiting Nurse, Cancer Society, Lung Association, Heart Association, Diabetes Association, etc.
6. Develops, maintains, and utilizes records and files pertinent to the patient education program.
7. Keeps the Director of Inservice informed of progress by oral and/or written reports on a monthly basis.
8. Reviews Standards of Care for inclusion of patient learning needs.
9. Reviews Patient Care Plans for patient learning needs.
10. Serves as a member of the Staff Development Committee.
11. Serves as chairperson of the Steering Committee for Patient Education.

Minimum Requirements

Graduate of an accredited school of nursing
Current license as Registered Nurse in the state
Baccalaureate Degree in Nursing. Additional work in education, clinical nursing, human relations preferred
Successful experience in nursing service and/or nursing education with demonstrated leadership ability

TWO REQUESTS FOR PATIENT TEACHING

I would like my patient, patient's family _____
                                                        name
to have information about diabetes, including:
____ Diet, calories _____
____ Insulin injections
____ Urine checking ____ Diastix ____ Testape ____ Clinitest ____ Ketodiastix
____ Physiology
____ Foot care
____ Exercise
____ All of the above

I would, would not, like to preview printed information.

My expectation for this patient is _____ tight control, urine 0-¼%, BS 70–120;
_____ Moderate control, urine ¼-½%, BS 120-200; or _____ loose control, urine
     ¾-1%, BS less than 350.
Weight: _____ lb gain _____ lb loss _____ stable
Other _____   _____M.D.

I would like my patient _____
                                              name
to have the information included in the Coronary Rehabilitation Program.
(anatomy and physiology, risk factors, activity, diet, warning signs, and take-
home medications)
Exceptions: _____
I would, would not, like to preview printed hand-outs.
My expectation for this patient is _____ gradual return to normal activity _____
coronary bypass surgery _____ indefinitely restricted activity or _____
        (The above is solely to provide consistency with your care plan and will not
        be conveyed to the patient by the nurse.)

_____ M.D.

Barbara J. Stevens

The Director of Nursing Service as Facilitator of Patient Teaching

How does the Director of Nursing influence patient education?
How can the Director of Nursing assure that patient teaching will occur through-
out an organization?

Patient teaching, as well as many other aspects of quality patient care, seems to
occur most often when the administrator stresses its importance. Thus, the role
of the Director of Nursing will influence the type and extent of patient teaching
that occurs in the entire organization. The Director of Nursing does not do
patient teaching itself, but rather makes certain decisions based on a philosophy
of management and teaching. The following chapter describes how the
philosophy of the Director of Nursing affects patient teaching activities. Exam-
ples are provided that illustrate how an administrator's philosophy can translate
into the day-to-day activities of patient teaching. The inquiring attitude is
stressed as a means to provide answers to yet unsolved problems in teaching
patients in the acute-care setting.
  Information in this chapter should help the reader to

1. *Describe the administrative implications of a philosophy of patient teaching*
2. *Identify whether patient teaching is a specialty function or a generalized*
   function
3. *Describe the inquiring attitude necessary for an organization to solve patient*
   teaching (and other) problems

If patient education is to be successful in a nursing department, planning for that function must begin at the top, with the Director of Nursing. First, the Director must have a well-thought-out philosophy of patient education; second, he or she must systematically see that this philosophy is implemented throughout the department.

This chapter is an exploration of a personal philosophy of patient education and the implications that philosophy would have were it to be implemented in an acute-care setting. This exercise is given, not as a recommendation of the "right" philosophy of patient teaching, but as an example of the kind of interplay that must take place between *any* philosophy of patient education and its implementation. Other philosophic positions on patient teaching may be equally good and would be likely to lead to different administrative decisions. The important point is that a philosophy of patient education should be held, examined, and implemented in administrative planning if the philosophy is to have an impact on patient education.

The first concern in developing a philosophy of patient education is to ask why this aspect of nursing care receives so much attention as compared to other aspects of nursing-care delivery in the acute-care setting. Is patient teaching such a large component of nursing care that it deserves this attention? Or has patient teaching been exaggerated beyond its inherent importance as one component among many others in nursing care? The attention given to patient teaching probably *is* disproportionate to its importance; surely other components of acute-care nursing are equally significant. The concentration given to patient teaching, however, is *not* disproportionate to its complexity. Patient teaching is a difficult task that raises significant issues in nursing.

SIGNIFICANT ISSUES

The first issue raised in relation to patient teaching is whether patient education is a routine nursing function or a specialized function to be managed by specially prepared nurse practitioners. Arguments can be offered for both of these positions. The argument for patient education as a routine nursing function is that nursing, as a health profession, has an inherent responsibility to guide the health practices of its clients under all circumstances; such guidance necessarily involves teaching. The argument for patient education as a specialist function centers on the complexity of the teaching act. Education, this argument asserts, is a separate profession in its own right; it is unrealistic to expect every nurse to be both a professional nurse and a professional teacher.

The Director of Nursing's basic philosophy of patient education will affect how he or she organizes the nursing department. If patient teaching is seen as a routine nursing function, the Director will provide experts to assist staff nurses in learning how to teach; if patient teaching is seen as a specialized function, the Director will provide experts for direct patient teaching.

This author believes that teaching must be an intrinsic part of the basic nursing role, even if the teaching function must be placed in the hands of an inexpert teacher. This position is valid for several reasons. First, nursing is accountable for the constellation of care offered to a patient. If nursing is divided into a series of specialty functions, the Gestalt "view of the whole" of the patient's care trajectory is lost. This danger is greater than that represented by the presentation of materials by an inexpert teacher.

Second, it is difficult to believe that a teaching specialist is able to identify all the patient's significant teaching needs. Many teaching needs are discovered by the staff nurse incidentally during the course of other nursing activities. Also, patients may need to reach a certain degree of rapport with a nurse before they can reveal their teaching needs; they may be unwilling to voice such needs to a specialist whom they view as an outsider.

Finally, a patient who is motivated to learn some particular thing can learn it from an inexpert teacher if that teacher has the right knowledge. Conversely, the patient is unlikely to learn from the best of teachers if he or she is not motivated to learn the particular thing under consideration.

Perhaps yet another suspicion lurks behind this philosophy of staff nurse teaching. It seems that when any aspect of nursing care gets labeled as a specialty area, the staff nurse soon develops an inability even to recognize the need for that sort of care. Discharge planning exemplifies this pattern: where a discharge planner exists, nurses often abdicate any and all responsibility for a "future orientation" in patient care.

Given these philosophic predilections, a Director of Nursing will provide experts to teach nurses how and what to teach but will not let the experts absolve the staff nurses of their teaching responsibilities. No methodologic skill can substitute for just plain knowledge. One simply cannot teach what one does not know, no matter how skilled at the teaching craft, no matter how versed in adult education, no matter how versatile, clever, creative, innovative. Staff nurses should become competent in basic teaching arts, but it is more important that they know the content required before tackling any teaching task.

The next issue in patient education is a need to differentiate between needs for education and needs for information. Often these are treated as if they were the same. The term *teaching* should be used only when acquisition of the information, skill, or attitude by the patient requires a sustained and organized effort on the part of the nurse. *Information sharing,* in contrast, can be accomplished by a single telling (for most patients). To consider all information sharing, however vital, as patient teaching makes the situation more complex than it need be. To say that information giving differs from patient teaching, however, does not absolve the nurse of an obligation to see that a patient receives all information vital to his or her recovery or future functioning.

What does the nurse *really* need to learn about teaching in the acute-care setting? First, she needs to learn how to recognize a learning need. Learning needs, not teaching acts, should become the focus of patient education, and developing a sensitivity in recognizing the veiled learning need of a patient is a skill the nurse needs to develop. Second, the nurse needs to learn to gauge a patient's learning potential. The nurse must learn to gauge the patient's ability to learn *today,* while he or she is in this psychic state, while he or she is under these pressures. If nurses were to study learning curves in relation to patients' illness trajectories, they might discover optimal times for learning or they might identify specific variables that indicate learning readiness. Third, the nurse needs to make the material meaningful for the patient. The nurse must focus on how the patient will *apply* the learning rather than on the mere *acquisition* of facts or skills. The learning that counts in patient care is the learning revealed in action. In most cases, this means that attitude is a key factor. Attitude determines acts to a greater degree than does cognitive knowledge (however essential that prerequisite knowledge be).

Attitudinal factors (present and known or future and unpredictable) confound the teaching situation in the acute-care hospital. But even without the affective element, such teaching presents difficulties. Teaching for future action in a different place is a little like assuming a would-be pilot can safely and competently take to the air after practice on a ground trainer. Unfortunately, though the trainer may be great, there is no substitute for training in the place where the action really will take place.

ADMINISTRATIVE IMPLICATIONS

What are the administrative implications of these beliefs about patient teaching? First, the resources that are used in teaching the nursing staff how to teach must be carefully selected. One cannot rely heavily on persons whose only teaching experiences are with well students. Persons who are able to recognize the subtleties and complexities of teaching and learning in the acute-care hospital are desirable. Also, one should probably look for an educator with a healthy sense of doubt about the efficacy of teaching in the acute-care setting. A person should look to the *results* of patient education rather than be a zealot about the *issue* of patient teaching.

The managerial staff should hold the nursing staff accountable for teaching *and* for inquiring about the efficacy of that teaching. Managers should seek to answer the many open questions about patient education in the acute-care setting. The managerial staff should be economical in the use of resources for delivery of cognitive content and skill building. Where it can be predicted that large numbers of patients will require the same knowledge or identical techniques, the managers should develop (or have developed) economical modes of patient education, such as group teaching, programmed study units, media presentations, or whatever works effectively and economically.

NURSING OPPORTUNITIES

In an era when nursing is endeavoring to advance its professional status, attention inevitably focuses upon those nursing actions that allow for optimal independent judgment and action. Patient teaching is such an arena. It has potential for decision-making concerning (1) what is to be taught, (2) how it is to be taught, and (3) who should be the pupil.

The subject matter of patient teaching has two major sources: (1) those aspects of self-care dictated by the course of the illness or injury and its anticipated aftermath, and (2) those aspects of self-care related to hygiene and health in general. Teaching usually involves immediate self-care, self-care needs for home, or ongoing convalescent or permanent care needs. Basic hygiene and health has long been the teaching domain of nursing, but care related to illness or medical/surgical physician intervention is not entirely secured as nursing's teaching domain. Some aspects of this teaching still are reserved by medicine in general or by individual physicians as their domain.

In some cases, nursing has lost ground to physicians in the teaching activity by failing to keep up with the changes in medical/surgical therapy. For example, the nurse who has a single teaching plan for the patient with a spinal fusion is overlooking advanced technologies in which fusions done in different ways create different teaching needs. The nurse is better off to do no teaching than to offer teaching that contradicts the physician's communications to the patient. A Director of Nursing will want nurses to know what to teach. This calls for close collaboration and mutual respect between nursing and medical staffs. Frankly, this cannot be achieved by a focus on interpersonal relationships. It only happens when physicians really learn to respect a given nurse as excellent in his or her field. Hence, the best of clinical nurses will be required, as part of their job description, to systematically build the necessary open communication lines with the medical staff to get the knowledge on which teaching plans may be predicated.

Many nurses prefer to derive nursing plans separate from the medical plan as a mode of asserting nursing's independence. However, knowledge of the medical/surgical events of a patient's case never demeans the independence of nursing. Indeed, knowledge of the physician's regimen and interventions is only one factor necessary for the development of a successful nursing plan. To consider the physician's therapy as a subelement in a nursing plan does not make nursing subservient to medicine. Indeed, one could as easily offer the opposite conclusion.

Further, a Director of Nursing will support the clinical staff and will run interference in those cases of specific physicians who withhold information from the nursing staff to prevent their teaching activities (or those who demand that nurses not teach *their* patients). Such physician behavior is usually exhibited by the worst, not the best, practitioners. The Director of Nursing should be willing to say that nurses cannot give *any* care to patients when they must function in ignorance or with their lips arbitrarily sealed. That mode of functioning simply is not intrinsically compatible with nursing.

When the best clinical nurses have derived appropriate teaching plans for given patient situations, these plans should be converted to formal teaching protocols to be shared with and available for the total nursing staff. There is no need for every nurse to reinvent the wheel, nor is every nurse capable of doing so. Formal teaching protocols give both direction and sanction to the teaching act. Protocols also increase the total amount and quality of teaching.

Further, formal teaching protocols can be the subject matter for those inquiries into teaching methodology. Audiovisual and other teaching aids can be developed for those teaching needs that are repetitive (and therefore have become the subject matter of formal protocols). The Director of Nursing should get a good sense of the growth and development of patient teaching activities by a simple quantitative count of the teaching protocols being developed or updated. The development of teaching protocols will be the responsibility of the managerial staff, guiding the clinicians in formalizing their knowledge. Teaching protocols will *not* be the responsibility of the nursing staff development department. Teaching protocols are primarily an outgrowth of clinical expertise, not of teaching expertise. Teaching expertise may be used as a secondary resource in finalizing a teaching protocol, but a teaching protocol begins and ends with clinical knowledge of what *content* is to be taught.

Patient education is an arena of nursing presenting both opportunities and problems. It is an area open for nursing inquiry, an area to be developed over time. At present, given the diversity of patients in the acute-care setting, we know little about *what* should be taught, *how* it should be taught, or *when* it should be taught. These are all arenas for inquiry.

The Director of Nursing will want a staff who seek to find the answers rather than a staff who see patient education as a settled issue. The Director will encourage the inquiring attitude in staff by focusing on patient education research and will insist that answers to patient education questions lie, not in what is said in some text, but in how patients respond to teaching plans. A teaching plan will be judged to be effective, not when a nurse "taught it well," but when a patient "learned it well," as reflected in changed activities.

The Director of Nursing will be cognizant of the knowledge needs of the nursing staff, recognizing that these needs precede patient education. The Director must set an administrative tone that makes clear that intellectual pursuit is an expected role function for the staff nurses—and every other nurse employed.

Finally, the Director must see that results-oriented patient learning is the focus of the patient teaching efforts by building patient learning goals into the quality evaluation tools and systems that serve as care control mechanisms. The control systems will enable the Director to convey success or failure judgments back to the managerial staff and will enable them to convey such judgments on to nursing staff. Special successes (as well as chronic failures) will be tied into the reward and punishment structure of the department. People need to know what efforts are required, desired, and respected. Hence, both quality assurance systems and performance appraisal systems will need to reflect the desired patient learning goals.

In essence, this managerial approach to patient education represents a multipronged approach rather than a direct and specialized approach. This approach makes control and implementation more difficult, but it is still the best choice. To isolate patient teaching from other components of the nursing care is undesirable. The Director of Nursing will want to build teaching excellence as a natural part of the nurse's role, and that cannot be done by separating that aspect of nursing care from the other aspects of care. Patient education is still an unsolved problem in the acute-care setting. The nursing department should be a tool in the inquiry that will ultimately give us knowledge about what is effective in patient teaching and patient learning.

Obtaining Physician Support

What can I do if the physician doesn't want the patient to be taught?
How can I get the physician to approve of patient teaching done by our staff?

The physician is at times described as the "Captain of the Ship" when it comes to the control of a patient's care. This control, however, may be viewed by other health-care professionals as hindering their own patient-care efforts, especially when independent functioning is held as a value.

It should be obvious that all health-care team members need to work together to coordinate all their efforts in the best interests of the patient. Thus, the nurse, as well as other team members, needs to attain and maintain an effective, supporting relationship with the physician in order to achieve optimum learning outcomes.

The following chapter describes some of the reasons why it is important to have a cooperative relationship with the physician, as well as some of the reasons why physicians may resent patient education done by nurses. Strategies that may be useful in avoiding or preventing physician's resistance are cited, and examples are used as illustration.

The information in this chapter should help the reader to

1. *Describe why physician support of patient education is essential*
2. *List reasons why some physicians may be unsupportive*
3. *Discover why a specific physician does not support the patient education program*
4. *Describe ways to avoid causing physician resistance*
5. *List strategies for turning physician detractors into supporters*

Many members of the hospital's medical staff will encourage your efforts to instruct patients. Others, however, will be detractors, harshly critical of the idea and the practice of patient education by nurses.

The reasons for resistance are many. A nurse educator using wrong approaches with physicians or patients can create resistance. For example, one nurse educator complained, "How can I do my work if the doctors won't let their patients attend the program?" This nurse's whining tone, the fact that her concern seemed to center on herself rather than the patient, and her concept that patient education is a "program" to be "attended" all turned the physician off completely. It is not really surprising that this nurse had difficulty obtaining physician support.

Another doctor does not use his hospital's patient education program anymore. He stopped when one of his patients with incurable cancer was told by a well-meaning student of Dr. Kübler-Ross's work, "But you aren't supposed to be happy. You're still in the anger stage!"

This chapter should help you select the right approach to obtaining physician support.

WHY IS IT ESSENTIAL TO WORK WITH THE DOCTORS?

Surely no one would think that effective patient education could exist without physician involvement. Yet some nurses seem to think, "I know as much as the doctor does, and I'm going ahead with him or without him!" Don't let critical and obstructionist physicians force you into this error. There are substantive reasons why the physicians' role is important.

"This is My Patient." Patient education in the hospital setting is not going to be effective until we resolve the "my patient" issue. First of all, we must concede that the doctor has a point, considering the patient's total life and not just the brief hospital or clinic visit experience. This perspective helps us understand why the physician feels so strongly that "This is my patient." He may have seen the patient and several other family members through many medical problems over a long period of time.

Then we must help physicians understand that during a patient's hospitalization the doctor visits "his patients" only briefly during the day. The nurses and other hospital personnel are *also* entitled to think of "my patient" within the context of the current hospitalization. Hopefully, better understanding of what we both mean by "my patient" will lead us to speak of "our patient."

The Physician Writes the Order Sheet. The physician is the primary decision-maker in the care of an individual patient and is entitled to expect that hospital personnel will respond to his or her direction. The physician needs to be shown the value of your instructional activities because he or she controls when the patient will be discharged. Otherwise, the doctor may send the patient home before you are ready *or* before the patient is ready.

The Doctor is a Good Resource. Nurses always want to know, "Where can I find more patient education resources?" Usually they are thinking about audiovisual materials, brochures, and instruction booklets. Take advantage of the resources at hand! Experienced clinicians on the hospital's medical staff may be excellent resources, and their knowledge of clinical content is just the beginning. From years of practice in the community, they might help you modify clinical content to fit the needs of a particular patient population.

Some Facts of Life. You need the doctor's support. For one thing, you need the administration's support for your patient education activities because it controls the budget, and the administration needs the physician's support because the doctor decides which hospital to use. Thus, the doctor is a valuable advocate in obtaining administrative support. In addition, you will often need approval from the hospital's medical staff executive committee and from clinical department chiefs. For example, new patient record forms should be approved by the medical staff executive committee.

Remember the Patient. If the patient's doctor and the patient's nurses are not communicating about what the patient is being told, he or she will be confused. In the hassles of the real world, it will be easy to forget your main goal. Remind yourself daily that our purpose is truly effective education for the patient.

You May Underestimate the Physician. When a doctor says, "I'll instruct the patient in my office," the hospital nurse tends to assume that it will not be done. But many doctors have good rapport with patients and are effective patient educators. Do not assume that every physician ignores this important part of patient care just because some do. And do not make the error of assuming that if there is no formal program, then there is no effective patient learning.

WHY DO SOME DOCTORS RESIST PATIENT EDUCATION BY NURSES?

The following list can be used to help you discover the reasons for objection by a specific physician. The final section of this chapter will suggest some possible approaches to relieving these objections.

1. The doctor may be genuinely concerned about your ability and knowledge. He or she may believe that your clinical knowledge is superficial and that you may not be effective as an instructor.
2. The doctor may think your program is too standardized. He or she knows that effective patient instruction means putting the information in terms each patient can understand and making it relate to each individual patient's specific fears and questions. The doctor may be afraid you will teach what you are determined to teach rather than what the patient needs to learn.
3. The doctor may be *unaware* of what the patient needs to know.

4. The doctor may not trust the continuity of nursing care. Doctors see their responsibility as constant and yours as limited to one shift. The doctor wonders what happens when the nurse is not there. (Of course, there is an answer. But have you made sure the doctor knows the answer?)
5. The doctor may think nurses ought to be doing something else. Most doctors do not understand (indeed, are threatened by) the changes occurring in nursing.
6. The doctor may be responding to "the wrong approach." This can mean either the wrong approach to patient education or to the physician himself. Two examples of the wrong approach to patient education are given at the beginning of this chapter. The wrong approach to the physician, put simply, means that some nurses come on too strong. They act as if they want to replace the physician rather than to assist him or her and work in collaboration. They seem to enjoy "invading" many traditional physician prerogatives. Those nurses may have substituted personal goals for the goal of effective patient education.
7. The doctor may feel a threat to the "mystique of medicine." He or she may think, "The more the patients know, the less they will need me." The doctor, like everybody else, requires reassurance that he or she is needed.
8. The doctor may think patient education will make malpractice worse; "The more patients know, the more likely they are to find something to sue about." Actually, malpractice experts state that lack of rapport is a major cause of malpractice. Making the effort to help the patient understand his or her illness should decrease the incidence of malpractice suits.
9. The doctor's attitude may be a function of his or her specialty. A pediatrician knows the parent must understand that cough medicine should not be expected to completely suppress the cough. The better the parent understands, the fewer nuisance phone calls the doctor will get. The surgeon, on the other hand, may feel that removing a diseased organ solves the medical problem, and it is unimportant for the patient to understand how. But it is dangerous to generalize. And it is dangerous to assume that a gruff exterior precludes inner sensitivity. Some surgeons take a great deal of time to provide patients with an understanding of the nature of their illness, operation, and aftercare, and would do so even without legal emphasis on informed consent.
10. You may be experiencing one component of the doctor's reaction to the hospital. Many doctors are convinced that the government and the hospital are in a conspiracy to control his or her practice. For instance, third party reimbursement agencies may insist that the hospital provide information about the doctor's practice under threat of withholding payment from the hospital. And now you, a hospital nurse, want to come between the doctor and the patient! Demonstrate to the doctor that your interest in the patient is professional, not political.

HOW TO AVOID OR ELIMINATE THESE PROBLEMS

Identify and Work with Cooperative Physicians. Learn the attitudes of individual physicians. Do not try to save the world by being determined to convert the "hopeless" physician. Forget about him or her. Go ahead and work with the cooperative members of the hospital's medical staff. Even if the unsupportive physician is chief of the department, your best bet is still to work with cooperative physicians who will eventually either change the attitude of, or overrule, a truly recalcitrant chief.

Be Sure You and the Doctor Mean the Same Thing by "Patient Education." Are you both including all of the following in your definition?

1. Hospital procedure and routine
2. Nature of the illness
3. Expectations (prognosis)
4. Instructions for self-care
5. Level of activity
6. All aspects of medications, including purpose, consequences of not taking, how to obtain refills, and how long to take
7. What signs and symptoms should be reported to the physician
8. Follow-up instructions: When and where is the patient to talk to the physician next
9. Any special instructions to family members
10. Informed consent prior to an operative procedure
11. Special diets
12. An opportunity for the patient or family to ask questions.

Learn to Phrase Key Questions. If the physician objects to patient education, is he or she objecting to all the above components, or just to certain parts? Why does the doctor think some of these areas should be left up to him or her? Does he or she appreciate that certain areas, such as obtaining informed consent, cannot be left completely up to you?

Invite Input to Educational Content. Resolution of many problems begins when doctors become more familiar with your instructional activities—or, better yet, participate in development of content and methods. If audiovisual aids from outside sources are used with patients, there should be frequent opportunity for physicians to preview them. New materials should be selected jointly by physicians and nurses.

Content should be tailored to the individual physician and the individual patient. Those providing patient instruction should ask each physician, "What patient questions are the biggest problem for you? What would you like us to tell your patients?"

Provide Feedback from the Educational Session to the Physician. The physician should receive a written summary of the patient instruction provided, including notes about any specific questions that the patient asked and how they were answered.

Clarify What Requires an Order and What Does Not. One of the biggest helps in getting patient education started is to make the use of the program optional. Some nurses do not like the idea that an order is required for patient education, but an order is probably the best way to start. Then, as acceptance increases, the medical staff should support requiring a specific order that instruction *not* be given. (From the beginning, clarify that instruction about nursing care is a nursing function and does not require a doctor's order.)

Don't Be a Know-It-All. The doctor will feel more comfortable with your competency and professionalism if you exhibit a willingness to say, "I don't know." Those are hard but useful words.

Identify and Avoid "Red Flag Words." Find out what words are "red flags" to your doctors. Believe it or not, some physicians who are resistant to a "patient education " program, may agree to a " patient instruction" program. "Educating" the patients sounds too academic to them. "What my patient needs is simple instruction, not a complex lecture on pathologic physiology, differential diagnosis, and an update of current research efforts in the field."

You will notice that this chapter avoids the term patient education program. That term may lead us to compartmentalizing patient education—"Now it's time to be admitted. Now it's time to be operated on. Now it's time to be educated."

Patient education is not a program to be attended. All of us are imparting knowledge and attitudes to the patient whether we mean to or not. Doctors want you to be aware of this.

Be Consistent. If the doctor expects his or her patient to get certain information through the previously agreed-upon patient instruction activity, see that the patient gets it. If the doctor has a problem in the office because the patient did not receive information he or she counted on you to provide, that doctor may become a skeptic and a critic.

Emphasize Advantages to the Physician. Emphasize that effective patient instruction

1. Reduces legal liability
2. Helps the physician have good rapport with his patient
3. Reduces nuisance phone calls
4. Frees the physician's time for other uses
5. Reflects favorably on the physician as one who cares about his or her patients

Suggest Ways the Doctor Can Be Helpful. Some doctors might want to be supportive without knowing exactly how to be. The physician can demonstrate support by explaining to patients that teaching activities are shared by all health-care team members, including the nurse in the physician's office. Support is further demonstrated when the physician encourages other physicians to consider the importance of instruction given by nursing staff.

Learn the Right Organizational Approaches. Here is an example of a poor organizational approach that ended in disaster. The medical staff of a hospital was asked to approve a "patient discharge summary form for the nurses." The reason given was that it would help the nurses do what they had to do for the Joint Commission on Accreditation of Hospitals (JCAH). In the ensuing 40-minute discussion, more than one physician expressed his displeasure at this further attempt by the nursing staff to usurp physician prerogatives. More than one physician also objected to such a standardized approach when patient care is clearly an individualized activity. The key argument that defeated the proposal was that "the JCAH and the nurses aren't going to tell us how to practice medicine."

The following errors (at least) were made.

1. No nurse was present to emphasize that the form was not just a requirement but a helpful patient care aid.
2. There apparently was no physician input into the design of the form, and no attempt was made to acquaint at least a few supportive physicians with the form prior to the meeting.
3. The form was misnamed. A "discharge summary form for the nurses" is a red flag. The Discharge Summary, a summary of events during the hospitalization of an individual patient, has always been the physician's prerogative. Had the form been titled Patient Instruction Summary, the result might have been different.
4. It was not clarified that use of the form would be optional.
5. There was no indication in the presentation that modification to fit the habits and beliefs of specific physicians was possible.

A supportive physician can suggest proper organizational approaches to the medical staff.

Finally, Ask Instead of Telling. Few people fail to respond cooperatively to the right approach. Instead of telling the doctor "We're entitled to do this if we want to, you know," ask:

Doctor, I wonder if you are aware of some of the things we include in our patient instructions?

Doctor, do you think that if Mrs. Jones understands how to change her wound dressing, it might reduce the possibility of a wound infection?

Doctor, if we help your patient understand how to refill her prescription, do you think that might save you some nuisance phone calls?

Fine, doctor, we won't instruct your patient. By the way, I just wonder how you plan to get this information to the patient?

Doctor, I wonder if you know that your patient in the semiprivate room, whom you asked us not to instruct, is asking why her roommate is getting instruction and she is not?

IT'S A NECESSITY

Knowledge of educational theory and clinical content are not enough to implement effective patient education. You must also understand possible reasons for physician objections and be willing to work toward the goal of obtaining physician support.

David K. Solomon

19

The Role of the Pharmacist in Patient Teaching

Does the pharmacist have a role in systematized patient education programming?

How can the pharmacist help achieve patient learning outcomes?

Almost all patients who enter the health-care system have medications ordered for them. Regardless of whether the patient goes home with a prescription drug in hand or just takes medications while in the hospital, the patient needs to understand what he or she is taking and why. The patient who does need to continue drug therapy after discharge, however, has an even greater need to understand the chemical regimen that has been prescribed. The following chapter describes why the pharmacist is the most appropriate health-care professional for teaching patients about their medications. Various methods and techniques for patient medication counseling are presented, including an illustration of a Medication History form. Goals of medication counseling are presented, as well as a description of the types of information recommended for inclusion in counseling. Techniques and guidelines for medication counseling service illustrate how the pharmacist may accomplish counseling goals for patients as well as doctors, nurses, and other health-care professionals. Illustration of a medication counseling service is provided for three different settings, and several implications of the pharmacist's role in patient teaching are presented.

The information in this chapter should help the reader to

1. *Describe the responsibilities of the pharmacist in teaching patients about safe and effective use of medications*
2. *List elements of the patient's medication history*
3. *List the goals of medication counseling*

227

4. List areas of drug information recommended for inclusion in medication counseling
5. Describe techniques for counseling patients regarding drug therapy
6. Describe the role of the pharmacist as a resource for other health professionals
7. Describe how medication counseling can be conducted in various health-care settings
8. List three implications of the pharmacist's role in medication counseling

PHARMACISTS AND PATIENT TEACHING

Pharmacists, like all health-care professionals, are challenged to meet societal needs for effective and efficient health care. The National Center for Health Services Research and Development, Department of Health, Education, and Welfare stated in a report by its Task Force on the Pharmacist's Clinical Role that "the pharmacist is a health resource whose potential contribution to patient care and public health is grossly underdeveloped and which, thereby, is used ineffectively" [52]. This statement is amplified by Goddard [18], a physician who states, "I see the pharmacist as a professional resource person whose full potential is not being realized at the present time. . . . I strongly believe that the modern practice of medicine demands greater utilization of the knowledge and skills which only the pharmacist can offer."

In recent years there has been a trend to expand and increase the professional contributions of the pharmacist beyond his role as a dispenser of medications. If the thesis is accepted that drug therapy has been for some time and continues to be the prime modality of treatment for the ill, the pharmacist has a considerable responsibility to the patient to assure safe and effective use of medications.

One wonders how effective the medications are that physicians prescribe and pharmacists dispense if there is insufficient understanding on the part of the patient regarding the safe and effective use of these medications. This point is illustrated by the following situation: A physician presented a patient with five prescriptions and went over each one (not the name, just the directions). When the medications were dispensed by the pharmacist, all were labeled "Take as directed" [55]. Such experiences continue to occur more frequently than most physicians and pharmacists would care to admit. Too often the physician assumes that the pharmacist has discussed medications with the patient, and the pharmacist assumes the physician has already discussed medications. As a result, the patient receives little information, if any, and is poorly informed about his drug regimen.

Potential consequences of inadequate medication information provided to patients include noncompliance to drug regimens, increased morbidity and mortality, and increased patient readmissions to hospitals.

The literature is replete with studies documenting the failure of patients to comply with prescribed medication regimens. In a review article on the subject, Stewart and Cluff [66] reported the percent of patients failing to take their medications as directed, with a few exceptions, ranged from 20 to 82 percent.

Regarding efforts to increase patient compliance, various methods and techniques have been tried such as pill calendar dispensers and medication monitors [41, 42]. However, perhaps the most logical method is patient education. Unless a patient understands the importance of drug therapy and the correct methods of administration, he or she will likely feel that the drug regimen is an annoying factor that interferes with normal activities. On the other hand, if the patient becomes an active participant in the drug therapy, he or she is more likely to follow the prescribed regimen and make fewer medication errors [14]. Other sources have also advocated patient education specifically related to drug regimens as a remedy for noncompliance [20, 38].

The understanding the patient has concerning prescribed drugs and their correct administration is often directly related to patient progress subsequent to discharge from a hospital. Indeed, the entire efforts of the health team may be futile if the patient fails to take medications correctly while at home.

The Task Force on the Pharmacist's Clinical Role [52] has indicated that the pharmacist should consult with patients to review instructions for proper home use of medications. The American Society of Hospital Pharmacists indicates that "pharmacists, as well as other health professionals, have a responsibility to properly inform patients about their drug therapy" [65].

The Dichter Study reports a strong desire on the part of patients for the return of the personal pharmacist and the reestablishment of a professional relationship between the pharmacist and the patient [10].

METHODS AND TECHNIQUES FOR PATIENT MEDICATION COUNSELING

Medication History

The first function prior to providing drug information to patients via consultation is to obtain a thorough and accurate medication history. The purpose of the history is to review current and past (over the previous six months) use of both legend and over-the-counter (OTC) drugs. Specifically screened are drug allergies, drugs that may interact with projected medication regimens or procedures, and compliance to medication regimens.

A simple format is best (see the Patient Medication History Form in the Resource Materials section) and this information should then become a part of the patient's chart. When questioning the patient for past and current drug use, the pharmacist may find that a body systems approach works well. The pharmacist asks if any medications are taken for the circulatory system, the respiratory system, or the sensory organs. Care should be exercised to probe for use of OTC drugs; due to their common usage and widespread availability, many patients do not consider preparations such as aspirin, antacids, and cough-cold combinations to be drugs. However, they are drugs in every sense of the word and have the potential, as with prescription drugs, to generate beneficial as well as detrimental effects.

The medication history provides baseline information to facilitate further treatment with drug regimens and is an aid to the medication counseling process to help individualize the information provided to patients.

Patient Medication Counseling

Simply defined, patient medication counseling is a pharmacist or other health professional meeting the medication and health related informational needs of a patient by communicating with that patient. The goals of medication counseling are to:

1. Instill in the patient the importance of taking medications as prescribed
2. Convey to the patient pertinent information with regard to medications he or she will be self-administering
3. Establish a good relationship with the patient as a foundation for future interaction and consultations
4. Attempt, by the above measures to increase compliance and patient drug knowledge regarding a medication regimen, thereby minimizing drug related problems and therapeutic failures

What Information to Share

Information provided to patients should address the following areas of drug information as outlined in the "Statement on Pharmacist-Conducted Patient Counseling" [65]:

1. Name (trademark, generic, common synonym or other descriptive name)
2. Intended use and expected action
3. Route, dosage form, dosage and administration schedule
4. Special directions for preparation
5. Special directions for administration
6. Precautions to be observed during administration
7. Common side effects that may be encountered, including their avoidance and action required if they occur
8. Techniques for self-monitoring of drug therapy
9. Proper storage
10. Potential drug-drug or drug-food interactions or other therapeutic contraindications
11. Prescription refill information
12. Action to be taken in the event of a missed dose
13. Any other information peculiar to the specific patient or drug

Who Should Receive Counseling and When Counseling Should Be Conducted

Every patient who receives medication as a part of his or her treatment regimen should be counseled regarding that medication. In the case of new prescription medications for patients, all pertinent information about the drug should be provided in a comprehensive manner. In the case of refilled prescription medications a thorough yet briefer consultation may be indicated in order to review information previously discussed. The time of prescription renewal provides the pharmacist with the opportunity to follow patient progress through evaluation and assessment of drug effectiveness, observation for side effects, and compliance to the regimen. This is advantageous in the case of patients with chronic disease states who have only infrequent physician appointments yet are maintained on drug regimens for months.

In the case of patients being discharged from the hospital, if the pharmacist has shared information with the patient during the hospital stay, at discharge a summary, preferably in the privacy of the patient's room, will suffice.

If it is not possible to counsel each patient due to staffing or workload demands, a selective technique may be utilized to counsel patients who are self-administering a new prescription drug; potent drug entities such as digitalis preparations, anti-coagulants, and steroids; medications with complicated dosage regimens; and a large number of concurrent medications (prescription or OTC).

Portions of the previously mentioned 13 areas of drug information do appear on the prescription label; however, this information alone has proven inadequate and has been documented as a source of misinterpretations by patients. On occasion, this has been a contributing factor to noncompliance, therapeutic failure, and drug toxicity [3,17,19,34,35,50,55].

When counseling patients regarding drug therapy, the pharmacist should be a good communicator and a good listener. In addition to communicating verbally, the pharmacist should interpret nonverbal communications of the patient such as tone of voice, posture, and facial expressions. Of primary importance is the establishment of a positive "therapeutic climate." This may be achieved in part by maintaining an active, alert interest in what the patient says and does. The patient should feel the pharmacist is interested in him and what he has to say; such interest creates a situation in which it is easy for the patient to talk. Looking at the patient and maintaining eye contact is one way of showing interest. Other qualities the pharmacist should demonstrate include tactfulness, consideration, empathy, and kindness. Maintaining confidentiality of patient information is also necessary. These actions on the part of the pharmacist will help to foster a mutual relationship with the patient built upon understanding and trust [11,22,29,70].

The excessive use of medical and pharmacy terminology should be avoided when counseling patients concerning drug therapy; lay terminology should be used when possible. Also, in explaining instructions to patients about how and when to administer medications, the pharmacist should take care to observe the patient's everyday schedule and habits, for example, his work routine and when or how often he eats meals. The pharmacist should use his or her knowledge of drug absorption rates to arrange medication schedules that will better assure compliance and provide maximum benefit of the drug.

There are several methods of providing drug information to patients including verbal communication, audiovisual materials, printed materials, and written instructions. Audiovisual cassettes and graphics should be reinforced with verbal communication and patient feedback to ascertain patient comprehension of information. Advantages exist in combining some of these methods. Verbal information (see Sample Notes for Verbal Consultation in the Resource Materials section) can be supplemented and reinforced with written information (see the Sheet for Written Reinforcement in the Resource Materials section) which in turn may be retained and referred to at a later time by the patient [6,25,37,40,54,67,71,72]. Since the consultation should not be one way only, the pharmacist should allow and even encourage questions from the patient. It may be advantageous at times to involve family members of the patient in the consultation in order to better assure proper understanding of the information provided. When counseling, the pharmacist should remain flexible and experiment with various approaches to convey needed information to patients.

THE PHARMACIST AS A RESOURCE FOR NURSES, PHYSICIANS, AND OTHER HEALTH PROFESSIONALS

The pharmacist has an opportunity and indeed a responsibility to interface and assist with inservice education programs for other health practitioners that will facilitate promotion of the safe and appropriate use of drugs in the treatment of patients [4]. Linton has described an educational program model to assist with providing inservice education to health professionals [28].

As a result of changing roles and responsibilities in the health professions, more hospital personnel are becoming involved in the solution of drug-related problems. Physicians' assistants, nurse practitioners, nurses, respiratory therapists, and intravenous therapists are among those whose need for formal drug-related education is now recognized by accrediting bodies within these professions, by governmental licensing and regulatory agencies, and by internal institutional requirements [2].

Pharmacists have been involved with multidisciplinary educational approaches to chronic disease states. Respiratory therapy services as well as treatment of chronic obstructive pulmonary disease (COPD) have received attention. With one program involving COPD, the respiratory therapist provides instruction for proper use and maintenance of oxygen equipment and in the safe handling of medical gases used in the home for respiratory therapy. The pharmacist conducts a medication history, consults with the patient, and monitors drug therapy. The physical therapist gives instructions on techniques for deep breathing and coughing and for postural drainage. The social worker plans with other health professionals to help the patient and family cope emotionally, socially, and economically with the chronic illness [39].

Basically, throughout the hospital the pharmacist should participate as a resource for development of drug related educational programs for health professionals and patients.

ENVIRONMENT FOR MEDICATION COUNSELING AND PATIENT TEACHING

Medication counseling and patient teaching may be conducted in various practice settings and at multiple levels of patient care—from inpatient through ambulatory status.

Inpatient Care

Self-medication programs for patients with various disease states are currently underway in a variety of institutional settings, and the pharmacist can assist by coordinating these activities. Self-medication programs have been instituted for psychiatric [21,24], rehabilitation [23,51], long-term care [27,32,53], cardiac [5,62], obstetrics [30], postsurgical [45], epileptic [44], and spinal-cord injury [58] patients. Advantages for such programs include:

1. Saving time for pharmacists, physicians, and nurses and convenience for patients
2. Teaching patients about medications and proper administration in a controlled institutional environment
3. Building self-confidence in patients by increasing responsibility for themselves

Discharge Planning

It is not uncommon for the typical patient being discharged with medications from a hospital to make his way to the pharmacy, pick up his discharge medications, which have been neatly placed in a bag, and go home. On arriving at home, the revelation when opening the bag may be very confusing to the patient as to which medicine to take first, which to take before or after meals, and so on.

Additionally, with progressive drug distribution systems such as unit-dose, the inpatient receives medications almost automatically, yet he is expected to duplicate these oftentimes complex regimens on his own, when he makes the transition into self-care.

Patient instruction at the time of discharge is easier in the hospital environment when the pharmacist has access to the patient's medical chart. The pharmacist in consulting with discharge patients should

1. Review the patient's chart (note discharge summary, recent lab tests, nursing notes, and other pertinent information)
2. Compare orders for medications to be sent home with nursing notes or pharmacy patient medication profile to note changes in regimen
3. Use data collected as a baseline; then proceed with individualized discharge patient medication consultation

Home Health Care

Home health services can best be described as an extension of institutional care to the patient's home. Home health nurses are responsible for executing treatment plans in much the same manner as for hospitalized patients, except that nursing care is performed in the patient's home on an intermittent basis.

Pharmacists may provide services directly to home health patients or indirectly through the visiting nurse. One study documented a need for comprehensive services such as medication dispensing, discharge medication consultations, and medication profile maintenance [63]. Some reports have also outlined responsibilities of the pharmacists in providing services to home-care patients and personnel [1,8,13,16,63]. Others have described an ongoing drug information consultation service and inservice education regarding pharmaceuticals for a visiting nurse association [8,10].

Ambulatory Care

Pharmacists provide services to ambulatory patients through outpatient clinics, primary care clinics, and health maintenance organizations. In the course of these activities, medication consultations are conducted with patients. There are several descriptive articles in the literature that outline medication consultation programs for ambulatory patients [7,26,49,52,61,69].

Studies have shown that providing medication information and consultation to ambulatory patients can increase compliance and reduce the incidence of medication errors [9,12,31,48]. Two controlled investigations showed that private medication consulting, including verbal and written information by a pharmacist, reduced medication misuse significantly and that the pharmacist had a real impact on improving patient understanding of the medication regimen [33,64]. Another study with antibiotic regimens demonstrated that those patients who received written information on an auxiliary label and a one page fact sheet from a pharmacist were significantly more compliant than those patients who did not receive this information [60].

IMPLICATIONS

Costs and Reimbursement

In this era of cost-containment, it is incumbent upon all health practitioners to provide services in a cost-effective fashion. Costs for patient education functions of the pharmacist are variable but dependent primarily upon the time spent with patients per consultation [36,43]. As previously discussed, patient understanding of medication regimens can improve compliance, reduce hospital readmissions, and decrease drug related problems. Failure to follow through by the patient in these areas can be expensive. Research has shown that pharmacist-patient counseling can, in fact, result in significant cost savings to the patient [57,95].

Pharmacist reimbursement in the majority of cases is associated exclusively with dispensing an actual drug product and not with provision of services such as patient consultation. However, some third party payers are now realizing the cost benefit of pharmacists providing such services. Reimbursement methodologies have been developed for recognizing the patient education functions of the pharmacist for patients with medical problems ranging from hemophilia to home parenteral hyperalimentation [15,47,68].

Pharmacolegal

It is expected that as the pharmacist assumes additional responsibilities and functions for the care of patients, his or her liability will increase proportionately as will the sequela of malpractice litigation.

The ramifications of patient package inserts (PPIs) for drugs is yet unclear. The PPIs do imply informed consent on the assumption of three responsibilities: the drug manufacturer has the responsibility to supply the PPI; the pharmacist has the responsibility to dispense the PPI; and the patient has the responsibility to read the PPI. The list of drugs that require dispensing with the PPI undoubtedly will grow in the future. While the PPI constitutes a method of informing the patient about a particular medication, experience as well as the literature indicates that verbal and other reinforcement methods are needed to properly educate patients concerning their medications [46,73]. Already several states require by law that pharmacists consult with patients regarding their drug therapy when prescriptions are dispensed.

Staff to Conduct Patient Medication Teaching

It is clear that there is a need for greater collaboration among health professionals to more effectively accomplish the goal of having patients more knowledgeable regarding their drug regimens. In the case of pharmacy specifically, it will be necessary for pharmacists to more effectively utilize supportive personnel such as pharmacy technicians to enable pharmacists to do more in the area of patient education.

REFERENCES

1. Baumgartner, R. P., et al. Home health agencies and the pharmacist. *Journal of the American Pharmaceutical Association,* NS14 : 7 : 355, 1974.
2. Beste, D. F., et al. New services generate teaching role—pharmacy. *Hospitals,* 47 : 141, 1973.
3. Brands, A. Complete directions for prescription medications. *Journal of the American Pharmaceutical Association,* NS6 : 634, 1966.
4. Britton, H. L. The pharmacist's role in inservice education programs. *Hospital Formulary Management,* 33 (Oct.), 1973.
5. Buchanan, E. C., et al. A self-medication program for cardiology inpatients. *American Journal of Hospital Pharmacy,* 29 : 928, 1972.
6. Burkhart, V. P., and Lamy, P. P. Patient education using audio-visual aids. *Hospital Formulary Management,* 30 (Jul.), 1973.
7. Canada, A. T., and Iazzetta, S. M. Pharmacy care for ambulatory patients. *Journal of the American Pharmaceutical Association,* NS14 : 1 : 18, 1974.
8. Cardoni, A. A., et al. Drug information consultation services for visiting nurses. *American Journal of Hospital Pharmacy,* 31 : 1057, 1974.
9. Chubb, J. M., and Winship, H. W. The pharmacist's role in preventing medication errors made by cardiac and hyperlipoproteinemic outpatients. *Drug Intelligence and Clinical Pharmacy,* 8 : 430, 1974.
10. Communicating the Value of Comprehensive Pharmaceutical Services to the Consumer. A Motivational Research Study by the Dichter Institute for Motivational Research. Commissioned by the American Pharmaceutical Association, 1973.

11. Covington, T. R., and Whitney, H. A. K.   Patient-pharmacist communication techniques. *Drug Intelligence and Clinical Pharmacy,* 5 : 370, 1971.
12. Dickey, F. F., et al.   Pharmacist counseling increases drug regimen compliance. *Hospitals,* 49 : 85, 1975.
13. Eastman, P. F.   Pharmaceutical services for home health agencies. *Journal of the American Pharmaceutical Association,* NS11 : 7 : 391, 1971.
14. Franke, D. E., and Whitney, H. A. K.   *Perspectives in Clinical Pharmacy.* Hamilton, Ill.: Drug Intelligence Publications, 1972. Pp. 37–59.
15. Fudge, R. P., and Vlasses, P. H.   Third party reimbursement for pharmacist instruction about antihemophilic factor. *American Journal of Hospital Pharmacy,* 34 : 831, 1977.
16. Gerson, C. K.   The team approach to home health care. *Journal of the American Pharmaceutical Association,* NS18 : 11 : 37, 1978.
17. Gibson, M.   Patient instruction by private consultation. *Journal of the American Pharmaceutical Association,* NS6 : 636, 1966.
18. Goddard, J. L.   University of Michigan Annual Pharmacy Lecture, 1967.
19. Greiner, G.   The pharmacist's role in patient discharge planning. *American Journal of Hospital Pharmacy,* 29 : 72, 1972.
20. Hecht, A. B.   Self-medication, inaccuracy, and what can be done. *Nursing Outlook,* 4 : 30, 1970.
21. Henderson, J. H.   Self-medication in a psychiatric hospital. *Lancet* 1 : 1055, 1967.
22. Ivey, M., et al.   Communication techniques for patient instruction. *American Journal of Hospital Pharmacy,* 32 : 828, 1975.
23. Johnson, E. W., et al.   Self-medication for a rehabilitation ward. *Archives of Physical Medicine and Rehabilitation,* 51 : 300, 1970.
24. Lacerva, S. P., and Kennard, E. A.   Self-medication: Another step toward self-responsibility. *Mental Hospital* 11 : 43, 1960.
25. Lamy, P. P.   Audio-visual aids in patient instructions. *Journal of the American Pharmaceutical Association,* NS11 : 9 : 486, 1971.
26. Lesshafft, C. T.   An exploration of the pharmacist's role in outpatient clinics. *Journal of the American Pharmaceutical Association,* NS10 : 4 : 205, 1970.
27. Libow, L. S., and Mehl, B.   Self-administration of medications in hospital or extended care facilities. *Journal of the American Geriatric Society,* 18 : 81, 1970.
28. Linton, C. B.   An educational program model for hospitalwide education. *Southern Hospitals,* 16 (Mar.–Apr.), 1974.
29. Love, D. W., et al.   Teaching interviewing skills to pharmacy residents. *American Journal of Hospital Pharmacy,* 35 : 1073, 1978.
30. Lucarotti, R. L., et al.   Pharmacist-coordinated self-administration medication program on an obstetrical service. *American Journal of Hospital Pharmacy,* 30 : 1147, 1973.
31. Ludy, J. A., et al.   The patient pharmacist interaction in two ambulatory settings—it's relationship to patient satisfaction and drug misuse. *Drug Intelligence and Clinical Pharmacy,* 11 : 81, 1977.
32. Madaio, A., and Clarke, T. R.   Benefits of a self-medication program in a long term care facility. *Hospital Pharmacy,* 12 : 72, 1977.
33. Madden, E. E.   Evaluation of outpatient pharmacy patient counseling. *Journal of the American Pharmaceutical Association,* NS13 : 437, 1973.
34. Malahy, B.   The effect of instruction and labeling on the number of medication errors made by patients at home. *American Journal of Hospital Pharmacy,* 23 : 283, 1966.
35. Mazzulo, J. M., et al.   Variations in interpretation of prescription instructions—the need for improved prescribing habits. *Journal of the American Medical Association,* 227 : 929, 1974.
36. McGhan, W. F., et al.   Cost-benefit and cost-effectiveness methodologies for evaluation of innovative pharmaceutical services. *American Journal of Hospital Pharmacy,* 35 : 133, 1978.

37. McKenney, J. M.   Counseling techniques on the use of home care medications. *The New Environment of Pharmacy*, p. 8 (Jan.–Feb.), 1977.
38. Melmon, K. L., and Morrelli, H. F.   *Clinical Pharmacology*. New York: MacMillan, 1972. Pp. 555–577.
39. Miller, M. B., and Conrad, W. F.   Pharmacist involvement in an education program for patients with chronic obstructive pulmonary disease. *American Journal of Hospital Pharmacy*, 32 : 909, 1975.
40. Morris, R. W., et al.   Technical and theoretical aspects of patient counseling using audio-visual aids. *Drug Intelligence and Clinical Pharmacy*, 9 : 485, 1975.
41. Moulding, T., et al.   Supervision of outpatient drug therapy with the medication monitor. *Annals of Internal Medicine*, 73 : 559, 1970.
42. Moulding, T., et al.   Vertical pill calendar dispenser and medication monitor for improving the self-administration of drugs. *Tubercle*, 48 : 32, 1967.
43. Munzenberger, P. J., et al.   A cost impact analysis of selected clinical pharmacy function in three hospitals. *American Journal of Hospital Pharmacy*, 31 : 947, 1974.
44. Nelson, W. J., et al.   Comprehensive self-medication program for epileptic patients. *American Journal of Hospital Pmarmacy*, 35 : 798, 1978.
45. Newcomer, D. R., and Anderson, R. W.   Effectiveness of a combined drug self-administration and patient teaching program. *Drug Intelligence and Clinical Pharmacy*, 8 : 374, 1974.
46. Newman, D.   Pharmacists: The next deep pocket: malpractice mania hits pharmacy practice. *American Pharmacy (Washington)* NS18 : 11 : 14, 1978.
47. Nold, E. G., and Pathak, D. S.   Third-party reimbursement for clinical pharmacy services : Philosophy and practice. *American Journal of Hospital Pharmacy*, 34 : 823, 1977.
48. Paulson, P. T., et al.   Medication data sheets—an aid to patient education. *Drug Intelligence and Clinical Pharmacy*, 10 : 448, 1976.
49. Plant, J.   Educating the elderly in safe medication use. *Hospitals*, 5 : 97, 1977.
50. Powell, J. R., et al.   Inadequately written prescriptions: "As Directed" prescriptions analyzed. *Journal of the American Medical Association*, 226 : 999, 1973.
51. Reibel, E. M.   Study to determine the feasibility of a self-medication program for patients at a rehabilitation center. *Nursing Research* 18 : 65, 1969.
52. Report of Task Force on the Pharmacist's Clinical Role. Drug Related Studies Program, National Center for Health Services Research and Development, Health Services and Mental Health Administration, Department of Health, Education, and Welfare, Rockville, Md., *HSRD Briefs* No. 4 (Spring), 1972.
53. Roberts, C. J., and Miller, W. A.   Clinical pharmacy, self-administration, the technician drug administration services in a 72-bed hospital. *Drug Intelligence and Clinical Pharmacy*, 6 : 408, 1972.
54. Romankiewicz, J. A., et al.   Development of patient medication instruction cards. *American Journal of Hospital Pharmacy*, 33 : 928, 1976.
55. Rosenburg, S. G.   A case for patient education. *Hospital Formulary Mangement*, 6 : 14, 1971.
56. Ruzevick, M., and Trudeau, T. W.   Dealing with patient medication noncompliance through drug counseling. *Hospital Pharmacy*, 12 : 295, 1977.
57. Ryan, R. B., et al.   Economic justification of pharmacist involvement in patient medication consultation. *American Journal of Hospital Pharmacy*, 32 : 389, 1975.
58. Sather, M. R., et al.   Educating patients on a spinal cord injury unit for self-medication. *Hospital Pharmacy*, 11 : 14, 1976.
59. Schneider, P.   The pharmacist's role in inpatient and home care hyperalimentation programs. *Hospital Pharmacy*, 13 : 71, 1978.
60. Sharpe, T. R., and Mikeal, R. L.   Patient compliance with antibiotic regimens. *American Jouranl of Hospital Pharmacy*, 31 : 479, 1974.
61. Smith, D. L., et al.   A patient information system in an out-patient clinic. *Canadian Journal of Hospital Pharmacy*, 165 (Sept.–Oct.), 1974.

62. Soflin, D., et al.   Development and evaluation of an individualized patient education program about digoxin. *American Journal of Hospital Pharmacy,* 34 : 367, 1977.
63. Solomon, D. K., et al.   Pharmaceutical services to improve drug therapy for home health care patients. *American Journal of Hospital Pharmacy,* 35 : 553, 1978.
64. Solomon, D. K., et al.   An improved utilization of the pharmacist in ambulatory health care. Presented at the 10th Annual Midyear Clinical Meeting, American Society of Hospital Pharmacists, Washington, D.C., Dec. 10, 1975.
65. Statement on Pharmacist-Conducted Patient Counseling: American Society of Hospital Pharmacists. *American Journal of Hospital Pharmacy,* 33 : 644, 1976.
66. Stewart, R. B., and Cluff, L. E.   A review of medication errors and compliance in ambulant patients. *Clinical Pharmacological Therapy,* 13 : 4, 1972.
67. Temkin, L. A., et al.   Communicating information to the ambulant patient. *Journal of American Pharmaceutical Association,* NS15 : 9 : 488, 1975.
68. Touquan, S.   Clinical pharmacy and blue cross plans: Reimbursement and support of innovative pharmacy programs. *Hospital Pharmacy,* 12 : 22, 1977.
69. Weibert, R. T., and Dee, D. A.   A successful program for patient drug education. *Hospital Formulary Management,* 110 (Feb.), 1977.
70. Welk, P. G., et al.   The technology of patient counseling. *Hospital Pharmacy,* 9 : 224, 1974.
71. Welk, P. G., et al.   A comparison of methods to educate patients. *Hospital Pharmacy,* 10 : 240, 1974.
72. White, S. J., et al.   Teaching patients to administer their own eye, ear, and nose medications. *Hospital Pharmacy,* 9 : 149, 1974.
73. Willig, S. H.   Legal considerations for the pharmacist undertaking new drug consultation responsibilities. *Food, Drug, Cosmetic Law Journal,* 25 : 10 : 444, 1970.

Resource Materials

WRITTEN MEDICATION INSTRUCTIONS*

1. Patient Medication Instruction Cards, Department of Pharmacy, The New York Hospital, Cornell Medical Center, 525 East 68th Street, New York 10021.
2. Medication Instruction Cards, Department of Pharmacy, Rhode Island Hospital, Providence, Rhode Island.
3. Medication Instruction Sheets, Department of Pharmacy, University of Kansas Medical Center, College of Health Sciences and Hospital School of Medicine, Kansas City, Kansas 64108.
4. Medication Instruction Cards, Ambulatory Patient Pharmacy, Sunnybrook Hospital, 2075 Bayview Avenue, Toronto, Ontario M4N 3M5.
5. Prescription Warning Labels, Pharmasystems, 1 Jasper Avenue, Toronto, Ontario M6N 2M9.
6. Monthly Medication Instruction Sheet, Adria Laboratories of Canada Ltd., 4500 Dixie Road, Mississauga, Ontario L4W 1V7.

*The author acknowledges the assistance of Dorothy L. Smith, Pharm.D.; Assistant Professor of Clinical Pharmacy, University of Toronto and Coordinator of Ambulatory Pharmacy Care, Sunnybrook Hospital, in compiling this list.

7. Drug Consultation Guide-III, Drug Intelligence Publications, Hamilton, Illinois 62341.
8. Medication Instruction Sheets, Manitoba Pharmaceutical Association, Winnipeg, Manitoba

BROCHURES AND BOOKLETS

1. "Department of Pharmacy Services," Departmant of Pharmacy, Lakeside Hospital, Kansas City, Missouri 64131.
2. "Pharmacy Services St. Joseph's Hospital," Department of Pharmacy, St. Joseph's Hospital, 350 N. Wilmot Road, Tuscon, Arizona 85711.
3. 24-page brochure intended to acquaint the patient with the hospital, Department of Pharmacy, Temple University Hospital, Philadelphia, PA 19140.
4. "Understanding Your Prescription," American Society of Hospital Pharmacists, 4630 Montgomery Avenue, Washington, D.C. 20014.
5. "Help Your Physician Help Your Breathing Problems," Dr. C. C. Gray, Executive Medical Director, Ontario Thoracic Society, Toronto, Ontario.
6. "Ambulatory Patient Pharmacy"
   "How To Use Your Medications Safely"
   "Drug Therapy in Rheumatoid Arthritis"
   "Drug Therapy in Diabetes Mellitus"
   "Drug Therapy in Hypertension"
   "The Safe Use of Nonprescription Drugs"
   Ambulatory Patient Pharmacy, Sunnybrook Hospital, 2075 Bayview Avenue, Toronto, Ontario M4N 3M5.
7. "Consumer's Guide To Self-Medication," Sarnia Pharmacy Limited, 206 Maxwell Street, Sarnia, Ontario.
8. "Patient Medication Information," Department of Pharmacy, Medical College of Virginia Hospitals, Richmond, Virginia.
9. "Your Good Health and the Pharmacist In Your Hospital," American Society of Hospital Pharmacists, 4630 Montogomery Avenue, Washington, D.C. 20014.
10. "Read The Label on Home Medicines," The Proprietary Association, 1700 Pennsylvania Avenue, N.W., Washington, D.C. 20006.
11. "The Medicines Your Doctor Prescribes—A Guide For Consumers," Pharmaceutical Manufacturers Association, 1155 Fifteenth Street, N.W., Washington, D.C. 20005.
12. "Anticoagulants, Your Physician And You," American Heart Association, 7320 Greenville Avenue, Dallas, Texas 75231.
13. "Hard Shell Facts About Your Medicine," Consumer Health Education Department, Perth Amboy General Hospital, 530 New Brunswick Avenue, Perth Amboy, New Jersey 08800.

FOREIGN LANGUAGE TRANSLATIONS

1. Spanish-English Phrase Book, Lillian Butovsky, Language Training Advisor, Citizenship Branch, Parliament Bldgs., Queens Park, Toronto, Ontario M7A 2R9.
2. Common Foreign Label Instructions, Canadian Pharmaceutical Association, 175 College Street, Toronto, Ontario M5T 1P8.

AUDIOVISUAL PROGRAMS

1. Digoxin Education Program (Slide/tape audiovisual presentation). Inpatient Pharmacy Services, University Hospital, University of Nebraska Medical Center, Omaha, Nebraska.
2. Common Prescription Drugs: Instructions for Patients, Medical Audiovisual Service, Arizona Medical Center, University of Arizona, Tuscon, Arizona 85724.

PROGRAMMED INSTRUCTIONS

1. "Care and Treatment of the Diabetic, A Programmed Instruction Text for Pharmacists and Other Health Professionals," Continuing Pharmacy Education, University of Minnesota, Minneapolis, Minnesota.

BOOKS AND BIBLIOGRAPHIES ON PATIENT COMPLIANCE AND PATIENT EDUCATION RELATING TO MEDICATIONS

1. Sackett, D. L., and Haynes, R. B. *Compliance With Therapeutic Regimens.* Baltimore: The Johns Hopkins University Press, 1976.
2. Smith, D. L. *Medication Guide For Patient Counseling.* Philadelphia: Lea and Febiger, 1977.
3. Sackett, D. L. *Workshop/Symposium On Compliance.* Hamilton, Ontario: McMaster University, 1977.
4. Davis, R. L. *Patient Education Workshop: Summary Report.* Atlanta: Center for Disease Control, Community Program Development Division, Bureau of Health Education, 1977.
5. *Patient Education Resource List.* Chicago: American Hospital Association, 1976.
6. Griffith, H. W. *Instructions for Patients.* Philadelphia: Saunders, 1975.
7. The Pharmacist's Role in Patient Compliance, Pharmacy Intelligence Center, American Pharmaceutical Association, Washington, D.C., 1977.
8. Burgess, G. D. Patient Health Education—A Bibliography, Veterans Administration Center, Temple, Texas, 1976.
9. *Medication Teaching Manual: A Guide For Patient Counseling.* Washington, D.C.: American Society of Hospital Pharmacists, 1978.
10. Strauss, S. *Patient Dosage Instructions.* Ambler, Pa.: Lea Publications, 1973.

Le

The Role of the Pharmacist 241

BOOKS ON TECHNIQUES OF PATIENT INTERVIEWING

1. Bernstein, L., Bernstein, R. S., and Dana, R. H. *Interviewing: A Guide For Health Professionals* (2nd ed.). New York: Appleton-Century-Crofts, 1974.
2. Froelick, R. E., and Bishop, F. M. *Medical Interviewing—A Programmed Manual* (2nd ed.). St. Louis: Mosby, 1972.
3. Johnson, M. A. *Developing The Art Of Understanding* (2nd ed.). New York: Springer, 1972.
4. Purtilo, R. *The Allied Health Professional And The Patient.* Philadelphia: Saunders, 1973.
5. Orlando, I. J. *The Dynamic Nurse-Patient Relationship.* New York: Putnam, 1961.
6. Enelow, A. J., and Swisher, S. N. *Interviewing And Patient Care.* New York: Oxford University Press, 1972.
7. Ujhely, G. B. *The Nurse And Her Problem Patients.* New York: Springer, 1967.

SAMPLE NOTES FOR VERBAL CONSULTATION

Hydrochlorothiazide (Oretic)

Hydroclorothiazide is a diuretic/antihypertensive medicine. Diuretic means that it is a medicine designed to help lose excess accumulations of fluids from the body. It produces the desired effect by acting on the kidneys to cause the excretion of more than the usual amount of fluid. Antihypertensive means that it is a medicine helpful in lowering the blood pressure of people with hypertension, which is high blood pressure. The dosage of Hydrochlorothiazide must be individualized to meet your needs. Therefore you must follow directions very closely to obtain the safest and best results. This medicine has been prescribed for you to take because of one or both of its actions, and if it is taken as prescribed, it should be safe and effective in treating your condition.

1. Hydrochlorothiazide should be taken by mouth with meals or shortly after meals to avoid stomach distress.
2. Take only the amount of medicine your doctor has prescribed for each dose. Never take more than the prescribed dose. (Explain dose)
3. Take each dose at the time interval prescribed to obtain the best results. (Explain time)
4. Occasionally, while losing extra fluid, the body may also lose too much potassium. To keep your body from becoming too low on this important chemical you should eat foods with high potassium concentrations such as oranges, grapefruit, bananas, and apricots. Or your medication can be taken with a glass of orange juice. (Does not apply to the patients receiving adequate potassium supplement by prescribed medications).
5. If while taking this medicine you experience muscular weakness, dryness of the mouth, thirst, drowsiness or restlessness, muscle pains or cramps, or if you feel dizzy when you stand up, contact your doctor.
6. If your urine output drops below what you are accustomed to passing on any day, *stop* taking Hydrochlorothiazide and notify your doctor at once.
7. Do not give any of your medicine to other people.
8. Store this medicine in a cool and dry place in the container you received from the pharmacy, safely out of the reach of children.

SHEET FOR WRITTEN REINFORCEMENT

Date _____

Name _____
Medicine (name) _____
For (purpose) _____
How much (dose) _____

When to take medicine _____
_____
_____

Storage _____

Refill information _____
Remarks _____
_____
_____
_____

Contact your pharmacist or physician if you have any problems or questions about your medicine.

Pharmacist _____

PATIENT MEDICATION HISTORY FORM

Patient name _____
Medication allergies and hypersensitivities (name of drug and nature of reaction)
_____
_____
_____

Current prescription medications self-administering (include dosage)
_____   _____
_____   _____

Current OTC medications self-administering (include dosage)
_____   _____
_____   _____
_____   _____

Impressions and comments
_____
_____
_____

Pharmacist _____

Rebecca R. Martin
Sen Yee

20

The Librarian and Patient Education

What do I do if a patient wants to go to the hospital's medical library?
Does the hospital's librarian have any role in patient education programming?

The library is one of the most important adult education institutions in the United States. Benjamin Franklin established one of the first subscription libraries in this nation in 1731 (The Library Association of Philadelphia), and since that date it has been relatively easy to walk into any library and find not only a source of entertainment but also a resource for solving almost any of life's problems. Once the patient enters the hospital, however, this life-long avenue for self-directed learning is usually closed to him. Hospitals often spend large amounts of money to provide a reference library to staff, but prevent patients from using this resource simply by establishing policies that patients are not allowed in the medical library. Thus, an avenue that many adults have utilized in the past is closed simply because they now carry the stigmatized label "Patient." The following chapter describes various elements of library services that impact on patient education, either through staff or patients themselves.
  Information in this chapter should help the reader to

1. *List four ways in which librarians may contribute to patient education programming*
2. *List library services that may be made available to staff and patients*
3. *Describe prototype library patient education programs*

The traditional role of the librarian in the hospital has been described as an informed intermediary between the health professional and the information he or she requires [2]. In the health-care setting, the librarian often acts as a bridge across the gap between the wealth of knowledge gathered over the years in the health-care field and the day to day activities of providing patient care. This role has been expanding in recent years to include an active involvement in the hospital's education programs and the coordination of library resources with other eductional programs such as media production and inservice education [6]. The demands of burgeoning hospital patient education programs are also beginning to be felt by the library, and they should be supported at the same level and with the same quality of information services provided to other educational programs in the hospital.

The current rise in the development of patient education programs has created a new clientele for many hospital librarians: the patients. Although library services for patients have been established in some hospitals for many years, these programs are the exception rather than the rule. In most hospitals where patients' library services have been developed, their emphasis has been primarily on recreational or rehabilitative materials and programs. The emergence of the librarian as a member of the health-care team has raised many questions for both the librarian and the health practitioner, particularly in the area of providing information to the patient regarding his or her health care. Despite the ambiguities, many of which are allayed once the librarian becomes involved in actual patient education activities, the library has much to offer to both the professional conducting patient teaching and to the patient seeking health information.

Harris [8] suggests that librarians should contribute to patient education programming "their expertise in the fields of information gathering and dis-semination, in other words, using what is already defined as their function in the hospital environment." She divides these contributions into four areas: (1) the provision of information from the health-care literature to patient education planners; (2) the assessment of existing resources in the hospital and commu-nity; (3) the procurement of teaching materials; and (4) the storage, classification and organization of these materials. Patient education also creates a demand for an array of health information services that varies in many ways from those provided to health-care providers as delineated above. Most of these new services are involved in some way with providing health information directly to the patient. The following chapter will discuss these elements of library services in patient education in detail.

SERVICES TO STAFF

The librarian should be involved from the outset in planning patient education programs in the hospital. As a resource person, he or she should be included as an active member of the patient education committee as well as an advisor to informal specific-subject planning groups. The materials already available in the hospital library can yield much valuable information to the patient education planner when utilized effectively.

Published information on patient education has expanded rapidly over the past several years as formal programs are first developed and then described in the literature. Whenever possible, a comprehensive search of the literature should be one of the preliminary steps in developing a patient education program. The library can provide information on model programs, guidelines and protocols for program development, teaching techniques, assessment and evaluation tools, and much more. Especially in hospitals with limited staff resources allocated to health education, building on the experience of others can save a great deal of time and energy.

Patient teaching is a new field for many health practitioners, and the level of formal preparation in this field varies widely within each discipline and from one discipline to another. Patient education is now being included in the curricula of many health-care training programs, but this has not always been the case. Many studies indicate that often the health professional does not feel adequately informed about teaching techniques to provide patient education [4]. Those staff members identified as possible teachers may require inservice training in this area, and there is a growing body of educational material for staff addressing this very topic that should not be overlooked.

Once the patient education program has been established, it is equally important that the educator keep abreast of new trends and developments in the field. Library resources and current awareness services can again influence and support such areas as program innovations, record keeping requirements, evaluation techniques, and quality assurance.

As plans for the patient teaching program progress, it will become necessary to assess the availability of existing resources that might support the developing program. Potential sources of material both in the hospital and in the surrounding community should be considered. The librarian will of course be in the best position to identify useful educational materials in the library's collections. In addition, he or she may be able to identify educational materials being used throughout the facility or in departmental collections elsewhere in the hospital.

In developing a hospitalwide patient education program, it may be advisable to survey all teaching materials in use, both to avoid future duplication and to assess the level of resource support in existing programs. Often this activity provides the added benefit of identifying human resources as well. The materials so identified may become the base of a centralized collection of patient education resources, to be expanded as the program develops.

Hospital librarians are also active members of resource sharing networks involving a variety of health-care institutions, and very often they provide one of the strongest links between hospitals with similar interests. Using these contacts, they can identify both materials and programs in other hospitals that may be of use in the local program.

A word about the use of professional information in the medical library as a resource for patients might be appropriate here. In most hospitals the medical library is the most well-developed source for health information, and may be looked upon by some as a resource for patients as well as staff. With the assistance of the librarian, it is sometimes possible to locate appropriate information for the lay person in the medical library collection. For the most part however, this material is widely scattered and once located, of varying suitability to the purpose at hand. The librarian who is willing to conduct such a search must spend a great deal of time gathering together the materials and then translating and reformating the information before effective communication with the patient can begin [10]. Though the medical library collection can be utilized to answer occasional patient questions, this is a limited source at best and one which will not adequately support a full-scale teaching program.

While patient education has been developing into an integral part of many health-care delivery programs, publishers and producers have aptly identified this field as a new market for their wares. Recent years have seen a mushrooming of activity in this area, with a great deal of material being rapidly introduced into a field that had been neglected for some time. The quality of these materials varies widely, and thus choosing appropriate teaching aids and other informational sources for the patient can be a difficult task. Limited funds for such items make wise selection procedures even more important, especially as many programs are quite expensive. The selection of relevant materials is an area very familiar to the hospital librarian and one in which he or she has formal training and extensive experience.

The first step in building a collection of resource materials in patient education that will be useful to the patient seeking information and to the practitioner providing information is to define the specific needs of both groups. Plans for specific teaching programs should be reviewed to identify topics requiring resource support and the type of support desired. Decisions should be made as to how resource materials will be used (to instruct, illustrate, reinforce, or elaborate). The educational setting should be considered, since a different program might be selected for group versus individual use. Preferred format of the material, whether print or nonprint, pamphlet, model, or audiovisual program, should be identified. The characteristics of the intended audience should also be considered, with particular attention given to educational level, age, perception or language problems, and anticipated level of patient motivation. Areas of possible patient initiated inquiry should also be considered for resource support, again taking into account the elements listed above.

Resource materials for patient education come in a wide variety of formats, including pamphlets, books, models, charts, films, slides, audiocassettes, and videocassettes, to name a few. When chosen carefully, these all can be effectively used to support a teaching program. The specific attributes of these different types of media are addressed elsewhere in this book and therefore will not be discussed here. It should be stressed, however, that it is advisable to build a collection that is made up of a combination of these formats rather than a concentration of a single type of media [11]. This flexibility will allow for the varying needs of individual patients and programs utilizing the materials. It should be noted here that as useful as many of these educational materials are, they should never be substituted for direct patient teaching, but should be used to supplement the interaction between the patient and the health professional.

Sources for patient education materials are as diverse as their types and purposes. They can be divided roughly into five main groups: commercial publishers and producers, voluntary health organizations, pharmaceutical companies, professional health organizations, and individual health-care delivery programs. To date, this information has not been gathered into a single source listing. A comprehensive clearinghouse for patient education materials is a project under consideration by the Bureau of Health Education [13]. In a feasibility study prepared for the Bureau by the American Hospital Association, the urgent need for an organized source of such information was clearly identified. This study proposed a design for a Patient Education Materials Clearinghouse. As of this writing, plans for the possible development of this clearinghouse are in the formative stages [12]. Various agencies have developed clearinghouses for information on specific health problems, such as the Cancer Information Clearinghouse and the Diabetes Clearinghouse at the National Institutes of Health. In addition, a number of source lists have been developed by individuals and organizations involved in health education; one such listing is found at the end of this chapter in the section entitled Resource Materials. As valuable as these source listings and clearinghouses may be, there is still no central location or tool for identifying all patient education materials available. Until such a clearinghouse is developed, the process of identifying appropriate materials for patient teaching programs will be both lengthy and complex, entailing a comprehensive search of numerous sources, preferrably by an individual trained in such information retrieval.

Once possible materials have been identified to support a specific program, careful evaluation for content and quality is imperative. This is particularly true in the case of audiovisual materials, where the investment can be quite high and prudent purchase is especially necessary. Moreover, the varying philosophies and modes of treatment in many fields make it essential that local practices be reflected in all resource materials selected. If practitioners do not agree with the information presented in a piece, they will not use it, nor will they wish their patients to have access to it.

Many producers of audiovisual programs make them available for previewing by the prospective buyer, either free of charge or for a rental fee. Previewing even when a charge is involved should be included in the planning stage of every patient education program; this is an important step in developing a teaching plan with resource support. All programs should be reviewed for technical quality by the librarian or media staff and for content by the subject specialists who will ultimately be responsible for teaching patients in these areas. This review may also extend to printed materials, though very often the librarian working with the health-care team will develop enough knowledge of program needs to make these selections in all but the most controversial areas. It has been our experience and that of others [4] that the use of subject specialists for previewing is preferrable to a preview committee. Utilizing the individuals directly involved in the teaching program as reviewers results in the selection of many relevant materials for that area and helps to stimulate patient referrals and use of the resource materials once the program is underway.

The desire for hospital-produced materials tailored to specific programs is likely to be encountered repeatedly in the development of resource support for patient teaching programs. Any proposal for such a venture should be evaluated critically in terms of the time, cost, and facilities required for a production of significant quality. A complete search for available materials from other sources should be made before serious consideration is given to any local production. Many times this search will turn up a suitable item at a much lower overall cost to the institution. When the decision is made to develop an item locally, whether it be an instruction sheet, a pamphlet, or an audiovisual program, the librarian should be a member of the multidisciplinary committee planning the production. Based on his or her familiarity with the range of patient education materials in many areas of health care, the librarian involved in patient education can offer advice on the most effective format, level of presentation, and informational approach for such materials.

The storage and organization of educational materials falls more within the purview of the traditional function of the librarian, and patient education resource materials should be no exception. Centralization of these materials in the library, media center, or other information source provides many benefits to the health-care provider and the patient education program as a whole. It provides a focus for patient education activity within the hospital, bringing together at one point both the diversity of teaching activities and the resources that support them. The need for duplication of materials is frequently eliminated, and a single access point to patient education information for both staff and patients will ensure wider utilization of available materials.

The librarian can also provide meaningful organization of this material and a system of access to the information contained therein, which will be of use to both the health professional teaching patients and the lay person seeking information. The primary users of the collection should be considered when such a system is designed, since the system used in the medical library for information access by health professionals will be too detailed for many lay persons. A center staffed by a professional librarian will have the advantage of a full range of library services. This librarian can provide knowledge of the resources available, a system for control of their use, and a special ability to match questions with appropriate resources.

Finally, the librarian in such a setting can furnish evaluators of patient teaching programs information on the use of educational materials and, for some special studies, can gather initial reactions from patients using specific items. As the Joint Commission on Accreditation of Hospitals now requires patient education in a number of clinical areas [9], documentation that such teaching is taking place is necessary. Such documentation is being initiated in part by the librarian in some programs [3,4,8] for inclusion in the medical record.

SERVICES TO PATIENTS

The librarian also has a great deal to offer to the patient. Most patients come to the hospital because they have been made aware of symptoms that are indicative of physical or mental problems. Upon entering the hospital, many factors will cause anxiety, fear, and doubt in the patient. For some patients, the loss of self-identity has been characterized as one of the most difficult aspects of hospitalization [16]. The library will very often provide a positive or more familiar setting for the patient within the larger hospital environment. The librarian may be one of the few staff members the patient will see who does not wear a uniform. This favorable image the patient may have of the library may encourage him or her to seek health information from this source, and this may be an important factor in the patient education process.

The motivation of the adult learner and the importance of providing teaching when the patient is receptive to learning have been discussed elsewhere in this book. The salient point here is that if the patient "recognizes a need to learn, and asks the librarian to help him meet that need, he must be helped at that time—the teachable moment; otherwise, the need will dissipate and not come back" [1]. Stated in another way "it is important to recognize the patients' curiosity and self inquiry as positive and necessary components of the health education process" [4]. For many, the library may be the most accessible source of health information, since the physician or other health-care provider may often seem too busy to be approached with questions. The librarian who can effectively provide the inquiring patient with information that will facilitate the patient teaching process is making a valuable contribution to patient education.

To meet these demands for health information, whether they come from a patient referred to the library by a health-care provider or one approaching the library independently, the resources of the librarian must be well developed in several areas. As previously indicated, an established collection of health infor- mation materials designed for the lay person and coordinated with the hospital's programs is of primary importance. Secondly, the librarian must be a working member of the health-care team, with knowledge of the hospital's treatment programs, philosophies, and practices. The role of the librarian providing infor- mation to patients is supportive of those providing care in the institution; he or she should not substitute for the health professional and either diagnose or interpret that information [17].

Perhaps the most important resource the librarian has to offer the patient is his or her professional ability to match the information needs of the patient with the appropriate materials. Librarians have received formal training in an area that they call reference, which is the function of first defining what information the library patron actually needs, and then identifying resources at hand that will meet this need. The basic problem of specifically identifying the exact question being asked is in this situation complicated by the foreign nature of medical terminology to patients. Furthermore, the anxiety and tension that often sur- round key topics related to an individual's health can make posing direct questions difficult. Librarians may find this to be one of their biggest problems in providing service to patients, but those actively involved in patient education programs are effectively overcoming these barriers.

Family members should also be considered logical recipients of patient educa- tion, and in many cases it is they who best utilize the resources of the librarian. Particularly in the instance where a family member will be providing specialized home care, information on dietary modification, exercises, and aids for the handicapped are most useful. Referrals to groups or publications that provide support for the relative may also be helpful.

It should again be emphasized that in all of these activities, the librarian is acting as a member of the health-care team. Communication with the health-care provider following contact with a patient is an important element in this process. The patient with further questions regarding his or her particular situation should always be referred back to the health-care professional. The resources and services of the patient education library cannot stand alone in the patient teaching process.

The role of the librarian in providing health information to patients should be well defined by the patient education committee or planning group. The issue of whether resource materials will be made available to all patients, or only to those with referrals or prescriptions from health professionals should be decided early in the planning process. Whatever this role might encompass, "the establishment of a definite policy regarding the responsibility for instructing the patient and disseminating the [educational] material . . . is the province of the individual institution" [16]. Such a policy will serve both the librarian and the health professionals by avoiding confusion as to the librarian's involvement and establishing for him or her a legitimate place on the health-care team.

LIBRARY PATIENT EDUCATION PROGRAMS

The prototype for patient education library programs is the Health Library at the Kaiser-Permanente Medical Center in Oakland, California. Established in 1969, this library is based at a large, prepaid group practice facility in an urban ambulatory care setting [3,17]. It performs all of the functions described here and also acts as a health education resource for the community at large. Anyone may use the library and its materials on an unrestricted basis or when referred by a health professional. The emphasis is on audiovisual programs, although there is also a large assortment of pamphlets and books. All materials are reviewed by a committee composed of physicians, nurses, health educators, resource staff, and potential veiwers, and consensus is required on each item before it can be added to the library. A number of programs and support materials have been developed internally at the request of staff members. Since its inception the Health Library staff has grown from one librarian to two librarians, a library assistant, and two clerks, although some of these positions are part-time. They provide a full range of library services, are experimenting with outreach programs, and are providing consultation services to other facilities in their system.

The Health Library is well utilized, averaging 875 visitors per month, primarily health plan members. Less than one-third of these are referred by a physician and most are seeking information about their personal medical problems. On entering the library, each person registers at the counter, is informed about the library services and pertinent supplementary materials and is then directed to an audiovisual program. A registration form is used to gather data on all visitors, for the dual purpose of feedback to the health care team and subsequent program evaluation. The library records on health plan members are punched for statistical tabulaton by a computer and routed to the chartroom for insertion into each patient's chart. This system ensures follow-up information to the health-care team.

This model program has stood the test of time, having been in operation for over ten years. During that time it has increased in both financial support and scope of programming and has become an integral part of this health-care delivery system.

Over the past several years the Veterans Administration Library Network, consisting of libraries in 175 medical centers, has made a strong commitment to providing resource support to patient education. In response to the interest and demand for health information programs in the hospital setting, some type of patient education material has been incorporated into most patient and medical libraries in the VA, and major library programs have been developed at several facilities [15]. The Patient Education Resource Center at the VA Medical Center in San Francisco, California, was based in large measure on the Kaiser model. This program has been designed to meet health information needs of the medical center's patients in both the inpatient and outpatient setting. Many of the Center's materials were selected to support specific teaching plans, and in some cases are written into treatment protocols.

Like the Kaiser Health Library and many other health education programs, the Patient Education Resource Center emphasizes the use of audiovisual materials. The Center also offers a wide array of models, charts, books, pamphlets, and displays. Easy access to medical information designed and approved for patients is stressed, and individuals are served on a drop-in as well as a referral basis. Patients who are unable to come to the center are provided with information at the bedside, through the use of mobile audiovisual carts. Since opening in 1977, the Patient Education Resource Center has served over 6000 patients and family members. The librarian who staffs this Center, acting in a role similar to the Kaiser librarians, now spends the majority of her time assisting patients in their use of the Center. In the developmental years of the hospital patient education program, she was instrumental in the formation of teaching plans and protocols, and in the coordination of activities in this area.

Library services in patient education need not always operate at the sophisticated level of these two programs. Many have evolved within the current parameters of the hospital library. A good example of this is the book cart service provided to patients at the Paoli Memorial Hospital in Paoli, Pennsylvania [18], in which a small collection of health information printed materials is made available to patients on ward visits by the hospital librarian. This type of library programming is taking place at many small hospitals with budding patient education programs. Librarians involved in clinical librarianship programs are also being called upon to provide information to patients [14] and are developing support services through this channel.

Public libraries are beginning to become involved in health information as well. Two notable examples of successful cooperative efforts between public and hospital libraries in this field are the Community Health Information Network (CHIN) in Cambridge, Massachusetts, and the Consumer Health Information Programs and Services (CHIPS) in Los Angeles County, California [5,7]. These concentrate primarily on the health-care information needs of the consumer, but also furnish patient educators with valuable resources and services.

As these programs illustrate, the potential for library participation in hospital patient teaching programs is great. This is a resource that is currently underutilized by many patient educators, yet with the limited means available to many of them, it is one they cannot afford to overlook. We hope that this delineation of the role of the librarian in patient education will serve to alleviate the confusion that often surrounds the librarian's involvement in this field. It is as a resource person, rather than as a teacher, that the librarian can best support patient education programs. As an active member of the patient education team, the librarian can provide valuable support in reaching that team's most important goal: quality health care for the patient.

REFERENCES

1. Bille, D. A.   The librarian as facilitator of patient education. *Hospital Libraries,* 1 : 6, 1976.
2. Bloomquist, H., et al.   *Library Practice in Hospitals: A Basic Guide.* Cleveland: The Press of Case Western Reserve University, 1972.
3. Collen, F. B., and Soghikian, K.   A health education library for patients. *Health Services Reports,* 89 : 236, 1974.
4. Elsesser, L.   *Patient Education Continuing Education Syllabus.* Chicago: Medical Library Association, 1978.
5. Gartenfeld, E.   The community health information network. *Library Journal,* 103 : 1911, 1978.
6. Gold, R. A., et al.   The health information specialist: A new resource for hospital library services and education programs. *Bulletin of the Medical Library Association (Chicago),* 62 : 266, 1974.
7. Goodchild, E.   CHIPS—Consumer Health Information Program and Services—Los Angeles. *California Librarian,* 39 : 19, 1978.
8. Harris, C. L.   Hospital-based patient education programs and the role of the hospital librarian. *Bulletin of the Medical Library Association (Chicago),* 66 : 210, 1978.
9. Joint Commission on Accreditation of Hospitals.   *Accreditation Manual for Hospitals, 1979 Edition.* Chicago: The Commission, 1979.
10. Kelly, M.   The consumer and health information. University of California, Berkeley, M. L. S. thesis, 1977.
11. Kucha, D.   *Guidelines for Implementing an Ambulatory Consumer Health Information System.* Fort Sam Houston, Texas: Army-Baylor University, 1973.
12. Lee, E.   Center for Health Promotion, American Hospital Association. Personal communication, May 21, 1979.
13. Llewellen, P.   *Feasibility Study: Patient Education Materials Clearinghouse.* Chicago: ITT Research Institute/American Hospital Association, 1978.
14. Marshall, J. G., et al.   The clinical librarian and the patient: A report of a project at McMaster University Medical Centre. *Bulletin of the Medical Library Association (Chicago),* 66 : 420, 1978.
15. Martin, R. R.   The role of the librarian in patient education efforts. Paper presented before the 2nd Annual National Symposium on Patient Education, San Francisco, Oct. 21, 1978.
16. Phinney, E.   *The Librarian and the Patient.* Chicago: American Library Association, 1977.

17. Quay, C. The role of the librarian in patient education efforts. Paper presented before the 2nd Annual National Symposium on Patient Education, San Francisco, Oct. 21, 1978.
18. Rickards, D. J. Providing health care information to patients in a small hospital. *Bulletin of the Medical Library Association (Chicago)*, 66 : 342, 1978.

Resource Materials

SELECTED RESOURCE LISTS

1. Ash, J., and Stevenson, M. *Health: A Multimedia Source Guide.* New York: Bowker, 1976.
   An annotated alphabetical guide to publishers, audiovisual producers and distributors, libraries, government agencies, societies, pharmaceutical companies, and research institutions that deal with health education materials.
2. Medical Media Directory: Programs and Producers. *Biomedical Communications* 7, March 1979.
   An extensive annual compilation of audiovisual programs and producers arranged in alphabetical order by medical specialty.
3. Medical Library Group of Southern California and Arizona. *Directory of Health Education Sources.*
   An alphabetical listing of agencies primarily located within Southern California and Arizona that offer health education materials free of charge or for under $25.
4. Duke, P. Audiovisuals: Patient Education. *Journal of Biocommunication* 5 : 18, 1978.
   An annotated list of sources of media for purchase or rental.
5. American Hospital Association. *Patient Education Resource List. Sources of Patient Education Videotape Programs.*
   Two listings of patient education materials suppliers and the types of resources that they provide.
6. Library of the Health Sciences, University of Illinois. *Sources of Health Information for Public Libraries,* 1976.
   A selective list of health related agencies and private companies.
7. Welch Medical Library. *A Guide to Medical Media Producers and Distributors.* Baltimore: Johns Hopkins University, 1977.
   An alphabetical listing of over 500 names and addresses of media producers and distributors of patient and health science education materials.
8. Yakote, G., and Homan, M. *Patient Education: A List of Societies, Companies and Institutions with Audiovisuals for Sale, Rent or Loan.* Los Angeles: Biomedical Library, Center for the Health Sciences, University of California, Los Angeles.
   A guide to sources of audiovisuals including types of media offered, costs, and subjects covered.

CLEARINGHOUSES

Cancer Information Clearinghouse
  Office of Cancer Communications
  National Cancer Institute
  7910 Woodmont Ave., Suite 1320
  Bethesda, MD 20014
High Blood Pressure Information Center
  Landau Building
  120/80 National Institutes of Health
  Bethesda, MD 20014
National Clearinghouse for Alcohol Information
  PO Box 2345
  Rockville, MD 20852
National Clearinghouse for Drug Abuse Information
  P.O. Box 496
  Kensington, MD 20795
National Clearinghouse for Mental Health Information
  Parklawn Building
  5600 Fishers Lane, Room 11A-33
  Rockville, MD 20857
National Clearinghouse for Poison Control Centers
  Division of Poison Control
  Bureau of Drugs
  Food and Drug Administration
  Room 1345
  5600 Fishers Lane
  Rockville, MD 20857
National Clearinghouse on Aging
  Administration on Aging
  Department of Health and Human Services
  Washington, D.C. 20201
National Diabetes Information and Education Clearinghouse
  National Institute of Arthritis, Metabolism, and Digestive Diseases
  National Institute of Health
  Westwood Building, Room 628
  Bethesda, MD 20205
National Nutrition Education Clearinghouse (NNECH)
  Society for Nutrition Education
  2140 Shattuck Ave., Suite 1110
  Berkeley, CA 94704
Office on Smoking and Health
  5600 Fishers Lane
  Parklawn Building, Room 158
  Rockville, MD 20857

Cathie E. Guzzetta

21

Can Critically Ill Patients Be Taught?

Are critically ill patients able to learn?
What is the role of the critical care nurse in patient teaching—if any?

Physical readiness to learn can be a factor in determining how effective a patient's teaching-learning program is in achieving learning outcomes. It may be easy, therefore, for the health-care professional to assume (though incorrectly) that the critically ill patient cannot learn. The following chapter disputes the widely held belief that patient teaching cannot be effective in a critical care unit. Various types of data, obtained through assessment of body, mind, and spirit, are described, and suggestions are offered for adapting the steps of the teaching-learning process to the critical care setting.
   Information in this chapter should help the reader to

1. *Describe various stressors faced by the patient in a critical care setting*
2. *List the elements included in the teaching plan in critical care*
3. *Describe how the steps of the teaching-learning process can be adapted in the critical care setting*
4. *Compare and contrast the* products *versus the* processes *of patient education programming, especially in a critical care setting*

"Everyone knows that patients cannot be taught anything during their stay in the ICU." "Don't begin teaching until the patient is transferred out of the CCU." "Patients won't remember anything in the MICU. They're too sick. They're not interested. They're too anxious. They don't listen."

Sound familiar? These attitudes have dominated the concept of the teaching-learning process of the critically ill. Perhaps we have tended to overemphasize the impossible task of trying to educate the critically ill patient without thoroughly investigating the variables, characteristics, and parameters related to the problem. The popularity of and need for critical care areas has grown rapidly in the past decade. To a great extent, this growth has been a function of the many research studies that have been directed toward this area. Extensive research, based on the medical model, has sought to answer questions related to new monitoring techniques, diagnostic procedures, emergency therapeutic treatments, and methods of care. The advantages and benefits of critical care areas have been evaluated in terms of patient mortality, morbidity, and prolongation of life. Research based on the holistic approach to care of the critically ill has been undertaken to identify stressors and the psychophysiologic stress response.

Unfortunately, in our flurry to study critical care, we may have in fact neglected, bypassed, or perhaps prematurely ruled out some areas of investigation that could prove useful in guiding the practice of nursing. Patient education of the critically ill may be one of these areas.

Shortly after the advent of the critical care unit, nurses identified the need for patient teaching. Researchers placed the teaching-learning process of the critically ill within the theoretical framework of learning theories and teaching strategies, investigated the problem, and quickly discovered, they thought, that patients simply do not learn while in the acute care setting. We accepted this information and incorporated it into our practice. As a result, we have concluded that educating the critically ill patient is an impossible feat. We have abandoned further research related to the teaching-learning process and its development.

If this area is indeed exhausted, why pursue it? The argument in this chapter is based on the author's strong conviction that critically ill patients *can* be taught. The problem of teaching the critically ill patient will be examined first in terms of a traditional mode of thinking and the logical inadequacies of that approach will be pointed out. Then a body-mind-spirit approach will provide the theoretical framework for why critically ill patients can and must be taught. From this framework, the discussion will continue by providing assessment parameters for teaching, by examining traditional and innovative methods of teaching, and by describing evaluation techniques.

The author wishes to gratefully acknowledge the following persons for their contributions in the development of this chapter: Dr. Ethel Tatro, Associate Professor and Chairperson of Adult Nursing, Medical College of Georgia School of Nursing at Augusta; Dr. Jean Morse, Associate Professor and Coordinator of Curriculum in Education Research and Development, Medical College of Georgia; Em Olivia Bevis, R.N., F.A.A.N., M.A., Professor and Coordinator, Medical College of Georgia, School of Nursing at Savannah; and Susan Davis, R.N., ICU-CCU Assistant Unit Coordinator Northside Hospital, Atlanta, Georgia.

THE THEORETICAL FRAMEWORK FOR TEACHING THE CRITICALLY ILL

Perhaps we have approached the teaching-learning process of the critically ill from the wrong perspective. If our investigations are resulting in useless answers to guide the practice of nursing, perhaps we are asking the wrong questions. What is our orientation to the teaching-learning process?

We can probably agree that our orientation is derived from information tested and evaluated from teaching-learning theories. We have set up protocols to teach critically ill patients those things that we believe they should learn and only occasionally include those things they are interested in learning. We have evaluated the process by determining what the patient remembers, how much he understands, and how well he incorporates the principles into his behavior.

This orientation has dominated our traditional framework of patient care. The Cartesian habit of viewing the human being as divisible into parts, body and mind, has been enormously useful in the growth and development of science. It has allowed scientists to investigate impartially the human organism without having to worry about the soul [14]. When Descartes masterfully defined the human being as divisible into two parts "as if" the individual were both a body and a mind, a prolonged confusion arose over the centuries until the "as ifness" of the body-mind duality was lost. Both nursing and medicine have become heirs to this gradual change. The primary assumption guiding most current nursing and medical care is that essentially it is the body that becomes sick. The mind may, of course, be secondarily involved, but is generally the etiologic factor only in rather unusual cases.

Our therapies, procedures, drugs, surgeries, and much of our research are body oriented. These methods of therapy and investigation are extremely successful and viewed as monumental achievements compared to those of a century ago. Although bodily ailments may be eradicated with body-oriented therapies, the patient's psychological response to disease may impair his ability to return to full function and may actually interfere with the healing process [8].

Replacing the old duality that has divided the patient into convenient, separated, and disconnected compartments of mind and body is difficult after the traditional framework has dominated our thinking, theory, and research for over 300 years. Viewing the patient in the "new" way, however, would permit the introduction of positive change in the practice of professional nursing. Viewing the mind and body as operating on a continuum allows the patient to be seen and cared for as a biopsychosocial unit. Disease is seen, therefore, as a process involving the whole patient.

The interconnections of mind and body, then, are reflected in changes of emotion and physiology. These associations may operate at conscious and unconscious levels and will be considered in detail as scientific evidence of this interrelatedness later in the discussion. If we continue to revamp our thinking, we may further begin to hypothesize that if the mind is educable, so must be the body. This point of view is fruitful because it enlarges the nurse's options for effective therapy. Because the body-mind continuum exists, therapeutic measures may include much more than medications, treatments, and surgical procedures. The nurse's contributions toward patient education can result in "body effects" that are as real as those achieved by traditional forms of therapy.

As we deviate from the traditional orientation of these theories, we might view teaching as a process that incorporates all aspects related to the care of the critically ill. If we can adjust our concept of patient teaching to incorporate it within a holistic approach to patient care, we can begin to realize that the *process* of teaching has value because of its impact on the learner. This approach is quite different from viewing the value of teaching from its outcomes, its *product*.

The implications of this orientation are enormous. Within the holistic framework, each nurse-patient encounter has therapeutic value and worth. Each time the patient and nurse interact, the nurse is meaningfully affecting the patient's body-mind-spirit. Each time she identifies and meets a patient's need her response affects the whole patient. The nurse who responds to the physical needs of her patient realizes the action being taken affects much more than the patient's physical function. Each encounter with the patient is a teaching-learning experience. This exchange may not be remembered by the patient three weeks or even three minutes later. The experience, however, has a biopsychosocial impact.

The outcomes of this process may or may not lend themselves to scientific inquiry. As we allow ourselves to be open to different ways of thinking, however, we must not forget that science is *one* way of thinking. We can no longer allow ourselves to regard it as the *only* way of thinking, for in doing so we begin to appear not as scientists, not as the patient's advocate, but as dogmatists seeking a position that is antithetical to the precepts of science itself.

No patient teaching encounter is a neutral event. It is a phenomenon always affecting both the patient (body-mind-spirit) and the nurse. The effect may be dramatic and measurable or it may be subtle; but something—either positive or negative—always occurs [14]. This theoretical formulation thus provides the basis for critical care teaching.

ASSESSMENT

Assessment is a vital part of the teaching-learning process. Assessing the learning needs of the critically ill is a difficult and complex problem [24]. The assessment process can be divided into three major areas: (1) biopsychosocial assessment, (2) assessment of stressors, and (3) assessment of readiness to learn.

Systematic assessment is both an initial and ongoing process. The analysis of such a process allows one to evaluate the patient's total clinical condition and should lead one to formulate hypotheses related to the patient's teaching needs (See Figure 5). The hypothesis can be tested, analyzed, and validated, thereby satisfying the demands of the scientific method (and the scientific minded).

Figure 5. Conceptual model for integrating the nursing process and the teaching-learning process. Steps of the nursing process are outlined, and teaching-learning activities and information are depicted.

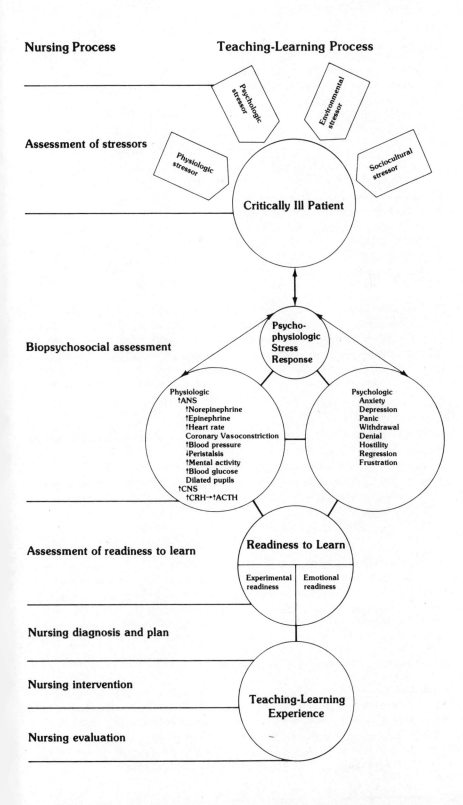

Nursing Process   Teaching-Learning Process

Assessment of stressors

Critically Ill Patient

Psychologic stressor

Environmental stressor

Physiologic stressor

Sociocultural stressor

Biopsychosocial assessment

Psycho-physiologic Stress Response

Physiologic
↑ANS
   ↑Norepinephrine
   ↑Epinephrine
   ↑Heart rate
   Coronary Vasoconstriction
   ↑Blood pressure
   ↓Peristalsis
   ↑Mental activity
   ↑Blood glucose
   Dilated pupils
↑CNS
   ↑CRH→↑ACTH

Psychologic
Anxiety
Depression
Panic
Withdrawal
Denial
Hostility
Regression
Frustration

Assessment of readiness to learn

Readiness to Learn

Experimental readiness   Emotional readiness

Nursing diagnosis and plan

Nursing intervention

Teaching-Learning Experience

Nursing evaluation

Biopsychosocial Assessment

The first step in the assessment process involves collecting information to formulate a complete database. A psychologic and sociocultural history is obtained to help identify the teaching needs of the patients. Pertinent information might also include:

1. What does the patient know or suspect about his condition? Some patients may be extremely knowledgeable about their illness and reasons for admission to the critical care unit, while others may have no idea what is going on.
2. What is the patient's level of education? Can he or she read and write?
3. What is the age of the patient?
4. Where does the patient fit in on the health-illness continuum? (For example, is the patient admitted in critical condition with severe respiratory distress or is he or she asymptomatic and admitted for elective cardioversion of a dysrhythmia?)

A physical assessment must also be accomplished and may frequently precede the interview and history as warranted by the patient's clinical status. The patient who is admitted to the unit in no acute distress will have different concerns and needs than the patient admitted with severe pain or in a medical crisis. The nurse would want to evaluate the following areas:

1. Is the patient in distress?
2. Does he have acute pain?
3. Is he conscious? What is his neurologic status? Orientation to time, place, and person? CNS intact?
4. Does the patient have respiratory difficulty?
5. Is his cardiac output normal? Is he cyanotic? Does he have a normal heart rate, blood pressure, normal urinary output, and peripheral pulses?
6. Is he sedated?
7. Can he see? Can he hear?

Abnormalities, concerns, and problems identified in the history and physical assessment are documented in terms of a problem list and plan of care (see Figure 5). This information is combined with the other two major areas of assessment to formulate a total clinical assessment of the patient's teaching needs.

Assessment of Stressors

The patient who enters the critical care unit is confronted with multiple factors that produce stress. The severity and duration of the stress in critically ill patients are usually greater in impact than in other types of medically or surgically ill patients. Factors that cause stress will produce psychophysiologic alterations in the individual. These alterations, in turn, will affect the patient's clinical status, his needs and concerns, and the teaching-learning process.

The relationship between psychologic manifestations and physiologic alterations has become an important area related to both an understanding of the patient as a biopsychosocial unit and in the development of a diagnostic classification system [9] used to generate a scientific body of knowledge in nursing. The interconnections of mind and body are reflected in changes of emotions and physiology, and these interconnections are felt to be invariable:

The psychophysiological principle, as we hypothesize it, affirms that every change in the physiological state is accompanied by an appropriate change in the mental/emotional state, conscious or unconscious, and conversely, every change in the mental/emotional state, conscious or unconscious, is accompanied by an appropriate change in the physiologic state. [12]

Nearly a century ago, Cannon found that an animal who was confronted with fear, pain, or rage responded with a set of physiological responses [6]. This response has been termed stress and has been described by Selye as "the state manifested by a specific syndrome consisting of all nonspecifically induced changes within a biological system" [22]. A stressor, on the other hand, may be defined as the thing that produces the stress [22]. A stressor, therefore, is an alarming stimulus that can produce physiologic, psychologic, chemical, or structural changes in the individual. The response occurs as a means of helping the individual adapt to the stressor.

The specific stressors that are capable of eliciting a psychophysiologic stress response are being investigated and appear to be physiologic, psychologic, environmental, and sociocultural in origin. When assessing stressors, we should consider the following:

1. What physiologic, psychologic, environmental, or sociocultural stressors are confronting the patient?
2. Are these stressors so intense that they have potential to block the teaching-learning process?
3. Is the focal stressor (generally the admission illness) so severe that it consumes all of the patient's psychophysiologic energy, leaving little in reserve to deal with and assimilate other information or potentially therapeutic encounters?
4. What stressors can be prevented, reduced, or eliminated?

If we can continue to identify, classify, and analyze the stressors present in our patients and relate these to the psychophysiologic stress response, we can, in turn, begin to evaluate nursing interventions that are useful in preventing, reducing, or eliminating the stressors as a means of reducing the stress response and controlling the outcome of patient care. The various types of physiologic, psychologic, environmental, and sociocultural stressors will be considered.

Physiologic stressors. The most obvious physiologic stressor, generally observed in all patients admitted to a critical care area, is the patient's admitting illness. This stressor may be termed the focal stimulus [19] and may range from a cardiopulmonary resuscitation, an acute burn, or acute renal failure, to mild congestive heart failure.

The focal stimulus will initiate the psychophysiologic stress response in an attempt to adapt or cope with the situation. The response or ability to adapt will be dependent upon the severity ·of the illness, the patient's previous state of health, any coexisting illness (contextual stimuli), the duration of the illness, and the patient's perceptions and previous experience with the disease (residual stimuli) [19]. Additional contributing and coexisting physiologic stressors related to the focal illness and the degree of severity include such things as pain, hypoxemia, hypercapnia, dysrhythmias, acidosis, leukopenia, infection, fever, convulsions, hypotension, abnormalities in fluid, electrolytes, or laboratory values.

Critically ill patients will respond to the focal stressor with their entire being. Their physiologic response and psychologic behaviors will be totally immersed in survival. This total involvement will leave virtually no energy for coping with other types of stimuli or stressors.

Psychologic stressors. Intense emotions can narrow the patient's responsiveness and ability to cope with situations. Psychologic stressors, particularly prevalent in the critically ill, might include such things as fear of death, weakness, loneliness, powerlessness, loss of virility, family conflicts, loss of peer respect, loss of or alterations in body image, inability to work, helplessness, and hopelessness.

Psychologic stressors (stimuli) will, of course, set off not only a physiologic response, as previously described, but also a psychologic response that may be exhibited in behaviors compatible with anxiety, depression, panic, withdrawal, denial, hostility, regression, and frustration (see Figure 5).

Environmental stressors. The critical care environment has not been adequately evaluated in recent years as to the impact it creates as a potential stressor, but there is a growing concern to manage and control environmental stressors as a part of nursing care.

The etiologic mechanisms are complex and confounding and include untidy surroundings, observation of other patients, lack of windows, clocks, and doors, lack of privacy, frightening noises and machines, multiple sounds, sleep deprivation, loss of territoriality, restricted visiting hours, lack of structure, and unpleasant odors.

The concepts of sensory overload or deficit have been analyzed. It would be wise to systematically investigate the problem (the primary factor and interacting factors) in terms of vision, hearing, taste, smell, touch, and position in space. Studies of isolated, sensory-environmental stressors dot the literature [5,10,13, 15,17,21,23].

Sociocultural stressors. Sociocultural stressors are capable of producing the psychophysiologic response to stress. Variables identified as specific to the sociocultural domain include age, sex, ethnic origin, economic status, religion, beliefs, attitudes, level of education, family, work, play, activity, and motivation. Stress in the critical care setting might be further reduced, eliminated, or controlled by restructuring nurse-patient interactions based on a nursing diagnosis of the various sociocultural stressors. Within a holistic framework, structural inconsistencies in the relationship can lead to problems in nurse-patient interactions that result in high levels of stress for patients. The results of a limited number of sociocultural research investigations in the area of stress provide suggestions as to which parameters might be observed [7,11,20].

Assessment of Readiness to Learn

The importance of motivation or readiness to learn is a universally accepted ingredient in the success of the teaching-learning process. It has been recognized, however, that few areas related to nursing are as difficult to assess. The concept of readiness to learn is divided into two areas: (1) the level of "experimental readiness" to learn and (2) the degree of motivation or level of emotional readiness [18]. The first characteristic involves the patient's skills, beliefs, attitudes, past experience, and ability to learn the material that has been specified as important. When assessing experimental readiness, the nurse must consider the variables that may influence the evaluation process and ultimately affect the learning process. We need to determine if the patient has sufficient background knowledge to understand the information presented. We need to evaluate his past and present beliefs and attitudes. The nurse must be able to assess the patient's previous knowledge of the situation and identify misconceptions. Moreover, the nurse must assess whether or not the patient is capable of learning.

The second characteristic of readiness to learn deals with emotional readiness—whether or not the patient is willing to expend the necessary energy that is needed in the teaching-learning process. Obviously during the acute crisis, the patient is in the early (first) stage of adaptation and frequently exhibits behavioral manifestations consistent with anxiety, denial, and disbelief. The severity of these behaviors will, in part, be dependent upon the patient's self-concept, role concept, severity and duration of illness, and the meaning the patient and family attach to the illness. An important question to be asked is whether or not the patient desires to know any information. Nurses assume that the patient has a right to know information related to their illness and plan of care. They also assume that patients desire or want to know this type of information. This, however, is not always the case.

For most patients admitted to a critical care unit, the stress response is predictive. The severity, degree, or level of the response, however, has been almost totally neglected and certainly has never been correlated with the teaching-learning process in the acute care setting. Certainly, the current work in the classification of nursing diagnoses will provide important knowledge in this area [9].

Experimental readiness and emotional readiness are interrelated; therefore, the assessment of the two levels are frequently interdependent. If a patient does not believe he has had an acute myocardial infarction, for example, he will find it extremely difficult to understand and accept the nursing and medical regimen of the coronary care unit.

Information that is related to experimental and emotional readiness is incorporated with the findings from the biopsychosocial assessment and the assessment of stressors to obtain the completed evaluation of the patient's teaching-learning needs (see Figure 5).

CONTENT AND METHODS OF TEACHING

Teach What the Patient Wants to Know

After the patient's assessment, the critical care nurse can begin the teaching-learning process as soon as the patient is admitted to the unit. The acuteness of the patient's condition, however, frequently does not initially permit a thorough assessment of psychophysiologic parameters, stressors, and readiness to learn. During this crisis period, the nurse must be perceptive and sensitive to specific questions, fears, concerns, problems, or areas of interest that are voiced by the patient upon admission. Nursing intervention and patient teaching are critically interrelated during this time and have an enormous impact on how the patient will view and accept the next hour, next day, or duration of his hospitalization. When the patient's initial and pressing problems are left unsolved or questions left unanswered, communication becomes blocked, anxiety is increased, and any progress toward a trusting relationship is stunted. The patient's concerns are usually grave enough that all further focus of attention is lost until the specific need is met. Because admission to a critical care unit is not generally anticipated or planned, patients frequently need time and assistance in solving psychosocial matters of concern. A patient who is suddenly admitted from home to a critical care area, for example, may be extremely worried about contacting a spouse who is out of town or arranging for the care of children after they return home from school. Occasionally, the patient's initial and future concerns or questions may appear inconsequential when compared to the acuteness of the patient's condition. The patient, nevertheless, will view the problem as monumental. It will be useless to continue teaching efforts or even to render comfort until the concerns have been met to the patient's satisfaction.

Teach the Patient About the Environment and Procedures of the ICU

Environmental stressors can be a serious problem in the critical care area. The critical care unit should be explained to the patient and family. Because an understanding of the unknown can reduce fear, anxiety, and stress, the patient should be taught about the sights, sounds, and odors he may perceive while in the unit.

The cardiac monitor can frequently be a primary source of anxiety to the patient if he does not understand its purpose and function. Patients may be afraid to turn, sit up, or cough because they observe that such activity causes the digital heart rate to change, triggers the alarm system, or causes artifact MCL_1 or the electrocardiographic pattern to float up and down on the monitor. Changing the electrode placement from lead I to MCL_1 can be a terrifying experience for a patient who has been observing his cardiac rhythm; the patient must be informed that after switching leads, he can expect to see a change on his cardiac monitor.

A patient who does not understand the reasons for every two hour vital-signs check may become extremely worried about his condition. Other areas to be discussed with the patient include bedrest, passive and active range of motion exercises, oxygen therapy, IV and diet therapy, laboratory tests, ECG, EEG, and respirators. This information can be developed into a booklet for family members and patients in the ICU.

When possible, special procedures need to be explained to the patient and include such things as insertion of arterial lines, Swan-Ganz catheters, and temporary pacemakers, tracheal suctioning, endotracheal intubation, and weaning from the ventilator. The patient should be briefly told the purpose and reason for the procedure as well as the sensations, pain, and discomfort associated with the technique. Again the nurse must remember that the anticipation of such procedures may produce such high levels of psychophysiologic stress that very little information is actually transferred to the patient upon the initial contact.

Prepare the Patient for the Sick Role

The short-term teaching objectives of the critically ill patient will also include, at some point in time, information related to his primary illness and sick role. This area is generally one that is conjointly shared by the physician and nurse. The patient may inquire about his illness, prognosis, complications, reasons for admission to ICU; he may ask if he will die, when he can return to work, how long he will be hospitalized, and what his restrictions or limitations will be. Frequently, these questions can be answered; however, sometimes they cannot. Discussion and collaboration with the primary physician is absolutely essential for the nurse to deal with this area of teaching, support, and reinforcement.

Involve the Family

The family should be considered as members of the health team. When properly informed, they become an important support system and can help to validate and reinforce information presented to the patient. Family members, understandably, may be extremely anxious when a loved one is admitted to a critical care unit. They may display anxiety, anger, fear, confusion, denial, guilt, or hostility and may be emotionally disruptive to the patient. The nurse frequently needs to assist family members during this time of crisis, allowing them time to convey their story, fears, and apprehensions. When appropriate, the nurse can begin to discuss the patient's current status and what they can expect when they visit the patient. Other helpful information may include how the family can be notified of any change in the patient's condition, the patient's routine while in ICU, the visiting hours and restrictions, what items the patient is allowed to have in ICU, and the location of waiting areas and the dining room.

Family members frequently want to know how they can help the patient. To address the issue meaningfully, the families' strengths, desires, and needs must first be evaluated. From the evaluation, the nurse can help family members identify and plan their involvement in patient care that may include such things as holding the patient's hand, sitting at the bedside, discussing the events of the day, orienting the patient to time, place, person, news, and weather, or reading to the patient. Other family members may wish to feed, bathe, or ambulate the patient. Sometimes it may even be appropriate to teach the family more complex skills. Occasionally they may request patient involvement and help with mouth care, skin care, coughing and deep breathing, helping the patient to relax, range of motion exercises, suctioning, or colostomy irrigation. We probably do not permit family members to be involved with the patient as much as they desire, or as much as we could, nor do we probably appreciate the therapeutic impact of this involvement.

Family members are frequently afraid of the complex environment of the critical care unit. When a patient is connected to tubes and machines, it is no surprise the family might be terrified and receive the unwritten message when they walk into the patient's room: *Do Not Touch.*

Prior to a family visit, it is necessary for the nurse to prepare the family for the sights and sounds they will experience. Additionally, family members gain security and confidence when the nurse accompanies them to the patient's bedside, explains the patient's current status, and allows them time to express their concerns and ask questions.

The teaching role may be so simple in this situation as to pull up a chair to the patient's bedside, sit down, stroke the patient's hand, and inquire how he or she is doing. When we turn over our chair to the family and they follow similar actions, we succeed in tearing down the *Do Not Touch* sign and replace it with one that reads *You Can Help.*

Prepare the Patient for Transfer

The transfer process from the critical care unit to the floor may be a stressful experience for the patient. Frequently, a patient may be transferred unexpectedly to make room for someone "who really needs the bed." The patient should be prepared for the possibility of this situation and should be informed early in his stay that he will only temporarily remain in the critical care area. When appropriate, the nurse can point out advances in the patient's condition such as diet and activity progression, improvement in vital signs, and reduction of medications. This information is tangible evidence of improvement and can be used in the preparation for transfer.

Preparing the patient for transfer should include a gradual weaning from tubes, equipment, and machines. When possible, the cardiac monitor, IV, Foley catheter, arterial lines, and oxygen therapy should be discontinued while the patient is still in the unit to help alleviate feelings of loss of security, anxiety, and dependence on the equipment. The nurse can discuss differences between the unit and the floor with the patient.

When the actual transfer takes place, the nurse should accompany the patient to the floor and introduce him to the staff. The patient should be made aware that a complete and thorough report of his condition and care will be given to the floor nurse. Family members should be contacted and informed of the location of the room and the reasons for transfer. The patient should understand who or how to call in case of need and be given an explanation of any changes in hospital routine, visiting hours, meal times, physicians, medications, treatment, or activities. If the patient has been on a progressive activity, exercise, or diet program, this information should be carefully communicated to the floor nurse and should be continued accordingly.

The critical care unit care plan should accompany the patient to the floor. The floor nurses should be made aware of the short-term teaching objectives that were developed in the unit and of any misconceptions, areas for clarification, or information that still needs to be discussed. The patient who has already read, digested, and discussed a teaching booklet related to his illness, for example, will certainly have different types of future teaching needs than the patient who has asked no questions about his illness or who is still in a state of denial. This information is thoroughly discussed and included on his updated care plan. At this time, an outline of the patient's long-term teaching needs can be discussed.

Teaching Methods in the Critical Care Unit

When teaching the critically ill patient, nurses should keep all explanations brief and concise. They should explain ideas in terminology easily understood by the patient. They usually need to repeat, and then repeat again. The short-term teaching needs of the patient are, in fact, short term. The need to repeat and clarify does not indicate failure. It is simply a function of meeting the moment-to-moment needs of critically ill patients. Each encounter with the patient has meaning and impact—perhaps for only a moment—but the impact may be enormous and certainly is never a neutral event.

We have pointed out various strategies used in the teaching-learning process of the patient. If we are operating from a holistic framework of patient care, we must look at other methods to approach this process that are consistent with body-mind-spirit interrelatedness. Biofeedback [4], meditation [1,3,16,25,26], and relaxation techniques [2] are among the exciting alternatives.

Traditional and holistic therapies must be viewed as complementary methods of effective nursing function. Each method has its place in the total approach to patient care. They should not be seen as either-or choices because one approach may be more applicable than another in a given situation. It may also be found that a combination of various approaches for different patients and situations are beneficial.

EVALUATION

How do we evaluate the effects of the teaching-learning process on the critically ill patient? Some quantitative suggestions that will lend themselves to methodologic research might include the following:

1. Do our teaching efforts reduce the amount of physiologic, psychologic, environmental, or sociocultural stressors affecting patients?
2. Does an assessment of the psychophysiologic stress response indicate which patients are ready to learn?
3. Is the psychophysiologic stress response reduced as a result of our teaching?
4. Does teaching have any effect on the patient's morbidity, mortality, or length of hospital stay?
5. Does teaching help to reduce feelings of powerlessness, helplessness, hopelessness, loneliness, fear of separation, or alteration in self-concept?
6. Are biofeedback, meditation, and relaxation techniques effective in reducing perceived stressors or in decreasing the psychophysiologic stress response? Can these techniques be effectively taught to critically ill patients? Can these techniques be combined with traditional forms of therapies to achieve successful patient outcomes? What types of patients are most receptive?

It is generally accepted that an evaluation of the teaching-learning process is directed toward the effect of the teaching. We are, in fact, evaluating the product of the teaching. The usual scientific design is developed to gain information related to how much the patient remembers, understands, or how well he complies to a given regimen. These questions are concrete, and are certainly worth consideration.

When we teach a critically ill patient, however, many of the traditional criteria or measures generated from teaching-learning theories simply do not apply. If we attempt to measure the outcomes of the unmeasurable it should not be surprising that our findings have been as discouraging as they are. Such has been the case in research directed toward measuring the outcomes of patient teaching in the critically ill.

Perhaps the solution is that we need to redefine our ideas of teaching in the critical care situation and redirect our thinking in its evaluation. Each time a critical care nurse encounters a patient, the situation has potential for teaching. The teaching may meet a momentary need. The effects may not be quantifiable according to the principles of scientific inquiry and may not lend themselves to computerization and probability theories. The holistic framework, however, provides the theoretical basis that allows one to believe that each encounter has profound body-mind-spirit implications. If we continue to evaluate the *product* of our teaching we are, at this point in the sophistication of our knowledge, asking the wrong questions and evaluating the wrong parameters. The answer might be found in an evaluation of the *process* of our teaching rather than in the product. When we evaluate the process within a body-mind-spirit framework, we no longer need to derive our satisfactions from knowing our teaching has been successful. Rather, we can focus our attention on assessment methods and techniques of teaching that are therapeutic and have meaning for the patient. We succeed as nurses by practicing a holistic approach.

Yes, the critically ill patient can be taught. When a nurse encounters a patient, it is never a neutral event [14].

REFERENCES

1. Allison, J. Respiratory changes during the practice of the technique of transcendental meditation. *Lancet,* 1 : 833, 1970.
2. Benson, H. *The Relaxation Response.* New York: William Morrow, 1975.
3. Benson, H., Steinert, R. F., Greenwood, M. M., et al. Continuous measurement of O_2 consumption and CO_2 elimination during a wakeful hypometabolic state. *Journal of Human Stress,* 1 : 37, 1975.
4. Brown, B. B. *New Mind, New Body: Biofeedback.* New York: Harper & Row, 1974.
5. Bruhn, J. C., Thurman, A. E., Chandler, B. C., and Bruce, T. A. Patients' reactions to death in a coronary care unit. *Journal of Psychosomatic Research,* 14 : 65, 1970.
6. Cannon, W. B. *The Wisdom of the Body.* New York: Norton, 1932.
7. Croog, S. H., and Levine, S. Social status and subjective perceptions of 250 men after acute myocardial infarction. *Public Health Reports,* 84 : 989, 1969.
8. Frank, J. D. Mind-body relationship in illness and healing. *Journal of the International Academy of Preventive Medicine,* 2 : 50, 1975.
9. Gebbie, K. M., and Lavin, M. A. *Classification of Nursing Diagnosis.* St. Louis: Mosby, 1975.
10. Geertsen, H. R., Ford, M., and Castle, C. H. The subjective aspects of coronary care. *Nursing Research,* 25 : 211, 1976.
11. Gentry, W. D., and Haney, T. Emotional and behavioral reaction to acute myocardial infarction. *Heart and Lung,* 4 : 738, 1975.
12. Green, E., Green, A., and Walters, E. Voluntary control of internal states: Psychological and physiological. *Journal of Transpersonal Psychology,* 2 : 3, 1970.
13. Hackett, T. P., Cassem, N. H., and Wishnie, H. A. The coronary-care unit—An appraisal of its psychologic hazards. *New England Journal of Medicine,* 279 : 1365, 1968.
14. Guzzetta, C., Kenner, C., and Dossey, B. *Critical-Care Nursing: Body-Mind-Spirit.* Boston: Little, Brown, 1981.
15. Klein, R. F., Kliner, V. A., Zipes, D. P., et al. Transfer from the coronary care unit: Some adverse responses. *Archives of Internal Medicine,* 122 : 104, 1968.
16. Lown, B., Temte, J., Reich, P., et al. Basis for recurring ventricular fibrillation in the absence of coronary heart disease and its management. *New England Journal of Medicine,* 294 : 623, 1976.
17. Marshall, L. A. Patient reaction to sound in an intensive coronary care unit. In Marjorie V. Batey (Ed.), *Communicating Nursing Research.* Boulder, Colorado: Western Interstate Commission for Higher Education, 1972.
18. Redman, B. K. *The Process of Patient Teaching in Nursing* (3rd ed.). St. Louis: Mosby, 1976.
19. Riehl, J. P., and Roy, C. *Conceptual Models for Nursing Practice.* New York: Appleton-Century-Crofts, 1974.
20. Schachter, S. *The Psychology of Affiliation.* Stanford: Stanford University Press, 1959.
21. Sczekalla, R. M. Stress reactions of CCU patients to resuscitation procedures on other patients. *Nursing Research,* 22 : 65, 1973.
22. Selye, H. *The Stress of Life.* New York: McGraw-Hill, 1956.

23. Shannon, V. J.   The transfer process: An area of concern for the CCU nurse. *Heart and Lung,* 2 : 364, 1973.
24. Storlie, F.   *Patient Teaching in Critical Care.* New York: Appleton-Century-Crofts, 1975.
25. Wallace, R. K.   The physiological effects of transcendental meditation: A proposed fourth state of consciousness. University of California, Los Angeles, Ph.D. dissertation, 1970.
26. Wallace, R. K.   A wakeful hypometabolic physiologic state. *American Journal of Physiology,* 221 : 795, 1971.

Karen K. Sedlacek

22

Patient Teaching in the Pediatric Unit

Does patient teaching philosophy or methodology change in pediatrics?
Who is the focus of teaching in pediatrics?
How does the child's age affect the types of patient teaching he or she needs?

This text has thus far been discussing the teaching-learning process of adult patients. When the patient is a child, however, some adaptations may be required because of learning limitations imposed merely by age. Adult education theory does apply, however, when the pediatric patient's parents are the target of the teaching-learning process. The following chapter describes how the child's developmental stages influence the content and approach to patient teaching. Play is described as a means to portray feelings and express anxieties and questions. Approaches in teaching parents and several important teaching content areas are described. Suggestions are offered for preparing the child for surgery and for discharge from the hospital.

Information in this chapter should help the reader to

1. List the developmental stages a child moves through as he or she masters the stages in the human life cycle
2. Describe how the child's developmental stage effects the teaching-learning process
3. Describe how play assists the child's teaching-learning process
4. Utilize the teaching-learning process with a child's parents
5. List several important teaching areas when teaching a child and parents
6. Prepare a child and parents for an operation
7. Prepare a child and parents for discharge

Hospitalized children are in need of informed and skillful care. Their families need help, too, as the child goes through the signs and symptoms of his illness, the duress of hospitalization, the discomforts of diagnostic tests, the stress of surgery, and at last (one hopes) the pains of healing. All this is almost too heavy a burden for a small child.

ROLE OF THE PEDIATRIC NURSE IN PATIENT TEACHING

Through the patient teaching function, the pediatric nurse can do much to alleviate the stressors associated with hospitalization, both for the child *and* the parents.

The child and his or her parents should be seen as a dynamic unit in the planning of care, rather than two separate entities. When the nurse works with both child and parents, they learn from one another during the three-way transaction. This is particularly true of the parents, who may see for the first time what the child knows and does not know about what is going to happen as the nurse interacts with the child. Therefore, it is important to instruct the parent and the child together about preparation and support procedures during hospitalization [12].

In order to plan for child and parent education, the nurse must perform a thorough initial and ongoing assessment of the child's physical condition, developmental level, behavioral reactions and readiness for particular learning.

The family dynamics and parental responses, behaviors, and expectations related to the child, illness, and hospitalization must also be assessed. The nurse must observe the verbal and nonverbal cues of the child and his parents in order to determine what the needs, fears, and concerns are, and then intervene with the appropriate teaching.

DEVELOPMENTAL STAGES

In developing from the undifferentiated emotional state of the newborn to the highly integrated personality state of the adult, the child moves through a number of distinct developmental stages that involve particular crises (core problems), or developmental tasks. According to Erikson there are eight stages in the human life cycle [3]. The first five of these stages pertain to children and youth. In each phase the child must master the central problem before moving on to the next.

Each core problem or crisis has positive and negative counterparts. In the initial stage of psychosocial development, *infancy,* the negative counterpart of the core problem (mistrust) is conquered through a mutually satisfying mother-child relationship. The infant who finds that his needs for food and other kinds of comfort are consistently met learns that his world is a safe place and that he can trust others. As the child progresses through subsequent stages of development, his relationships expand, first to others within the family and then later to persons in the world beyond his home.

During the *toddler* stage, the child must acquire a sense of autonomy rather than shame and doubt. Toddlers who have learned to trust want to assert their

Table 7. The Eight Stages in the Human Life Cycle

Period of Life	Core Problem or Crisis
1. Infancy (from birth to 1 year)	trust vs. mistrust
2. Early childhood (toddler: ages 1–3)	autonomy vs. shame and doubt
3. Play age (preschool: ages 3–6)	initiative vs. guilt
4. School age (ages 6–13)	industry vs. inferiority
5. Adolescence (ages 13–18)	identity vs. identity diffusion
6. Young adulthood	intimacy vs. isolation
7. Adulthood	intimacy vs. self-absorption
8. Senescence	integrity vs. disgust

Source: Adapted from E. Erikson, "Youth and the Life Cycle," *Children*, 7 : 43–50, 1960.

growing awareness that their behavior is under their own control. "I can do it myself and that delights me" is the earmark of autonomy.

In the *preschool stage* the central task is to develop a sense of initiative rather than a sense of guilt. Preschoolers enjoy exploring what they can attain and create, and they enjoy seeing what they can do with the motor, language, interpersonal, and other skills of which they are becoming more capable.

The *school-age child* uses the physical, cognitive, and social skills he or she has brought from the preschool phase and now tries to learn what he or she must know in preparation for success in the adult world of facts and tools. The central task of this period as identified by Erikson is to develop a sense of industry rather than a sense of inferiority.

Adolescence is centered on the task of developing a sense of identity, with the undesirable alternative being role confusion or diffusion. Erikson describes the attainment of identity as the young person's coming to feel that his or her views of the self are internally consistent and consistent with others' views of him.

Successful conquering of the negative counterparts of each crisis (or core problem) prepares the child to undertake the next step in development. According to Erikson, "life is a sequence not only of developmental but also of accidental crises. It is hardest to take when both types of crisis coincide" [3]. One accidental crisis Erikson refers to is the crisis of illness. The pediatric nurse must be aware of the developmental problem that the child faces so that solutions of the problems can be effected.

TEACHING AND LEARNING IN CHILDREN

According to Holt [7], children naturally want to explore their surroundings:

The young child is curious. He wants to make sense of things, find out how things work, gain competence and control over himself and his environment, do what he can see other people doing. He is open, receptive, and perceptive. He does not shut himself off from the strange, confused, complicated world around him. He observes it closely and sharply, tries to take it all in. He is experimental. He does not merely observe the world around him, but tastes it, hefts it, bends it, breaks it. To find out how reality works, he works on it. He is bold. He is not afraid of making mistakes. And he is patient. He can tolerate an extraordinary amount of uncertainty, confusion, ignorance, and suspense.

He is willing and able to wait for meaning to come to him—even if it comes very slowly, which it usually does.

The hospital is not a place that gives much time, opportunity, or reward for this kind of thinking and learning. The nurse can help the child maximize learning by realizing that children learn best independently, not in groups; that they learn out of interest and curiosity, not to please or appease the adults in power; and that they ought to be in control of their own learning, deciding for themselves what they want to learn and how they want to learn it. This is the reason why children continuously ask *How?, When?, Why?* When the gap in understanding exists, they feel tension. When the gap in understanding is filled, they feel pleasure, satisfaction, and relief.

Nurses should adjust to the patients they teach by utilizing the foregoing methods of learning in children. Children in different developmental age groups perceive the world in different ways. The nurse's approach in giving an injection, for example, will vary according to the assessment of the child's level of biophysical and psychosocial development.

It is virtually impossible to prepare an infant for an injection with reasoned facts and verbal assurances. The nurse can help the infant cope with an injection by allowing his parents to be present, by handling him gently, and by talking quietly and continuously during the procedure. After the injection, the infant should be held and comforted by his mother or father. This provides the infant with a sense of well-being that is an essential component in his learning to trust.

The *toddler* may have difficulty understanding simple explanations before an injection. Although the toddler needs to assert himself and have control, his security is determined by the presence of his mother. Separation from his mother causes him undue stress and diminishes his ability to explore the world and develop autonomy; thus the nurse may suggest that the mother remain in the background during the injection, but be available to give support immediately after it has been given. It may be helpful to allow him to release his aggressions after the procedure, by pounding clay or splashing in water.

The *preschool child* may be able to cope with stress related to a threatening procedure by "playing out" his feelings and thoughts. Dramatic play—taking on roles and acting out reality and fantasy—is dominant during these years. It is through play that a child understands himself and his environment. A preschool child needs to feel and handle an object before he can understand it. Therefore, it is helpful to have him feel and use a syringe on a doll a few minutes before he receives an injection. After the injection, the child should be allowed to play with the syringe again and "give" the doll another injection if he desires. This gives the child a chance to feel control over the situation as well as to express feelings of aggression.

Since the preschooler is developing a conscience, he tends to view forms of aggression (like injections) as punishment for doing or thinking "bad things" [4]. An explanation should always be given using concrete and familiar words such as "the medicine will help keep your throat from hurting."

A preschooler is egocentric and fears bodily injury; thus he will need to know *how* a procedure will affect him. For example, the nurse can tell him that the injection will feel like a "pinch" and that he may say "ouch" or cry. Allowing him to put a Band-Aid on the injection site is a means by which he can maintain his body integrity.

In this age group, separation anxiety is a primary problem. Therefore, continuity of care should be stressed by limiting care and teaching to one person and by encouraging the parents to help care for their child as much as possible.

The *school-ager* is developing a sense of industry and is interested in learning how things work. His fear of the unknown may make him anxious; thus it is important for the nurse to take the time to explain *why* the injection is needed. He may also benefit from handling the equipment first. The school-aged child should be encouraged to talk about his feelings about the injection. By discussing these feelings, the nurse can help him discover that they are common to all youngsters and thus help him to maintain a healthy concept of himself [2].

For the school-ager, more sophisticated language and drawings can be used to explain the injection. Because he has a more mature concept of causality, he has the capacity to understand that neither illness or treatment is imposed on him because of his own misdeeds. He can cooperate better with treatment, can express his feelings in words, has a greater grasp of time sequence, and therefore can better tolerate separation. He enjoys praise, and the nurse can give it freely for something he does, such as holding still for the injection.

The *adolescent* striving for identity is trying to achieve socially responsible behavior. He may worry that he will break down when getting an injection and fear that others will discover his inadequacy. The nurse should listen to him and let him know that his fears are not uncommon.

The adolescent may benefit from role playing in preparation for an injection if he has not had one recently. A straightforward explanation of the procedure by the nurse can also be helpful. The adolescent may not specifically ask for an explanation about the injection, but he usually welcomes it. He is able to understand the relationship between receiving medication and getting well.

An adolescent may be modest during an injection. Whatever his behavior, it is important for the nurse to try to understand it and be accepting of it because the adolescent's self-image is based not only on how he perceives his own actions, but also on how others react to his body and his behavior [6].

A knowledge of growth and development is necessary for teaching in pediatric nursing. First, maturational readiness affects what can be learned and thus determines objectives and suggests teaching strategies that might be successful. Second, since illness and hospitalization can deprive children of activities central to their growth, it is necessary to think in terms of substitute experiences that might be provided to protect the growth potential.

Use of Play

Many possibilities for teaching young children center on play, the primary way in which children learn. Play is the process through which a young child comes to terms with his feelings and through which he is able to express all the anxieties and questions that adults are able to verbalize.

Table 8. *Teaching Approaches in Pediatric Nursing*

Age Range	Erikson's Stage*	Typical Behavior During Hospitalization	Recommended Teaching Approach
Infancy (birth–1 year)	Trust vs. mistrust	Under 7 months May cry more than at home Responds well to nurses Does not protest mother's leaving Over 7 months Cries more frequently Anxious and unhappy Clings to mother and cries when she leaves	Assign one primary nurse on each shift to care for infant and to work with mother Handle infant gently, communicate in soft, friendly tone of voice Encourage parents to participate in care as much as possible Support parents and educate them about the experience their infant is going through Allow security toy, pacifier, or blanket Provide infant with stimulation (mobiles, play simple games like Pat-a-Cake)
Early Childhood (1–3)	Autonomy vs. shame and doubt	Separation anxiety common May experience protest, denial, and despair Protest Urgent desire to find mother Expects mother to answer cries Frequently cries, shakes crib Rejects attention of nurses Despair Feels increasingly hopeless of finding mother Becomes apathetic May cry continuously or intermittently Denial Represses all feelings for mother Does not cry when she leaves May seem more attached to nurses Finds little satisfaction in relationships	Individual care by one nurse as much as possible Encourage parents to stay with child Utilize familiar stories or puppets in explaining procedures Give simple, direct, and truthful explanations about treatment or surgery just before it is to occur Allow toddler to play with equipment used in treatments to decrease anxiety Give child a choice to make if possible (i.e. choose which side for an injection) Allow parents to be present during painful procedures

Age	Psychosocial stage	Characteristics	Nursing interventions
Play Age (3–6)	Initiative vs. guilt	Separation anxiety continues Increase in anxiety and negativism Regression common (enuresis, evasion) Screaming and panic attacks may occur (especially when parents leave) Eating and sleeping disturbances common	Assign one nurse as much as possible to care for child Encourage parents' participation in child's care Use neutral words such as *opening, drainage,* and *oozing* instead of *cut* and *bleeding* in describing postoperative situation Encourage use of fantasy to "preplan" responses to a difficult situation Use a body outline or doll to describe treatment or surgical procedure Encourage play with equipment before and after a procedure Reassure that a surgical procedure will affect one part of body only Encourage dramatic play, puppetry, water play, etc. for ventilation and reality testing
School Age (6–13)	Industry vs. inferiority	May have insomnia, nightmares, enuresis Appears fearful, sensitive, modest Feels angry and hurt Feels responsible for own illness Alternately conforms with and rebels against adult authority	Assign one person to care for child consistently Continue with use of body outlines for explanation of anatomy and physiology and postoperative appearance Give logical explanation about *why* procedure is necessary Describe sensations that might be felt during a painful procedure (use *warm* and *hurt* rather than *hot* and *painful*) Encourage child to question, express feelings, and actively participate in teaching (he can reason, make generalizations, and can understand concept of time) Provide space, equipment, and give permission for child to indulge in physical activity as outlet for aggression Give praise freely (e.g., for holding still during a procedure)
Adolescence (13–18)	Identity vs. identity diffusion	Unstable emotionally—alternately happy and sad Wants to be independent, wants approval Fears loss of control Girls are concerned with bodily appearance Boys are concerned about virility and prowess and how mutilation of body will affect abilities	Assign one nurse to care for patient consistently Ask if patient wants parents present during teaching session and during painful procedures Use a body diagram to provide a scientific explanation of anatomy and physiology involved in surgery or treatment Ask if adolescent wants to see procedure or not Allow ventilation through art media, dramatic play, dialogue If loss of control seems inevitable, guarantee privacy so others do not see humiliation Give compliments freely

*Source: Stages are adapted from E. Erikson, "Youth and the Life Cycle," *Children*, 7:43–50, 1960.

The child may be inspired to learn through playing games, reading appropriate books or cartoons, or using puppets. Simple drawings, with explanations in appropriate language, may help explain a body part, a procedure, or what a medicine will do in the body. Role playing, dramatic play with dolls, painting, and sand play, are other ways the child can learn about new experiences in the hospital setting.

Thus, in teaching the child in the hospital, it is necessary to incorporate various play activities according to the child's developmental level.

TEACHING AND LEARNING IN PARENTS

The major goal in working with parents is to help them to increase their competence and confidence in meeting the needs of their children. It is clear that this goal can be achieved only through a relationship of mutual trust between parent and nurse. Because the establishment of trusting relationship takes time, health-care services should be planned to ensure continuity over time. As the parent and the nurse come to know each other better, both the communication process and the helping process will be facilitated.

It is necessary in the education of parents to consider each parent individually. The education level, cultural values, interpersonal and social norms, the family structure, and the ability to communicate and solve problems should be considered for each parent.

In order to provide the help and support parents in the pediatric setting need, the nurse should

1. Reemphasize, repeat, and simplify physician's explanation of the cause of illness, condition, and the child's proposed long-term or short-term treatment
2. Support mother and father as they learn (e.g., to give passive exercise, to care for corrective appliance)
3. Reinforce the need for the child's long-term treatment; involve the parents in planning as a means of increasing their committment and motivation
4. Help them verbalize feelings regarding ability to meet treatment demands (encourage exploration and venting of feelings)
5. Refer to social services or other appropriate community resources

IMPORTANT TEACHING AREAS

Disease Process

Teaching the child and family about the disease or accident process is a very important aspect of nursing care during episodes of acute or chronic illness. A mother may profit and learn by participating in some of the nursing assessment or in sharing some of the observations of the nurse. When the mother sees for herself the child's red throat or red ear, when she hears congestion in the chest, or when she feels enlarged nodes in the child's neck, her involvement helps to focus attention on the problem. Thus, understanding of the explanation and her motivation to participate in the child's care may be enhanced.

Parents should learn as much about the illness or injury as they can. Each of the measures used for relief and comfort by the nurse should be understood by the family in relation to a particular illness or symptom, and their own use of these measures should be encouraged in the hospital and later at home. Each of the alternatives the nurse uses in making a health-care decision should be shared with the whole family when feasible, and their participation in the decision encouraged. Thus, relevant learning is facilitated, and the family assumes a more integral participation in its own health care.

Preparation for Hospitalization

Hospitalization may evoke a variety of emotional reactions while the child is hospitalized, soon after discharge, or weeks after the event. For example, a child may not show his fears or have a problem sleeping while in the hospital, but after discharge, days or weeks later, the problem may become apparent.

Severe reactions may be prevented to some extent by properly preparing the child for hospitalization. The nurse can assist in preparing the child and support him or her in this new experience. Young children should be told simply and truthfully why they are going to the hospital. This explanation is best given to a child in the 2 year to 3 year age span a day or two before the event. Telling him too far in advance may produce undue anxiety. It is best to begin preparation for hospitalization four to seven days before admission if the child is 4 years or older. For the child over 7, a frank discussion a few weeks ahead and actual participation in the planning is advisable. A tour of the hospital prior to admission may also be a helpful learning experience for some children.

An adolescent should be told as soon as it is known about the need for hospitalization and his cooperation should be enlisted by sharing with him as much as he seems ready for. The nurse should sit down with the adolescent a few days before entering the hospital and discuss privately the reason for hospitalization. For example, he may be told that he is going to have tests done to help his asthma, that he will be able to be up and around on the unit, that he will be with other teenagers, that he will be hospitalized for about 3 days, and that his friends can call and visit him. The nurse should then listen to his concerns and offer additional support as needed.

Books and pamphlets have long been used as a means of preparing children for hospitalization. Murphy thinks that books can help children adjust to hospitalization, deal with personal problems, and grow socially, emotionally, and mentally [8]. Altshuler also thinks that books are an important avenue available to ease a hospitalized child's adjustment to the new environment [1]. (See the bibliography of children's hospital books at end of chapter, in the section entitled Resource Materials.)

Emotional Responses to Hospitalization

The young child may react to hospitalization in various ways. He may experience separation anxiety, regression, or become overly dependent. The nurse's main function in helping the child and his parents work through these problems is to provide emotional support from the moment the child is admitted to the hospital.

Separation Anxiety

Separation anxiety may occur when the child is removed from the supportive social network of his family and from the familiar surroundings of his home. The separation from family and home may interfere with a child's sense of accomplishment in the school-age period, for example.

The nursing intervention includes encouraging parents to visit their child at any time or to "room in" if possible. The nurse should explain the importance of parent's helping with the care of the child. Allowing the child to keep a favorite toy or blanket with him can also be helpful. Assigning the same nurse to care for the child as continuously as possible can assist the child in forming a trusting relationship and help him work through a separation from his parents. When parents are ready to leave the hospital, the nurse should encourage them to tell the truth to their child about where they are going and when they will return.

Regression

Regression may also occur in the child who is hospitalized. With regression, the child reverts to a behavior pattern that is compatible with an earlier developmental period in which he felt secure. Regression may take the form of losing recently acquired skills, becoming revengeful, or fearing strangers. The need most frequently not being met for a child who regresses is his need for love and security. The nursing approach to the child's regression is dependent on its cause and the need involved. The approach will also attempt not to reinforce the child's regressive behavior while reducing the cause and meeting his need.

Dependency

In illness the child may temporarily cease to function independently in many areas in which he had previously functioned on his own. Dependency is the result of many pressures, such as physical incapacity, restricted mental activity (as in fever), or fear of an unfamiliar hospital environment. If the dependency is great and extends over a long period of time, it becomes threatening and may prove extremely difficult for family members to keep up with the demands of the ill member. Whether or not a child actually learns and once again enjoys increasing independence or prefers to be dependent on others for his need satisfaction is the responsibility of those who control the child's environment. In the hospital setting the nurse is the primary person interacting with the child and the parents. The nurse can encourage independence by allowing the child to make some decisions about treatments being done to him, to help with procedures, or to do small tasks and errands on the unit. The nurse, through open discussions with the parents, can help them understand the child's need to be independent and assist them in achieving independence for their child.

There is no magic formula that will tell the nurse how much or what kind of information to give the pediatric patient. But as a rule of thumb the nurse should ask "What are his needs?" "What will be of concern to him?" "What will decrease his anxiety?" "What does he need to know so that he won't be surprised?" Brief clear answers will help him maintain his self-esteem and self-control.

Children have the ability to face and endure pain if they are adequately prepared for it. Their parents also should be informed of all aspects of the procedure.

Preparation for Surgery

Before an operation, the child must have an opportunity to make friends with the nurse who is to function with the parents in helping the child through the event. Preparation must be gradual, for the child can assimilate only *one* threatening concept at a time. The nurse must be ready to answer the same questions over and over again. Observation to see whether facts of preparation are accepted, denied, or misinterpreted is necessary to know the rate at which preparation can be given and what further help the child requires. Assuring the child that only *one* specific part of his body will be "fixed" may be helpful. Drawing a picture or using a doll as a model may help the child understand what will be happening in surgery. According to Gellert [5] and a more recent study by Smith [10], school-aged hospitalized children have meager knowledge about the organs and functions of the human body. Explanations for children must be individualized by the nurse to suit their understanding about their bodies. The standardized preoperative approach is not realistic.

Nurses can use a "hospital box" that contains real equipment: a stethoscope, blood pressure cuff, syringe, bandages, IV bottle and tubing, anesthetic mask, cap, gown, and mask to prepare the child for surgery. With these real "toys," the child and the nurse can act out the situation realistically. A visit by the anesthesiologist may be helpful along with a visit to the operating room and recovery room if permitted, prior to surgery.

Again, the nurse must keep parents informed of procedures, both preoperatively and postoperatively, so that they can give emotional support to the child.

Preparation for Discharge

The nurse who has had the greatest contact with the family and who has worked directly in helping the child with his feelings during hospitalization is in the best position to counsel parents in preparation for the kinds of behavior that might be seen at home. They need to know that phobias, nightmares, regression, negativism, and disturbances in eating and learning are common aftermaths of hospitalization and indicate unresolved difficulties. Parents' confidence can be increased when the nurse supplies guidelines for the management of regression. Some examples of guidelines to manage regression cited by Petrillo and Sanger [9] include the following.

1. Return the child to integrated family life as quickly as possible. (Give the child responsibilities equal to his abilities.)
2. Acknowledge the child's bravery but refrain from making him the center of attention because of his illness.
3. Be firm, kind, and consistent in the management of disciplinary problems.
4. Be truthful in order to preserve his trust.
5. Provide play materials such as clay, paints, doctor and nurse kits, and equipment given to him in the hospital. Allow the child to play on his own.
6. Permit the child to express his feelings regarding illness and hospitalization.
7. Avoid leaving the child for long periods or overnight until he is well adjusted and trusting of his safety at home.
8. Allow the child to visit the staff when in the hospital vicinity or after clinic appointments.

The nurse must also instruct the parents about the physical aspects of care upon discharge from the hospital. A written plan about a specific treatment, for example, may be helpful for the parents to refer to after the child returns home.

Throughout the child's hospitalization, the nurse will have observed the child interacting with the family and will have gathered information relative to learning needs, the meaning of the child's illness to the family, cultural patterns that will influence care-giving activities of the parents, interaction patterns within the family, the child's level of development, and the parents' level of understanding and coping capacities. The nurse should communicate this vital information in a written care plan. The plan should include provision for specific professional and supervisory services, referral services where appropriate, and specific provision for continued family support [11]. Such support will reduce parental anxiety when the child returns home, provides them with resources, and enables them to reorganize family functioning that was disrupted with their child's illness and hospitalization.

REFERENCES

1. Altshuler, A. *Books That Help Children to Deal With a Hospital Experience.* U.S. Department of Health, Education, and Welfare. Washington, D.C.: Government Printing Office, 1974.
2. Brandt, P. A., et al.   IM injections in children. *Nursing '72,* 72 : 1404, 1972.
3. Erikson, E. H. *Childhood and Society* (2nd ed.). New York: Norton, 1963.
4. Erikson, E. H. *Identity, Youth and Crisis.* New York: Norton, 1968.
5. Gellert, E.   Children's conceptions of the content and functions of the human body. *Genetic Monographs,* 65 : 293, 1962.
6. Hammar, S. L., and Eddy, J. A. K. *Nursing Care of the Adolescent.* New York: Springer, 1966.
7. Holt, J. *How Children Learn.* New York: Dell, 1967.
8. Murphy, D. C.   The therapeutic value of children's literature. *Nursing Forum,* 11 : 141, 1972.
9. Petrillo, M., and Sanger, S. *Emotional Care of Hospitalized Children.* Philadelphia: Lippincott, 1972.
10. Smith, E.   Are you really communicating? *American Journal of Nursing,* 77 : 1966, 1977.

11. Waechter, H., and Blake, B. *Nursing Care of Children* (9th ed.). Philadelphia: Lippincott, 1976.
12. Wolfer, A., and Visintainer, A. Pediatric surgical patients' and parents' stress responses and adjustment. *Nursing Research,* 24 : 244 (July–Aug.), 1975.

Resource Materials

CHILDREN'S HOSPITAL BOOKS

Bartosh, J. A. *Kenny Visits the Hospital.* Jericho, N.Y.: Exposition Press, 1956. (5–8 years)

Bemelmans, L. *Madeline.* New York: Viking Press, 1939. (3–9 years)

Children's Hospital of Philadelphia. . *Michael's Heart Test.* Philadelphia: Children's Hospital, 1967. (3–12 years)

Children's Hospital of Philadelphia. *Margaret's Heart Operation.* Philadelphia: Children's Hospital, 1969, (3–12 years)

Clark, B., and Coleman, L. L. *Pop-Up Going to the Hospital.* New York: Random House, 1971. (5–9 years)

Collier, J. L. *Danny Goes to the Hospital.* New York: Norton, 1970. (5–8 years)

Deegan, P. J. *A Hospital: Life in a Medical Center.* Mankato, Minn.: Amecus Street, 1971. (8–15 years)

Falk, A. M. *The Ambulance.* Toronto: Burke, 1966. (4–10 years)

Froman, R. *Let's Find Out About the Clinic.* New York: Franklin Watts, 1968. (5–9 years)

Greene, C. *Doctors and Nurses: What Do They Do?* New York: Harper & Row, 1963. (5–8 years)

Haas, B. S. *The Hospital Book.* Baltimore: John Street Press, 1970. (4–11 years)

Hallqvist, B. G. *Bettina's Secret.* New York: Harcourt, Brace & World, 1967. (8–13 years)

Kay, E. *The Emergency Room.* New York: Franklin Watts, 1970. (9–13 years)

Kay, E. *The Clinic.* New York: Franklin Watts, 1971. (8–12 years)

Pope, B. N., and Emmons, R. W. *Let's Visit the Hospital.* Dallas: Taylor, 1968. (3–7 years)

Rey, H. A., and Rey, M. *Curious George Goes to the Hospital.* Boston: Houghton Mifflin Company, 1966. (4–9 years)

Schima, M., and Bolian, P. *I Know a Nurse.* New York: Putnam, 1969. (6–9 years)

Shay, A. *What Happens When You Go to the Hospital.* Chicago: Reilly and Lee, 1969. (4–11 years)

Simmons, E. *I Went to the Hospital.* Ithaca, N.Y.: Tompkins Country Hospital Auxiliary, 1958. (2–5 years)

Stein, S. B. *A Hospital Story.* New York: Walker, 1974. (3–10 years)

Tamburine, J. *I Think I Will Go to the Hospital.* Nashville, Tenn.: Abingdon Press, 1965. (4–11 years)

Weber, A. *Elizabeth Gets Well.* New York: Crowell, 1970. (5–10 years)

Welzenbach, J. F., and Cline, N. *Wendy Well and Billy Better Say "Hello Hospital!"* Chicago: Med-Educator, 1970. (4–12 years)

Welzenbach, J. F., and Cline, N. *Wendy Well and Billy Better Visit the Hosptial See-Through Machine.* Chicago: Med-Educator, 1970. (4–12 years)

Welzenbach, J. F., and Cline, N. *Wendy Well and Billy Better Meet the Hospital Sandman.* Chicago: Med-Educator, 1970. (4–12 years)

Welzenbach, J.F., and Cline, N. *Wendy Well and Billy Better Ask a "Mill-yun" Hospital Questions.* Chicago: Med-Educator, 1970. (4–12 years)

ANNOTATED BIBLIOGRAPHIES OF CHILDREN'S HOSPITAL BOOKS

Altshuler, A. *Books That Help Children Deal With a Hospital Experience.* U.S. Department of Health, Education and Welfare. Washington, D.C.: Government Printing Office, 1974.
Flandorf, V. F. *Books to Help Children Adjust to a Hospital Situation.* Chicago: American Library Association, 1967.

FILMS ABOUT HOSPITALIZATION FOR CHILDREN

The People Shop. Education Films, Westport, Conn., 18 minutes. Introduces children to the hospital as an institution in their community and tries to dispel many of the fears children have of hospitals.
The Hospital. Encyclopedia Britannica Educational Corp., Chicago, 13 minutes. A dramatization of the hospital experiences of two children. Attempts to answer some questions and prompts children to ask other questions.
Puppet Preparation for Surgery. The Children's Memorial Hospital, Chicago, 12 minutes. Puppets are used to explain surgery to pediatric patients.
New World for Peter (Revised. Ithaca College Films, Ithaca, New York, 15 minutes. This film introduces children to the hospital by having 9-year-old Peter narrate the story of his operation.
Ethan Has an Operation. Case Western Reserve, Cleveland, 16 minutes. Ethan, a seven-year-old boy, narrates the story of his hernia operation.

Ann Marie T. Brooks

23

Patient Teaching in Psychiatric-Mental Health Nursing

What can I teach the psychiatric patient?
Can the psychiatric patient learn?

Many of today's theories of teaching and learning have their basis in psychotherapy. Theorists such as Freud and Carl Rogers did much in the way of promoting student-centered learning. Unfortunately, many staff in psychiatric wards and hospitals believe that they have no role in patient teaching, because, they think, their patients cannot learn. The following chapter describes patient teaching in psychiatric-mental health nursing. A foundation and framework for patient teaching are proposed. Three levels of prevention are described, and possible teaching content and approaches are suggested.

Information in this chapter should help the reader to

1. *Describe a foundation for patient teaching in psychiatric mental health nursing*
2. *List three levels of prevention in psychiatric-mental health nursing*
3. *Describe teaching-learning interactions that may be necessary in each of the three levels of prevention*

Patient teaching is an activity that is aimed at helping the individual adjust to the disruptions within the human system caused by physical and emotional illness. The goal of any educational effort by nurses is to facilitate the experience for the patient so that the knowledge gained will act as a stimulus for continued learning. This chapter will examine the role of the nurse in patient teaching in the practice of psychiatric-mental health nursing. A discussion of the role of the psychiatric nurse will also be included to provide a basis for the development of an approach that can be used by psychiatric-mental health nurses in all settings and treatment modalities to meet the changing learning needs of clients.

PSYCHIATRIC-MENTAL HEALTH NURSING PRACTICE

The practice of psychiatric-mental health nursing has been greatly affected by the major changes that have taken place in the delivery of mental health services. These advances since World War II coincided with other developments that were taking place in the nursing profession during the same period. The role of the psychiatric-mental health nurse changed during this time from primarily a custodian of a large number of patients to a role of more direct responsibility and involvement in the care and active therapeutic treatment activities of patients.

A major influence in psychiatric-mental health nursing practice has been the recognition of the importance of advanced education. The Nurse Training Act of 1964 is an example of major federal legislation that brought about significant changes for psychiatric-mental health nursing practice. It provided the funds for a large number of nurses who would be prepared to introduce new directions for practice. The advanced knowledge and skill obtained through this higher level of education resulted in the development of a new role for the psychiatric nurse. As mental health services shifted to more of a community health focus, nurses were also afforded an opportunity to establish new roles in the delivery of mental health services. Their skills in therapy and counseling were acknowledged by other disciplines, and their role became much more than the medication person. However, the number of nurses with baccalaureate, master's, and doctoral degrees in psychiatric-mental health nursing practice still falls short of the number needed to continue the development of role expansion and research in practice.

Terms now used to describe the role of the psychiatric nurse include primary nurse therapist, psychotherapist, primary nurse, psychiatric-liaison nurse, clinical specialist, independent nurse practitioner, and staff nurse. These roles occur in a variety of settings and are an integral part of many treatment modalities. Nurses in psychiatric-mental health nursing practice assume responsibility on consultation and liaison teams, child abuse teams, crisis intervention teams, and alcoholism treatment services. These roles provide the nurses with many opportunities for intervention and teaching. The exact role and function of the nurse is largely dependent on the specific type of service that is being offered but could be expanded as the need arises.

PATIENT TEACHING IN PSYCHIATRIC-MENTAL HEALTH NURSING PRACTICE

Increased recognition of the role of patient teaching in psychiatric-mental health nursing practice has been influenced by the standards of practice developed for this nursing specialty. According to the Standards of Practice for Psychiatric-Mental Health Nursing Practice developed by the American Nurses' Association, patient teaching is regarded as a necessary ingredient to assist individuals, families, and community groups achieve and maintain satisfying and productive patterns of living [1]. This standard, developed specifically to meet the needs of psychiatric patients, acknowledges the importance of patient teaching as the appropriate vehicle to aid the nurse in the delivery of quality patient care.

Several factors have contributed to the slow development of both formal and informal patient teaching approaches in psychiatric-mental health nursing practice. First, there has been an acknowledged difficulty in the identification of the content and the method that should be addressed in psychiatric patient teaching programs. Second, the confusion regarding the difference between psychotherapy and patient teaching has hindered the initiation of specific teaching programs. Third, there has been a lack of research to describe and evaluate the effects of patient teaching on the functioning of the psychiatric patient. Fourth, the psychiatric patient has been overlooked by many health-care personnel as a potential student and has not been viewed as an individual with intelligence, an ability to make decisions, or a motivation to learn.

Each of these factors has contributed to the delay in creation of patient teaching programs in psychiatric-mental health nursing practice. However, nurses now seem ready and motivated to move beyond these barriers and to initiate teaching programs based upon the needs of the patient and their own capabilities to enhance the learning process.

FOUNDATION FOR PATIENT TEACHING IN PSYCHIATRIC-MENTAL HEALTH NURSING PRACTICE

The basis for all patient teaching in psychiatric-mental health nursing practice is the establishment of the interpersonal relationship between the patient and the nurse. Travelbee [4] points out that both the nurse and the patient can learn from this mutual interaction. This interpersonal process is directed toward assisting the individual to cope with the experience of mental illness and suffering and to find meaning in these experiences.

If psychiatric-mental health nursing is viewed as an interpersonal process, then every interaction and encounter offers both the patient and the nurse an opportunity for learning and teaching. The focus of patient teaching is directed toward the establishment of an atmosphere in which the patient can be actively involved in determining the direction of this process. This relationship can be regarded as an opportunity for the patient to experience success in establishing a meaningful relationship with another individual. It can also be viewed as a chance for the patient to test new behaviors that will contribute to a more productive and meaningful style of living.

Patient teaching in psychiatric-mental health nursing is based on the same basic teaching principles used in other areas of nursing practice. According to Christman [3], if a patient is viewed as a vital link rather than a passive recipient of care, then the level of involvement for the patient will positively affect the patient's level of potential for learning. The responsibility for change still remains with the individual who has sought psychiatric help or has been placed in a psychiatric environment or treatment facility. The role of the psychiatric-mental health nurse is to aid the patient in developing new perspectives in dealing with problems. This would include identification of effective coping strategies that would allow for more self-directed and meaningful choices.

A PROPOSED FRAMEWORK FOR PATIENT TEACHING

As noted earlier, the practice of psychiatric-mental health nursing is not confined to one specific setting, type of patient, or role of the nurse. As psychiatric care has shifted from hospital settings to the community, nurses in psychiatric practice have assumed new roles in a variety of settings that have changed their availability and responsibility for teaching. There are many more opportunities for both informal and formal teaching depending upon the needs of the patient and the population that is being served.

The wide diversity of practice settings provides the rationale for the development of an approach to patient teaching in psychiatric-mental health nursing practice that would not restrict itself to one particular type of client or therapeutic treatment modality. The aim of such a framework would be to allow enough flexibility for nurses to plan for informal and formal teaching opportunities, yet not constrain the nurse from using all the resources available to devise effective coping strategies.

It is true that patient teaching requires a deliberate and comprehensive approach, but there are several methods in which the goals of patient teaching can be accomplished without restricting the creativity of either patient or nurse. The development and utilization of a broad framework for psychiatric-mental health nurses would also support the behaviors necessary to meet the criteria for the Standards of Psychiatric-Mental Health Nursing Practice developed by the American Nurses' Association that address the issue of patient teaching in practice.

One approach that can be used as an organizing framework for patient teaching in psychiatric-mental health nursing practice is a model based on the concept of prevention. This concept, which is drawn from the field of public health, is aimed at promotion and protection of the healthy aspects of the individual. Although there has been confusion regarding this concept and its definition in literature [12], it is still useful to examine patient teaching in relation to a prevention model.

Prevention has been of interest to health-care practitioners since the early 1900s, but acceptance and use of the three categories of prevention (primary, secondary, and tertiary) has been somewhat slower in the mental health field. Caplan (regarded as the father of prevention in the field of community mental health) has been a leading force in the examination of this concept. According to Caplan [3,12], the three levels can be defined.

Primary Prevention. The aim of primary prevention is to reduce the incidence of new cases of mental disorder by combating harmful forces that operate in the community and by strengthening the capacity of people to withstand stress.

Secondary Prevention. To reduce the duration of cases of mental disorder that occur in spite of the programs of primary prevention is the aim of secondary prevention. By shortening the duration of existing cases, the prevalence of mental disorder in the community is reduced.

Tertiary Prevention. The aim of tertiary prevention is to reduce the community rate of residual defect that is the sequel to mental disorder. It seeks to ensure that people who have recovered from mental disorder will be hampered as little as possible by their past difficulties in returning to full participation in the occupational and social life of the community [3].

Since patient teaching involves both healthy and unhealthy aspects of physical and emotional development, it seems most appropriate to view patient teaching as an integral and necessary part of prevention.

Use of a prevention framework for patient teaching by psychiatric-mental health nurses is helpful for several reasons. These reasons include:

1. providing clarification of goals in relation to patient education programs
2. providing motivation for development and refinement of patient teaching strategies and programs
3. promoting more responsibility and accountability for patient education by nurses

The following discussion of these three levels will include a brief definition and description of the level, implications for patient teaching by psychiatric-mental health nurses, and some specific patient situations and teaching strategies that could be employed as interventions.

Primary Prevention

The first level of prevention to be considered as part of a patient teaching framework for psychiatric-mental health nursing is primary prevention. It focuses on generalized health promotion as well as protection against disease [12]. In mental health this aim would be to foster the growth of positive personality development in individuals, families, and communities. This type of prevention activity may take place in the community, any type of health care facility, or completely outside the formal structure of an organization.

Although most individuals involved in the delivery of mental health services agree upon the importance of primary prevention to promote mental health and prevent disease, little attention has been directed toward research to validate the effects of primary prevention upon the avoidance of illness in the general population. In addition, many professionals—including nurses—regard their role as primarily illness-oriented rather than wellness-centered, which may impede efforts to promote and implement prevention activities and, therefore, overlook the importance of health teaching.

The role of the psychiatric-mental health nurse in primary prevention is exciting and challenging because of the boundless opportunities for interaction and health teaching that are available on this level. The areas of teaching range from how to cope with the stress of being a parent to the challenges of getting old. The methods available are quite varied and should be aimed at the promotion of health behaviors in a specific group or the general population. It is difficult to measure the effects of informal teaching efforts, but these methods have proved to be vital in helping individuals acknowledge and accept new ideas about health care. Informal teaching efforts also serve to promote independence in individuals regarding decision-making in their treatment.

Both formal and informal teaching-learning approaches can be used in primary prevention. These approaches may or may not fit the traditional model of teaching. The specific learning needs, readiness of the learner, and the anticipated learning outcomes will all determine the approach that should be used by the psychiatric-mental health nurse.

Examples of teaching-learning activities organized or initiated by the psychiatric-mental health nurse include: organizing a group of citizens to discuss the problem of the rising suicide rate in the adolescent population, forming a support group to work with bereaved parents and their children following a child's death, developing an in-service educational program to train volunteers interested in working on a community hotline, and presenting a program to inform citizens about the mental health services in the community.

Other topics or areas of concern that could be utilized as a jumping-off point for teaching and may be presented in a structured format include counseling parents how to identify teenagers with a drug problem, alerting the community to the social problems of venereal disease, or informing the elderly about what types of mental health services and programs are available. These specific topics provide entry for the nurse into several age groups and settings and, at the same time, address the specific health needs of the general population.

It is interesting to note that oftentimes the psychiatric-mental health nurse will discount the usefulness of informal teaching strategies that are an integral part of the nursing role. Helping an individual develop insight into his or her situation, developing support networks, and referring a teenager to a counselor for assistance in career decisions are all examples of teaching-learning situations that are not only difficult to measure but may seem insignificant when compared to dramatic cases of intervention.

The role of teaching by psychiatric-mental health nurses should not be underestimated. Utilizing resources and support systems properly as well as developing an ability to mobilize energy for action are definitely assets in dealing with the stress of everyday life.

Because the psychiatric-mental health nurse in the primary level of prevention is employed in a variety of settings (schools, public health departments, employee health clinics), the opportunities to promote healthy behaviors and prevent illness are boundless [9]. The nurse should take advantage of every opportunity to identify the health needs of individuals, groups, and communities, and work with other nurses as well as other disciplines in addressing these needs.

Secondary Prevention

Secondary prevention begins when a pathology is identified [12]. As a level of prevention it is aimed at early diagnosis and effective treatment of symptoms. The nurse's role and involvement in the delivery of mental health services on this level vary according to the role and the type of setting. The psychiatric-mental health nurse usually encounters the patient in an active treatment setting or program. The patient usually has entered the system because of an inability to cope with a particular problem, or is referred by another, erratic behavior, or the potential threat of harm to himself or others.

The nurse at this level of treatment and prevention may work as a staff nurse in a short-term acute inpatient setting, a member of an outpatient treatment team in a community mental health center, an independent practitioner who sees patients as a therapist, or a nurse employed as a member of a crisis team in a crisis intervention center. Although this list of roles for the nurse is not inclusive, it does in fact suggest that the psychiatric nurse is consistently involved in front-line assessment and intervention of patient's needs in conjunction with other mental health-care providers. It also suggests that major responsibility and accountability for the treatment of patients throughout their course of treatment is often assumed by the nurse.

The focus of patient teaching-learning activities in the secondary level of prevention by the psychiatric-mental health nurse is multidimensional. Teaching activities can address the acute educational needs of the patient and family as well as include the preventive educational needs.

Take, for example, the patient who is admitted to an inpatient acute psychiatric unit for repeated acts of violence at home. It would be somewhat foolish for the nurse to expect to change or eliminate violent behavior of the patient through a very structured teaching program about the evils of violence. It is realistic, however, to set limits with the patient; tell him or her that violence will not be tolerated and that he or she should concern himself with not losing control. It is reasonable to assume that after the patient has begun to trust the staff, it might be possible and helpful to examine the stressors that precipitate acts of violence and to discuss the possible harmful effects that these actions may bring about. This type of teaching-learning may also provide insight for the patient regarding feelings that he or she may have kept inside and is now ready to share. Development of alternative strategies to cope with feelings of anger, frustration, and guilt may contribute to the patient's feelings of inner control and reduce the need to act out. Using a punching bag, developing a physical exercise program, or talking about feelings of inner conflict and turmoil may provide acceptable alternatives and more appropriate channels for release of emotion.

Since the basic purpose of all patient teaching is to enhance the patient's level of functioning, it is imperative that a major goal is to promote learning that is both meaningful and is based on problems and situations that are perceived by the patient to be real. In an inpatient setting, the nurse can assist the patient to identify and assess the behaviors that have precipitated admission to the unit.

Using the process of communication as a tool, the psychiatric-mental health nurse can help the patient begin to examine his or her own situation and identify the behaviors that need changing. The relationship can also allow the patient to express a wide range of emotions—frustration, joy—and create an atmosphere that will promote learning.

However, the nurse-patient relationship and trust-building does not occur automatically, and the patient may in fact be unwilling to participate in any patient teaching-learning situation. The nurse should be patient and allow time for the patient to develop trust, motivation, and a readiness to learn. The nurse serves as a teacher, resource person, and facilitator of this process.

Although the majority of admissions to psychiatric treatment settings are voluntary admissions, this does not guarantee cooperation or development of trust in the staff. The nurse must orient the patient to the role of patient and help him overcome his fears about mentally ill individuals. The nurse should encourage the patient to participate in the varied activities offered as part of the treatment but should not force a depressed patient, for example, to take part in a lively game of bingo when the individual cannot tolerate it.

As mentioned earlier, the nurse should identify the specific learning needs, the readiness of the learner, and the anticipated learning outcomes. If a patient is acutely suicidal, it would be vitally important for the nurse to provide a safe environment while letting the patient know that he is a worthwhile individual and will be cared for during this difficult and trying period. As the acute suicidal crisis subsides, the patient may be more ready to learn about his inner controls and the alternatives available. The anticipated learning outcome is that the patient will be able to seek help before suicidal gestures are necessary. Other anticipated outcomes are that the patient will be able to develop a more positive self-concept and more effective support systems to cope with stress.

The nurse should utilize active therapeutic treatment as part of the educational process. Encouraging the patient in the beginning of treatment to take advantage of all opportunities available within the setting is a very basic and necessary part of the teaching role of the nurse. Participation in group therapy, occupational therapy, and assumption of responsibility in unit activities can be viewed as a learning experience for the patient and may contribute to an evaluation of positive progress for the patient. If the patient can begin to develop insight, translate the insight into action, and incorporate the insight into life experiences through a patient teaching-learning program, then the chances for long-term benefit to the patient are greatly increased.

Tertiary Prevention

The third level of prevention is the tertiary level. On this level, the goal is rehabilitation of the long-term disability of an illness. In mental health care, programs of aftercare, rehabilitation, and resocialization are aimed at the restoration of the individual to an optimum level of functioning in relation to the identified disability [12]. This type of prevention constitutes a large portion of the psychiatric services available today, although this number has been greatly reduced in recent years. Since the emphasis in mental health care delivery is to return the patient to the community, this third level of prevention has indeed demanded a new type of plan and provision of mental health services.

The role of patient teaching by psychiatric-mental health nurses at this level of prevention is primarily concerned with preparing the individual for his or her return to the community and assuming activities at a realistic level of functioning. Nursing care services at this level are most often rendered in long-term care facilities and aftercare programs including partial hospitalization programs, community mental health centers, and outpatient clinics. The nurse is involved in patient care at all levels and provides a vital link for the patient between the health-care setting, the family, and the community.

An example of an identified learning need for which a patient-teaching program could be developed would be the need to adhere to a medication regimen. The nurse could encourage learning on the part of the patient through creation of an atmosphere of trust and understanding regarding the usefulness of taking the prescribed medication. Using a variety of teaching aids, the nurse could explain the purpose, side effects, and dosage of the drug, and the time when it should be taken. This information should promote compliance to the medication schedule. A few trial runs and a follow-up by the nurse could also assist in a firm understanding and cooperation on the part of the patient.

Other learning needs may involve activities that most of us take for granted. Securing employment, obtaining housing, or setting priorities in the daily living routine may be foreign to patients who have been out of the mainstream for an extended period of time. It is up to the psychiatric-mental health nurse to identify the special strengths and needs of the patient and to develop specific teaching programs that will address these needs and reach the anticipated outcomes.

REFERENCES

1. American Hospital Association. *A Patient Bill of Rights.* Chicago, 1972.
2. American Nurses' Association. *Statement on Psychiatric and Mental Health Nursing Practice.* Kansas City, 1976.
3. Caplan, G. *Principles of Preventive Psychiatry.* New York: Basic Books, 1964.
4. Christman, L. Assisting the patient to learn the patient role. *Journal of Nursing Education,* 6 : 17–21, 1967.
5. Fralic, M. F. Developing a viable inpatient education program: A nursing director's perspective. *Journal of Nursing Administration,* 6 : 30–36, 1976.
6. Lee, E., and Garvey, J. L. How is inpatient education being managed? *Nursing Digest,* 6 : 12–16, 1978.
7. Lindeman, C. A. Nursing intervention with the pre-surgical patient. *Nursing Research,* 21 : 196–209, 1972.
8. Owens, J. F., McCann, C., and Huteimyer, C. M. Cardiac rehabilitation: A patient education program. *Nursing Research,* 27 : 148–150, 1978.
9. Perlmutter, F. D., Vayda, A. M., and Woodburn, P. K. An instrument for differentiating programs in prevention: Primary, secondary and tertiary. *American Journal of Orthopsychiatry,* 46 : 533, 1976.
10. *Report from the President's Commission on Mental Health.* U.S. Government Printing Office, Vol. II, Appendix p. 11. Washington, D.C., 1979.

11. *Report from the President's Commission on Mental Health.* U.S. Government Printing Office, Vol. II, Appendix p. 9. Washington, D.C., 1979.
12. Shamansky, S. L., and Clausen, C. L.   Levels of prevention: Examination of a concept. *Nursing Outlook,* 28 : 104, 1980.
13. Smith, B. O.   A Concept of Teaching. In B. Bandman and R. S. Guttchen (eds.), *Philosophical Essays on Teaching.* Philadelphia: Lippincott, 1969. P. 5.
14. Travelbee, J.   *Intervention in Psychiatric Nursing: Process in the One to One Relationship.* Philadelphia: Davis, 1969.
15. *Webster's New World Dictionary, College Edition.* New York: New World, 1979.

Epilogue

a charge for action

Information about health care (including diagnosis, prognosis, procedures, and all continuing health-care requirements following discharge from the hospital) is the right of the patient and his or her family and the responsibility of *all* health-care professionals that touch the patient.

Learning consists of knowledge, attitudes, and skills. Armed with the information and approaches discussed in this book, the health-care worker should now possess all the *knowledge* that is necessary to carry out teaching responsibilities. An *attitude* that patient teaching is necessary and accomplishable should be developed. The *skills* of patient teaching will only develop through practice, even though (at times) this practice may involve a trial-and-error approach. The reader has at this point, however, everything that is needed to get going and try.

One final belief must be added to the philosophy of adult education. Success as well as failure only comes from trying. All adults have the right to fail, to learn from failure, and to try again.

Appendixes

A Patient's Bill of Rights

The American Hospital Association presents a Patient's Bill of Rights with the expectation that observance of these rights will contribute to more effective patient care and greater satisfaction for the patient, his physician, and the hospital organization. Further, the Association presents these rights in the expectation that they will be supported by the hospital on behalf of its patients, as an integral part of the healing process. It is recognized that a personal relationship between the physician and the patient is essential for the provision of proper medical care. The traditional physician-patient relationship takes on a new dimension when care is rendered within an organizational structure. Legal precedent has established that the institution itself also has a responsibility to the patient. It is in recognition of these factors that these rights are affirmed.

1. The patient has the right to considerate and respectful care.

2. The patient has the right to obtain from his physician complete current information concerning his diagnosis, treatment, and prognosis in terms the patient can be reasonably expected to understand. When it is not medically advisable to give such information to the patient, the information should be made available to an appropriate person in his behalf. He has the right to know, by name, the physician responsible for coordinating his care.

3. The patient has the right to receive from his physician information necessary to give informed consent prior to the start of any procedure and/or treatment. Except in emergencies, such information for informed consent should include but not necessarily be limited to the specific procedure and/or treatment, the medically significant risks involved, and the probable duration of incapacitation. Where medically significant alternatives for care or treatment exist, or when the

Reprinted with the permission of the American Hospital Association.

patient requests information concerning medical alternatives, the patient has the right to such information. The patient also has the right to know the name of the person responsible for the procedures and/or treatment.

4. The patient has the right to refuse treatment to the extent permitted by law and to be informed of the medical consequences of his action.

5. The patient has the right to every consideration of his privacy concerning his own medical care program. Case discussion, consultation, examination, and treatment are confidential and should be conducted discreetly. Those not directly involved in his care must have the permission of the patient to be present.

6. The patient has the right to expect that all communications and records pertaining to his care should be treated as confidential.

7. The patient has the right to expect that within its capacity a hospital must make reasonable response to the request of a patient for services. The hospital must provide evaluation, service, and/or referral as indicated by the urgency of the case. When medically permissible, a patient may be transferred to another facility only after he has received complete information and explanation concerning the needs for and alternatives to such a transfer. The institution to which the patient is to be transferred must first have accepted the patient for transfer.

8. The patient has the right to obtain information as to any relationship of his hospital to other health care and educational institutions insofar as his care is concerned. The patient has the right to obtain information as to the existence of any professional relationships among individuals, by name, who are treating him.

9. The patient has the right to be advised if the hospital proposes to engage in or perform human experimentation affecting his care or treatment. The patient has the right to refuse to participate in such research projects.

10. The patient has the right to expect reasonable continuity of care. He has the right to know in advance what appointment times and physicians are available and where. The patient has the right to expect that the hospital will provide a mechanism whereby he is informed by his physician or a delegate of the physician of the patient's continuing health care requirements following discharge.

11. The patient has the right to examine and receive an explanation of his bill regardless of source of payment.

12. The patient has the right to know what hospital rules and regulations apply to his conduct as a patient.

No catalog of rights can guarantee for the patient the kind of treatment he has a right to expect. A hospital has many functions to perform, including the prevention and treatment of disease, the education of both health professionals and patients, and the conduct of clinical research. All these activities must be conducted with an overriding concern for the patient, and, above all, the recognition of his dignity as a human being. Success in achieving this recognition assures success in the defense of the rights of the patient.

Health Education
role and responsibility of health care institutions

INTRODUCTION

The following paragraphs from the AHA's *Policy Statement on Provision of Health Services* provide a foundation for the statement on health education.

"The system [for the delivery of health services] must be oriented to the maintenance of personal good health and to the prevention of illness rather than being primarily oriented to the treatment of illness after it becomes acute.

"The system must include financial incentives for keeping people well and, if they are ill, for making them well as soon as possible.

"Every individual shares a responsibility to protect his own health, and proper discharge of the responsibility will reduce the incidence of illness, disease, and injury. In order to encourage individuals to take care of themselves to the maximum extent possible, programs of education to teach people how to exercise this responsibility must be developed, conducted, evaluated, and maintained."

STATEMENT

Health education is an integral part of high-quality health care. Hospitals and other health care institutions, as focal points of community health care, have an obligation to promote, organize, implement and evaluate health education programs. As a part of this process, hospitals should plan with other health care institutions and community agencies to define each organization's role and responsibility in meeting the health education needs of the populations they serve.

In order to improve health and health care services, ongoing systems of health education must be planned, implemented, and documented. The maintenance of health and the prevention of disease can be achieved by a cooperative effort between knowledgeable and motivated consumers and health care personnel. Health education is a planned process that entails the joint identification of needs, the exchange of knowledge and concerns, and the clarification of personal responsibilities for health—all designed to encourage positive health practices and to improve the delivery of health care.

Hospitals and other health care institutions should recognize the opportunity to exercise a role of leadership in the health education of three specific audiences: the patient and his family; personnel, including employees, medical staff, volunteers, and trustees; and the community at large.

The major emphasis of health education is health promotion, which includes health maintenance, disease and trauma management, and the improvement of the health care system and its utilization. Through health education programs, hospitals and other health care institutions can contribute to important health care goals, such as improved quality of patient care, better utilization of outpatient services, fewer admissions and readmissions to inpatient facilities, shorter lengths of stay, and reduced health care costs.

A significant corporate commitment, including staff and financial resources, is essential if hospitals and other health care institutions are to fulfill their leadership role in health education. This commitment involves the acceptance and implementation of health education as an integral component of health care, the designation of specific responsibility for organizing and implementing health education programs, and continuing education. Programs to fulfill this commitment can be developed either independently by hospitals or other health care institutions or through collaboration with health professional groups, consumer groups, health associations concerned with specific diseases, and the educational community.

Financial responsibility for health education that is integral to the treatment and care of the patient is a legitimate part of the cost of caring for the patient. Health education that is designed to maintain the good health of the community at large and to prevent illness should be viewed as a service to the community. Such services are legitimate activities for hospitals and other health care institutions; however, efforts should be made to broaden the base of financial support for them by working collaboratively with other agencies and by seeking funding for health education programs.

White Paper
patient health education

The following White Paper addessses the issue of patient health education and the operational role which Blue Cross Plans can assume in this area. It finds that a patient education program, integrated into the routine services of the institution, offers the potential for both cost containment and improved quality of patient care. It concludes with the recommendation that Blue Cross Plans should encourage health care institutions to establish and operate programs in patient education and should support them financially through the existing payment mechanism.

The health care system is being challenged to improve its efficiency and effectiveness. Reforms in the system must forcefully address the need to contain rising health care costs and to assure the quality of health care services.

Given the complexity and the diversity of this challenge, no single response is appropriate. As one mechanism among many, patient health education may contribute to containing health care costs and enhancing the individual's understanding of and compliance with his treatment regimen. Patient education reinforces the patient's awareness of his responsibility for his own health, and self-responsibility is crucial for the ultimate effectiveness of health care.

Patient health education, for the present purpose, is a process comprising several elements: mutual identification of present and future health care needs by patient and professional, planning for the appropriate mix of professional and patient responsibility for meeting those needs, exchange of knowledge regarding the selected treatment regimen, motivation of patient and professional to perform their respective roles, and continuing evaluation of alternative methodologies. Patient education is part of the total process of patient care. As used here, patient education generally refers to hospital-based programs. However, the locus of the intervention is not as important as its nature.

The purpose of this statement is twofold: to examine the evidence on the impact of patient health education on the cost and quality of patient care and to recommend an operational course of action to Plans.

ISSUES

The concept of patient health education raises several issues. The principal questions which must be resolved, however, are:

1. Should Plans pay for patient education?
2. What kinds of criteria should be employed to determine the allocability of patient education expenses to Plan reimbursement?
3. What is the appropriate role for plans in patient health education?

The answers to such questions emerge from an evaluation of the impact of patient education on the cost and quality of health care.

EFFECTS ON COSTS

In examining the costs of patient care, one may adopt several perspectives: health care costs per capita in a given service area, costs per admission, costs per service unit, and costs per episode of illness. The development of valid and reliable measures is crucial to the proper evaluation of the patient education program.

Theoretically, patient education might contribute to reduced costs by decreasing the unnecessary utilization of health care services and by encouraging use of the most appropriate locus of care for health problems. These potential effects are critical to improving the efficacy of medical services.

Empirical evidence suggests that structured patient education speeds recovery in certain case types. For example, preoperative instruction has resulted in a significantly higher incidence of early discharge among those receiving intensive preoperative instruction and practice as compared to those not receiving such treatment.[1] Other studies have found similar results. Specific educational interventions can lead to reduced use of postoperative narcotics,[2] decreased emergency room utilization,[3] decreased readmissions and patient days for readmissions,[4] and reduced total admissions for a target population.[5]

[1]Healy, Kathryn M., "Does Preoperative Instruction Really Make a Difference?" American Journal of Nursing, January 1968, pp. 62–67.
[2]Egbert, Lawrence D., et al., "Reduction of Postoperative Pain by Encouragement and Instruction of Patients," New England Journal of Medicine, April 16, 1964, pp. 825–827.
[3]Miller, Leona, and Goldstein, Jack, "More Efficient Care of Diabetic Patients in a County Hospital Setting," New England Journal of Medicine, June 29, 1972, pp. 1388–1391.
[4]Rosenberg, Stanley G., "Patient Education Leads to Better Care for Heart Patients," HSMHA Health Services Reports, September 1971, pp. 793–802.
[5]Ibid.

Total health care cost for the individual may be reduced by substituting less expensive treatment modalities and loci of care for hospitalization and emergency room use. To assess whether such substitutions really do reduce *total* costs, total utilization of health services by specific groups over a given time frame must be calculated.

While not presenting conclusive evidence of reduced *total* costs of care for specific groups, some studies do suggest large cost savings as a result of changes in the pattern of utilization. For example, the Tufts-New England Medical Center research,[6] using a self-selected sample of male hemophiliac outpatients given postperiod instruction and practice in self-infusion, yielded the following pre-post comparisons: total inpatient days declined from 432 to 42, outpatient visits per patient decreased from 23.0 to 5.5, and total costs per patient went down 45% (from $5780 to $3209). At the University of Southern California Medical Center, a reorganization of the diabetic care system, incorporating a telephone "hotline" for information, medical advice, and the filling of prescriptions, counseling by physicians and nurses, and pamphlets and posters to promote the service, was associated with more than a 50% reduction in emergency room visits per clinic patient and the avoidance of approximately 2300 medication visits.[7] These findings suggest that certain types of patient education do promote the substitution of self-care and information-seeking for acute care services.

On balance, organized patient education has demonstrated its effectiveness in reducing the unnecessary utilization of certain health care services and in encouraging the use of the most appropriate, least-cost settings for care.

EFFECTS ON QUALITY OF CARE

Patient health education has also demonstrated considerable potential for improving the quality of care.

Several studies have demonstrated the beneficial impact of patient education on the *process* of patient care. The use of an interdisciplinary team to provide educationally oriented support to patients with congestive heart failure has resulted in increased knowledge among study patients in one sample regarding diet, medications, disease process, and, even more importantly, increased adherence to the treatment regimen.[8] Other research suggests that patient education enhances patient understanding of and compliance with the process of care.[9]

With respect to health care *outcomes,* studies have shown the quality-increasing effects of patient education. At the University of Southern California Medical Center, the reorganization of the system of diabetic care and the initiation of a multi-faceted program of patient education was associated with a reduction of approximately two-thirds in the incidence of diabetic coma from

[6]Levine, Peter H., and Britten, Anthony F., "Supervised Patient Management of Hemophilia," *Annals of Internal Medicine,* No. 78, 1973, pp. 195–201.
[7]See previous study by Leona Miller and Jack Goldstein.
[8]Rosenberg, Stanley G., "Patient Education Leads to Better Care for Heart Patients."
[9]Reported in: Green, Lawrence W., "Toward Cost-Benefit Evaluations of Health Education: Some Concepts, Methods, and Examples," pp. 36–37 (unpublished paper).

1968 to 1970.[10] Similarly, in another study, a significantly higher percentage of congestive heart failure patients receiving educational support improved in their ability to function, as measured by the American Heart Association classification. Also, recent work[11] at Massachusetts General Hospital has shown that the provision of intensive preoperative and postoperative information and guidance contributed to reduced pain among surgery patients. these studies point to the potential of patient education in enhancing health status.

CONCLUSION

The available information regarding patient health education indicates that, where conducted by a coordinated mix of educational and clinical specialists and directed to individual needs and capabilities, it both increases the quality of health care and presents potential cost savings to the health care system and to the public it serves. The Blue Cross system has consistently supported delivery and financing innovations which improve the system's efficiency and effectiveness. As such, patient health education efforts should be encouraged and supported, for they are one promising means of achieving these objectives.

Accordingly, Plans should encourage health care institutions to establish and operate programs in patient education and should support them financially through the existing payment mechanism. To realize its full potential for cost savings and quality improvement, it is critical that the patient education function be integrated into the total process of patient care. To assure that sound programs are developed and maintained, the following guidelines are suggested as criteria for determining payment for patient education programs. In applying these guidelines, the variation in programs and population needs for patient education should be considered. Accordingly, a flexible approach to their interpretation should be adopted.

GUIDELINES FOR PROGRAMS IN PATIENT EDUCATION

1. The purpose and operational objectives of the program should be clearly stated, and the techniques for meeting the objectives should be specified.
2. Patient education should be provided as an integral element of the total patient care process within a supportive organizational framework.[12] Existing hospital-based programs in patient education shall be reviewed by either the Joint Commission on Accreditation of Hospitals or the Bureau of Hospitals of the American Osteopathic Association.
3. Necessary and appropriate health education should be developed and financed as a routine element of the care of each patient.
4. Educational methodologies should be directed to specific case types and

---

[10]Miller and Goldstein.
[11]Egbert, et al.
[12]Examples of this organizational framework are the hospital, home care program, HMO, or community health education program.

desired behavioral changes and the results of such interventions as to cost and quality of care should be documented. As in other expenses, continuing management evaluation of the cost effectiveness of the service should be conducted. Programs should be revised over time to reflect the results of such evaluation.

It is appropriate that the Blue Cross system encourage the development of cost-effective programs in patient education. Where patient education is properly related to the other components of the total patient care process, there is clear potential for reduction of health care costs and improvement in the quality of health care processes and outcomes. Blue Cross Plans share responsibility with those providing patient education to ensure that this potential is realized. Accordingly, the Blue Cross System should play an active part in the development, implementation, and evaluation of sound programs in patient education.

Statement on Patient Education

Resolutions 37 and 41 (C-74) dealing with patient education were referred to the Board of Trustees for study and report at the 1975 Annual Convention.

Both resolutions called for planned programs of patient education developed and supervised by patient education committees whose membership would include health professionals, educators and consumers. Both would have required that such programs be prescribed by a physician and documented on the patient's charts, as a basis for third-party reimbursement.

The American Medical Association's Department of Health Education and Division of Medical Practice have been exploring the overall subject of planned patient education programs and have arrived at the following general findings and recommendations in response to Resolutions 37 and 41 (C-74).

DEFINITION AND ROLE OF PLANNED PATIENT EDUCATION PROGRAMS

It is recognized that increasingly complex patterns of health care, along with the patient's environment, attitude, lifestyle and cooperation, all play an important part in effective treatment. Informed, motivated and supportive participation in treatment by patients and their families can aid the recovery of the patient and enhance the quality of his health. Patient education, as an integral part of high quality health care, provides an avenue to such improved participation.

Education of the patient has always been part of the ongoing professional responsibility of physicians, nurses, dietitians, therapists and all other members of the health team. Health professionals have traditionally provided patients with some information about their illness and the prescribed course of treatment. Some health instruction has also been provided. In some situations, there is a need indicated for a structured educational effort beyond that which individual members of the team can provide. It is in these situations that planned patient education programs may be expected to serve.

The provision of patient education services, designed to assist the patient and his family in the effective management of individual health, is a shared and continuous responsibility of both the physician and the patient. Patient education directed toward the effective management of individual illness and maintenance of health commences with the patient's entry into the health services. A positive personal experience between the physician and the patient at first contact will greatly contribute to the success of an effective patient education program.

The following factors define planned patient education:

1. Programs are distinguished from general health education of the public in that they focus on individuals who present themselves for medical services in institutions and in physicians' offices.
2. Programs are directed at the patient's understanding of his specific disease entity or physical or mental disability.
3. Programs assist the patient (and/or sometimes family members) to cooperate in the treatment of the disease or disability.
4. Programs involve patients with diseases or disabilities in which there are substantial grounds for belief that the patient will be better able to participate in treatment and that the treatment will be more effective with such a planned program than without it.

It should be clear from these four factors that planned patient education programs are distinct from general health education programs for the public and from programs intended as education for prevention of disease or for health maintenance. The planned program is for patients under treatment.

As the relationship between the physician and the patient is established, the physician determines the patient's level of knowledge concerning his illness or health, and the patient's educational needs. In this relationship, it is incumbent upon the patient to provide the necessary health history and medical information, and to comply with the prescribed medical regimen. Adherence to a prescribed treatment program is dependent upon the patient's understanding and acceptance of his condition, recognition of the importance of his role in the daily management of his prescribed treatment and satisfaction with health services provided. It is in these areas that a planned patient education program can enhance quality care.

REIMBURSEMENT

Planned patient education is a legitimate reimbursable item of patient care, when prescribed by a physician, appropriate to the patient's condition and substantiated by entries on the patient record. Planned patient education should be eligible for reimbursement under the various health insurance and other third-party payment programs.

BENEFITS

Properly planned programs of this type will improve care and can reduce the overall cost of treatment. Enabling patients to play a greater part in their own treatment can reduce unnecessary utilization of trained health professionals and of health care facilities. However, potential benefits such as cost containment, shortened recovery time and improved patient morale may not be immediately achievable. Any new interdisciplinary program takes time to develop and to become effective.

CONTENT AND ORGANIZATION

Planned patient education programs should be based on identified objectives; should make use of sound educational methods; should have approved content that is scientifically accurate; and should be adaptable to the individual needs of patients.

Objectives need to be clarified at the outset along with specific criteria for measuring their achievement. The success or failure of the program should be determined by how well the objectives are realized.

RECOMMENDATIONS

The Board of Trustees believes the general findings and recommendations contained in this report respond to Resolutions 37 and 41, and recommends that the report be adopted and Association activities to improve effective patient education be continued.

Janice C. Colwell
Michael R. Ryan

V

Patient Teaching Resource File

Patient teaching at Mercy Hospital and Medical Center is part of the day-to-day delivery of nursing care. As a means of enhancing the teaching-learning process, the nursing staff identified the need for supplemental aids as a visual reinforcement for the patient and his family.

A committee composed of interested staff nurses, clinical specialists, supervisors, and clinical instructors was formed with the initial task of assessing the patient population, both adult and pediatric, to determine patient education needs. The assessment indicated that the majority of the patient teaching focused on the following illness areas and related interventions: (1) hypertension, (2) respiratory, (3) oncology, (4) diet, (5) ostomy, (6) cardiac, (7) diabetes, and (8) medication. Based on this assessment, letters of inquiry were sent to companies and health organizations known to have an interest in patient education. A list of recipients of the letter follows.

Abbott Laboratories
Public Relations Department
P.O. Box 68
North Chicago, Illinois 60064

Aims Instructional Media Service, Inc.
P.O. Box 1010
Hollywood, California 90028

American Cancer Society
Audiovisual Program Assistant
219 East 42nd Street
New York, New York 10017
(also, local branch)

American College of Obstetricians and Gynecologists
1 East Wacker Drive
Suite 2700
Chicago, Illinois 60601

American Dental Association
Bureau of Audiovisual Service
211 East Chicago Avenue
Chicago, Illinois 60611

American Diabetes Association
620 North Michigan Avenue
Chicago, Illinois 60605

American Foundation for the Blind
15 West 16th Street
New York, New York 10011

American Heart Association
National Center
7320 Greenville Avenue
Dallas, Texas 75231
(also, local branch)

American Hospital Association
840 North Lake Shore Drive
Chicago, Illinois 60611

American Journal of Nursing Company
Educational Services Division
10 Columbus Circle
New York, New York 10019

American Lung Association
(local branch)

Ames Company
Division of Miles Laboratories, Inc.
1127 Myrtle
Elkhart, Indiana 46514

Association Films, Inc.
600 Grand Avenue
Ridgefield, New Jersey 07657

Association Instructional Materials
A Division of Association Films, Inc.
600 Madison Avenue
New York, New York 10022

Ayerst Laboratories
685 Third Avenue
New York, New York 10017

BFA Educational Media
2211 Michigan Avenue
Santa Monica, California 90404

Carman Educational Associates, Inc.
Box 205
Youngstown, New York 14174

Central Press
P.O. Box 252
Milwaukee, Wisconsin 53201

Ciba Pharmaceutical Company
Public Relations Department
556 Morris Avenue
Summit, New Jersey 07901

Connecticut State Department of Health
Public Health Education Section
79 Elm Street
Hartford, Connecticut 00115

Ealing Corporation
2225 Massachusetts Avenue
Cambridge, Massachusetts 02140

Educational Television Division
1501 Health Sciences East
University of California
San Francisco Medical Center
San Francisco, California 94122

Eli Lilly and Company
Audiovisual Film Librarian
Indianapolis, Indiana 46206

Endo Laboratories, Inc.
1000 Stewart Avenue
Garden City, New York 11530

Epilepsy Foundation of America
1828 L Street, N.W.
Washington, D.C. 20036

Film Library
Lederle Laboratories
Pearl River, New York 10965

Geigy Pharmaceuticals
Division of Geigy Chemical Corporation
Ardsley, New York 10502

Foundation for Research & Education in Sickle Cell Disease
421–431 West 120th Street
New York, New York 10027

Johnson and Johnson
Consumer Relations Department
501 George Street
New Brunswick, New Jersey 08903

King Screen Productions
320 Aurora Avenue, North
Seattle, Washington 98109

Lifelong Learning
University Extension
University of California
Berkeley, California 93720

McNeil Laboratories, Inc.
Camp Hill Road
Fort Washington, Pennsylvania 19034

Mead Johnson and Company
Public Relations Department
Evansville, Indiana 47721

Merck, Sharp and Dohme
2010 Swift Drive
Oak Brook, Illinois 60521

National Clearinghouse for Drug Information
5600 Fischers Lane
Rockville, Maryland 20852

National Dairy Council
111 North Canal
Chicago, Illinois 60606

Nutrition Foundation
888–17th Street Northwest
Washington, D.C. 20006

Professional Research, Inc.
461 North LaBrea Avenue
Los Angeles, California 90036

Society for Visual Education, Inc.
1345 Diversey Parkway
Chicago, Illinois 60614

Sterling Communications, Inc.
309 West Jackson Boulevard
Chicago, Illinois 60606

United Ostomy Association
1111 Wilshire Boulevard
Los Angeles, California 90017

The patient education committee evaluated the available literature for suitability to the patient's level of understanding, range of information, and clarity of the subject matter. Needless to say, the committee had a wealth of material to choose from. The most pertinent pamphlets and booklets were selected for each of the eight sections.

About 50 percent of the materials selected were available at no charge. Several of the items ranged in cost from twenty-five cents to four dollars. Because the Administration of Mercy Hospital and Medical Center views patient teaching as an important facet of quality care, they agreed to establish a patient education account. All charge items are purchased from this fund; thus, there is no charge to the patient.

As a means of providing a concise and efficient system for the staff nurse to select pertinent supplemental resources, a Patient Education Catalog File was developed. The File is divided into eight sections as previously noted. A sample of each booklet was placed in the Catalog to facilitate the nurse's evaluation of its appropriateness for the individual patient. Each nursing unit received a Catalog to be used as a resource for staff members.

The pamphlets and books are stocked, distributed, and inventoried by our Supply, Processing, and Distribution Department (central supply). Each section of the catalog was assigned a corresponding number and each pamphlet for that section was assigned an order number. When the nurse selects the appropriate item, she can order it directly from the S.P.D. Department utilizing this system, for example, 5-2 Urinary Ostomies (see Figure 6). Because there is no charge to the patient for the booklets, several copies may be ordered and given to family members.

Since the development of the File, the materials have been periodically evaluated in an attempt to maintain the standards established by the committee. Staff suggestions for new material are reviewed by the members of the Nursing Education and Research Department.

The Patient Education Catalog File has been utilized for two years. The Nursing Staff of Mercy Hospital and Medical Center have found the catalog to be an effective resource in addition to, but not in place of, bedside teaching. The catalog's effectiveness has been determined by frequency of reordering materials and the verbal response of the staff and patients.

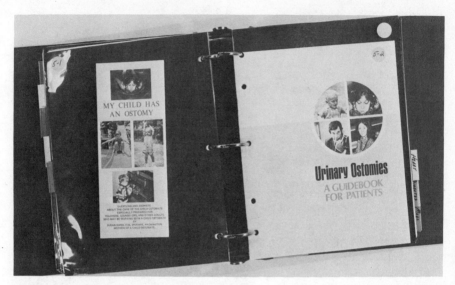

Figure 6. *Sample pages from the patient education catalog file. Booklets shown are from urinary ostomies. (Reprinted courtesy United Ostomy Association, 1111 Wilshire Boulevard, Los Angeles, Calif. 90017)*

At present our patient education endeavors are centered on exploring the use of other media as supplemental aids to the teaching-learning process for the patient.

Guidelines for Teaching Cardiac Surgery Patients

The following tools are utilized in the teaching program for patients about to undergo cardiac surgery. The tools illustrated include:

1. Preoperative information for cardiac surgery patients.
2. Documentation forms· entitled "Assessment and Teaching Record for Preoperative care."
3. Discharge information for cardiac surgery patients.
4. Documentation form entitled "Nursing Transfer/Discharge Summary."
5. Documentation form entitled "Initial Postoperative Clinic Assessment."

Sample documentation is added to illustrate the use of each of the forms.

PREOPERATIVE INFORMATION FOR CARDIAC SURGERY PATIENTS

This preoperative information will assist you to

1. Define the operative procedure
2. Identify the preparations necessary before your surgery
3. Recognize equipment and procedures necessary for immediate postoperative care

You have been admitted to this hospital for cardiac surgery that is to take place in the near future. Your doctors will discuss the exact problem you have and describe what your surgery will be. This information and diagrams will help you to understand your disease and surgery. If you have questions, please ask them.

FUNCTION AND STRUCTURE OF THE HEART

The heart is a hollow, muscular organ that pumps blood, enriched with oxygen and nutrients to all parts of the body. It lies in the center of the chest, slightly to the left, and is protected by the breast bone and rib cage. The structure is divided into four chambers, separated by valves that regulate blood flow through the heart.

Like all other parts of the body, the heart requires oxygen and energy to work. The heart muscle is nourished by its own blood supply that originates from the aorta, the RIGHT and LEFT CORONARY ARTERIES. These two main arteries lie on the surface of the heart and divide into smaller branches so the entire heart muscle is supplied with blood and nutrients.

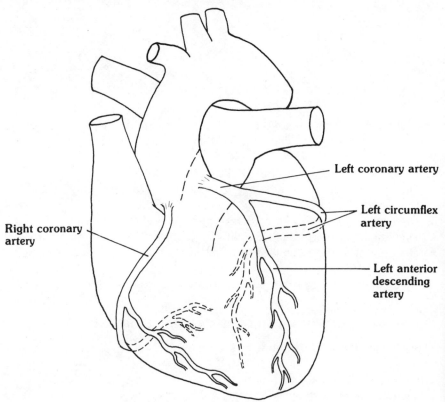

Right coronary artery

Left coronary artery

Left circumflex artery

Left anterior descending artery

HEART DISEASE AND RELATED SURGERY

Open heart surgery originally described procedures requiring opening the heart chambers to correct a defect. This term now applies to any procedure in which the heart-lung or bypass machine temporarily replaces the normal function of the heart. During the operation "the pump" will circulate and put oxygen into your blood and allow your heart to be at rest. When the operation is completed, your heart gradually resumes its work of pumping blood throughout your body.

Coronary Artery Disease is caused by atherosclerosis commonly called hardening of the arteries. In atherosclerosis the inner lining of the artery is thickened and made rough by fatty deposits of cholesterol. The passageway is narrowed like rust build-up in a pipe, and blood flow beyond the blockage is decreased.

We do not know why atherosclerosis develops but the following factors are more common in people with coronary artery disease.

Risk Factors

Smoking
Overweight
Stress or tension
Lack of exercise
High blood pressure
Diabetes
Family history of heart disease
Eating too much animal fat and cholesterol

Coronary artery disease is a mechanical problem due to the blockage of blood flow. This obstruction can be surgically bypassed to provide improved blood flow to the area of the heart below the blockage. One or more coronary artery bypass grafts may be used to add circulation to the heart muscle thereby relieving angina and improving the function of the heart.

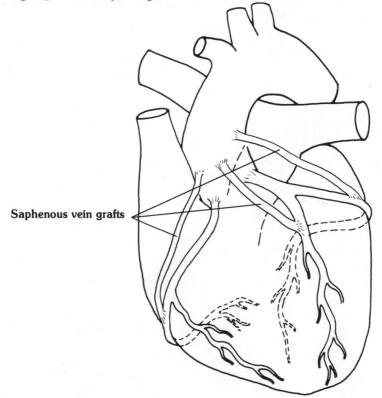

Saphenous vein grafts

Valvular Heart Disease exists when one or more of the chamber outlet structures are changed by birth defects, infection, rheumatic or scarlet fever. Such changes cause thickening and scarring which make opening or closing of the valve more difficult. Defective valves cause extra work for the heart. Repairing or replacing your damaged valve allows the heart to pump more effectively.

The damaged valve will be replaced by an artificial valve or a tissue valve. Following valve replacement it is very important that you follow specific recommendations for preventing infections that could damage the new valve. It will also be necessary for you to take medication to anticoagulate your blood. Clotting is a normal characteristic of blood but it can cause problems with certain types of artificial valves. Anticoagulants lengthen the time it normally takes for blood to clot and therefore reduce the possibility of clots forming inside a blood vessel. Additional information about infection and anticoagulants will be discussed with you after your surgery.

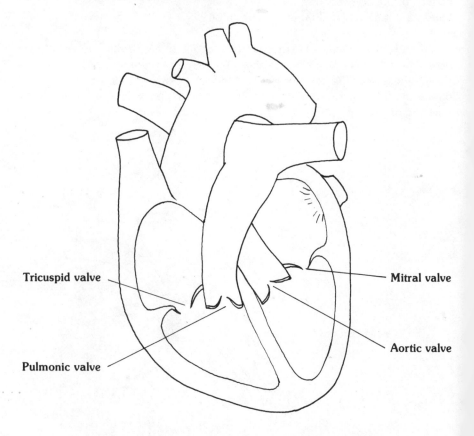

Tricuspid valve

Mitral valve

Aortic valve

Pulmonic valve

Regardless of whether you are having a valve replacement or artery bypass grafts, the procedures and care you will require are the same. It is important that you and your family have and understand this information.

Please ask questions about anything you do not understand!

PREOP PREPARATION

The day before surgery you will have x-rays, EKG, and blood drawn for laboratory work. You will meet many of the people—nurses, doctors, and technicians—who will be taking care of you after your surgery. The anesthesiologist, the doctor who puts you to sleep, will talk with you about how he will give you the anesthetic.

The evening before surgery you will take a shower using special soap to wash both your body and your hair. In the morning before surgery you should repeat the shower and shampoo. This decreases the bacteria on skin and hair and lessens the likelihood of infection.

After midnight you will not be permitted to eat or drink. This is to empty the stomach and decrease the possibility of vomiting during surgery.

A respiratory therapist will see and instruct you on the use of breathing treatments and exercises for use postoperatively. If you smoke, you will be advised to stop if possible or reduce the number of cigarettes you use. This is to prepare your lungs to function as well as possible after surgery and prevent an infection or pneumonia.

The afternoon before or the morning of surgery, a technician from the operating room will come to shave your skin in preparation for surgery. Your chest and abdomen will be scrubbed and shaved. If you are having a coronary artery bypass graft, both legs will also be shaved as the vein graft will be taken from one of the legs. After this prep you should shower again with the special soap.

INCISION

The chest incision will be a midsternum (breast bone) incision from the notch at the clavicle (collar bone) to below the end of the breast bone. Access to the heart is made by dividing the breast bone. If a vein graft is needed, an incision will be made in the leg from thigh to ankle to permit removal of a vein. Each incision will be covered by a dressing.

VALUABLES

Jewelry, wallets, eyeglasses, etc. should be given to the family if possible or may be sent to BMS to be locked in the clothing room. No personal belongings may be left in the room because you will go to the Intensive Care Unit (ICU) for several days and it is possible you may not return to the same room.

MEDICATIONS

Before leaving for the Operating Room, you will be given medication to help you relax before anesthesia is begun. You will leave your room approximately one hour before your surgery is scheduled to begin. This allows time for additional preparation in the operating room.

OPERATING ROOM PROCEDURES

After you are in the Operating Room additional procedures will be done. These include:

Intravenous. As many as five IV lines will be necessary to give you fluids, medications, and blood during the operation. These will be started in your arms during surgery and will be removed when they are no longer necessary, usually on the second or third day after surgery.

Nasogastric tube. The N-G tube will be inserted through your nose into your stomach to drain out gastric fluids that will accumulate during the operation and to decrease nausea and vomiting. This will be removed before you begin eating, usually on the second or third day after surgery.

Foley catheter. Will be inserted into your bladder so all urine produced can be measured and you need not worry about urinating while you are asleep. This will be removed when you are awake and able to urinate, usually on the second or third day after surgery.

Endotracheal tube. The E-T tube will be inserted, usually through the mouth and down into the windpipe. This allows air to be pumped into the lungs by a ventilator during the operation. While the E-T tube is in place, you will not be able to talk because the tube passes through the larynx (voice box). It will stay in place until you are able to breathe normally, usually 24 to 72 hours.

Chest tubes. Will be inserted under the incision area to allow drainage of blood and fluid that accumulates immediately after surgery. You may have one, two, or three chest tubes. These are removed when drainage has stopped, usually on the second or third day after surgery.

Pacemaker. Temporary pacing wires may be placed into the heart during the operation. These are connected to a small external pacemaker and may be used if the heart's rate is too slow. These are removed when the heart is stronger, usually on the second or third day after surgery.

While you are in the Operating Room, the Clinical Specialist will keep your family informed of your condition and progress. Upon completion of the operation, the doctor will want to talk with your family.

POSTOP CARE

You will be transferred from the Operating Room directly to the ICU. All staff in ICU are professional nurses and one nurse will be assigned to care for only you for the evening and night to provide the constant observation all cardiac surgery patients require.

After you arrive in ICU, it is necessary to complete many procedures including EKG, lab work, and x-rays and to attach the needed equipment to monitor your progress. It requires one to two hours to complete these tasks before your family will be permitted to visit for the first time. This is usually late on the afternoon of surgery. Most likely you will not really be awake or know that your family is visiting during the first evening.

PAIN

You will have pain postoperatively. Usually this is incisional pain and can be relieved by repositioning or medication. Pain medication will be given to you as you need it and the nurse will check with you frequently to determine if you are uncomfortable.

If you have coronary artery disease, you may experience some angina and nitroglycerine will be given for this pain.

VISITING AND WAITING AREAS

While you are in ICU your family may visit during the specified times. These visiting hours are posted on the doors to ICU.

Waiting areas for families are located on the sixth floor by the elevator and on the fifth floor near the chapel. The chapel provides a quiet area for meditation and waiting. If your family wishes to see a chaplain they need only to ask. Your family should advise the nursing staff of contact telephone numbers where they may be reached when away from the hospital.

ACTIVITY

Your activity will be increased as you can tolerate it after surgery. You will probably sit on the side of the bed the first day and be up in a chair on the second day after surgery.

Your stay in ICU will be dependent both on your progress and the availability of beds. The usual length of stay in ICU is three to five days.

You should review this information and share it with your family. The Clinical Specialist or Staff Nurse will discuss this with you and your family before your surgery. If you have any questions, please let us help you answer them.

ASSESSMENT AND TEACHING RECORD FOR PREOPERATIVE CARE

	Patient Instructed (Date)	Verbalized Understanding (Initial)
I. PreOp Care		
A. Type of anesthesia (local, spinal, general)	*by anesthesia*	*SF*
B. P.M. prep (shower, enemas, NPO)	*8/31*	*SF*
C. A.M. prep (shower, skin prep, NPO, care of valuables, prosthesis, on call med)	*8/31*	

	Patient Instructed (Date)	Verbalized Understanding (Initial)
II. Immediate PostOp Care		
A. Return to Unit, RR, or SICU	8/31	SF
B. Routine care and equipment (VS, IV, ET tube, NG tube, Foley cath., chest tube, dressing)	8/31	SF
C. Pain (medication, splinting wound)	8/31	SF
D. Family (visiting hours, time of surgery, waiting area)	8/31	SF

	Patient Demonstrated Ability to Do	
	(Date)	(Initials)
III. Special PostOp Care		
A. Ventilation (T, C, DB, Rebreather, Spirocare)	8/31	SF
B. Circulation (exercise extremities, i.e. isometrics, ROM, elastic stockings)	8/31	SF

IV. Comments (Narrative to include A. and B.)
A. Ability to explain anatomy and physiology
in relation to operative procedure
B. Reaction and response to surgery

Subjective: *Speaks with a calm and assured tone.*

Objective: *States he is prepared for his surgery. States the nature of his coronary artery disease and can identify by name the arteries to be bypassed, and describes the operative procedure using a saphenous vein graft. Admits that he is nervous, but feels better now that questions have been answered.*

Assessment: *Prepared for surgery in the A.M.*

Plans: *Support family with information during the course of the surgery and answer additional questions. Be available for first visit by the family in the afternoon.*

Sondra Ferguson, R.N.

DISCHARGE INFORMATION FOR CARDIAC SURGERY PATIENTS

This is a brief outline of your recovery period from the time of discharge until you return to clinic. It will help you to

1. Plan for going home
2. Recognize your tolerance for activity
3. Identify any problems with surgical incisions
4. State the name, dosage, and purpose of each medication
5. Plan for return visit to the clinic

By following these guidelines, using common sense, and setting realistic goals for yourself, you will attain maximum recovery.

After any type of surgery the recovery period may seem to pass slowly and you will have good days and bad days. Considerable psychological energy was used in preparing for surgery, and now you may experience a let down or depressed feeling. These feelings are normal and they should not be allowed to interfere with your recovery.

The normal recovery period is the first four to six weeks you are home. Muscle tone begins to return and you are able to resume normal levels of activity. It is important *not* to overdo. Rest when you are tired. Activities should gradually be increased each day.

Here is information to help answer questions you may have.

Going Home. Travel by car is best. You may stop frequently (every 1 – 2 hours) if the trip is long. Loose clothing is usually more comfortable than pajamas. Just before you leave the hospital you may want to ask for pain medication.

Bathing. Permitted when the stitches have been removed and there is no drainage from the incision. Wash gently with soap and water but do not scrub. Adhesive strips should be removed after bathing so they do not retain moisture and irritate the skin. Extremely hot water should be avoided as it may cause you to feel dizzy.

Diet. Eat a well balanced diet. If you were on a salt restriction before surgery, it is wise to continue the same degree of restriction in the first month after surgery. If you are to follow a special diet, the dietitian will discuss this with you before discharge. As before surgery, shortness of breath, ankle swelling, or rapid weight gain indicate fluid retention. This should be reported to your doctor and may indicate the need for reducing fluid and salt intake.

Drinking. If you enjoy a drink before or during your evening meal or at bedtime you may continue to do so after surgery. Do not drink alcoholic beverages if you are taking medication like tranquilizers or sleeping pills. Limit your drinks to one or two drinks a day during your recovery period.

Driving. You may not drive for at least six weeks after your surgery. In order to operate on your heart, the breast bone was divided. It is now wired together with stainless steel wires. These wires hold the bone firmly together so it can heal. It takes four to six weeks for the sternum (breast bone) to completely heal together. Other activities which could cause injury include riding bicycles, motorcycles, or horses.

Housework. You should not expect to resume total responsibility for household duties or meal preparation for four to six weeks. This includes vacuuming, unscrewing jar lids, opening heavy windows, or lifting more than 10 pounds. If you live alone, you should consider staying with a friend or relative for a short time.

Incisions. May be numb or sore for several weeks. This gradually decreases. Some redness is not uncommon. Changes in the weather, too much or too little activity and morning stiffness from sleeping in one position too long can all cause an incision to be uncomfortable. Allowing your shoulders to slump forward really does not help to make you more comfortable and certainly poor posture does not help your appearance. Maintain good posture and take your pain medication if necessary. If there is excessive or increased swelling, tenderness, or drainage from the incision, or if you have a temperature over 101°, call your doctor.

Medications. You may need to continue some of the same medications you were taking before surgery. Before discharge a nurse will discuss with you the purpose of your medications and when and how to take them.

Recreation. Do what you enjoy doing, but do not tire yourself. Spectator sports are best at first; then work more gradually into active forms of recreation.

Rest. Plan rest periods during the first week or two at home. It is not necessary to dress in pajamas or to go to bed. Try to get eight to ten hours of sleep each night and space your activities with rest periods to avoid extreme fatigue.

Sex. How soon you resume sexual activity will depend on you and your partner. Your desires and capacity to satisfy each other will be quite individual and should be discussed between the two of you. As with other activities, if you experience chest pain or discomfort, wait until you feel better and are more rested. Nitroglycerine may be prescribed for chest pain and can be taken prior to or during sexual activity if pain occurs.

Smoking. Increases heart rate, narrows blood vessels, raises blood pressure, and scars the lungs. It is very important that you stop. You were able to do without smoking for several days while in ICU and this is a good start toward breaking the habit. Stopping now can make you and your heart healthier.

Stairs. Climbing stairs requires more energy than walking. You may need to go slowly and rest if you become tired, dizzy, or short of breath.

Support stockings. May have been fitted immediately after your operation. They improve circulation and decrease fluid accumulation while you are less active during your recovery period. You may not require them. It is most important that you avoid crossing your legs as this causes pressure behind the knees and decreases blood flow to the legs. Elevate your legs when sitting and avoid standing in one position for lengthy periods of time.

Walking. The *best* exercise for you. It improves circulation, muscle tone, strength, and the way you feel. Walk daily and gradually increase the distance. Several short walks are better than one long walk. Extreme temperatures should be avoided, and it is easier to walk on flat surfaces as in shopping malls or athletic tracks.

Weight. Watch it carefully. Avoid excessive weight gains. Most likely you have lost a few pounds since your surgery. Do not worry about gaining it back unless you really need it. A weight gain of two to three pounds in one day is usually due to fluid retention rather than fat. If you are on a salt restriction and diuretics (water pills) you should weigh yourself regularly.

Work. The decision to return to work should not be made for at least six weeks, and your doctor may not release you until you have had a stress test, which is usually given at two to three months after surgery.

This information should be reviewed and discussed with you by the Clinical Specialist or Staff Nurse.

A clinic appointment has been made for you to see the doctor in the Cardiothoracic (CT) clinic on ————————————. If you are unable to keep this appointment call the hospital and ask for clinic scheduling to make another appointment.

MEDICATIONS FOR PATIENTS WHO HAVE HAD CORONARY ARTERY BYPASS

Multivitamin
  Dose:
  What it does: helps build you back up after surgery and may stimulate your appetite.
  Remember: Take only one tablet a day and eat a well balanced diet.
Iron (Ferrous sulfate or Ferrous gluconate)
  Dose:
  What it does: helps build your blood back up after surgery.
  Remember: It may upset your stomach so it is best to take with meals. It may make your bowel movements dark in color and tarry-like.
Aspirin
  Dose:
  What it does: decreases clotting mechanism of blood and lengthens bleeding time.
  Remember: May cause upset stomach, prolonged bleeding, ringing in the ears. DO NOT TAKE ANY ADDITIONAL ASPIRIN. If you have a headache or mild pain, acetaminophen (Tylenol or Datril) should be taken.
Persantine (dipyridamole)
  Dose:
  What it does: dilates coronary arteries to allow blood to pass more easily through newly grafted arteries.
  Remember: May cause headache or dizziness and stomach upset. Should be taken with meals
These medications are taken for approximately four to six weeks following surgery. You will be told when you no longer need them.

NURSING TRANSFER/DISCHARGE SUMMARY

Date & time of release: *9/12*
Destination: *Home*
Nursing referral: Yes *X* No
Condition at release: *Satisfactory*
Period of convalescence: *6 weeks*
Patient/family ability to provide care after discharge: *Independent in self-care activities*
Plan for medical follow-up (if discharged): *Cardiothoracic clinic in 2 weeks—10/1*

Prescriptions	Size and Dosage Form	Directions
Aspirin	*600 mg po*	*bid*
Dipyridamole	*50 mg po*	*bid*
Multivitamin	*1 tablet po*	*every day*
Ferrous Sulfate	*325 mg po*	*tid with meals*

SUMMARY BY PROBLEM TITLES (include special treatments/procedures, equipment being used by patient, patient/family teaching done, and response to teaching. Indicate if problem was resolved; if not, give specific recommendations for continuing nursing care.)
Coronary Artery Disease   → Surgery 9/1   ·

56-year-old man admitted 8/29 following 2 weeks work-up on medical service for CAD that did not respond to medical and dietary management. He had coronary artery bypasses to the right and left anterior descending arteries using saphenous vein grafts on 9/1. Post-op care included two days in SICU. On 9/4 he was transferred to 6-S. Cardiac monitor was d/c'd following no evidence of arrhythmias for 24 hours. IV antibiotics continued for 2 additional days and were stopped 9/6. He has been afebrile with stable B/P and pulse (B/P 116/70, apical pulse 86 and regular).

Ambulation is at will and he requires no motivation to be active. Sutures removed from sternal incision 9/8 and from right leg incision 9/11. Both incisions are clean, dry, and healing with no evidence of redness or edema.

Written discharge information sheets given to patient and wife. He is able to verbalize his understanding of discharge teaching including:

Activity limitations for 6 weeks—no driving or lifting
Dietary restrictions—continue on No Added Salt
Medications by name, dosage, and purpose
Return clinic appointment for follow-up care

PLAN: See in CT Clinic 10/1 for initial post-op visit.

Sondra Ferguson, R.N.

INITIAL POSTOPERATIVE CLINIC ASSESSMENT

Type of Surgery: *Coronary Artery Bypass*   Date: *9/1*   Surgeon: *Johns*

	Medications
Aspirin	*2 tabs (600 mg) twice a day*
Dipyridamole	*2 tabs (50 mg) twice a day*
Multivitamin	*1 tab each day*
Ferrous Sulfate (Iron)	*1 tab three times a day with meals*

Activity Tolerance/Limitations—*Walking around the block morning and afternoon. Has not begun to drive.*

Chest Pain and/or Use of NTG—*No angina requiring nitro. Some soreness along incision and side of chest.*

Diet—*Wife is preparing No Added Salt diet. Has gained 3 lbs. since discharge.*

Vital Signs—B/P *118/78*   T *98*   P *88* Ap.   R *20*   Wt. *176* lbs.

Edema—*1 + pedal on right leg below incision. Reminded this is not unusual and to keep legs elevated when sitting and to wear support hose.*

Incisions/Wound—*Sternal incision well healed. Leg incision tender to touch. No drainage. Steri-strips removed. Instructed to shower.*

ROM—*Full use of shoulder joints.*

Assessment: *Complying well with self-care instructions. He is pleased with his post-op progress.*

Plan: *See on return visit in one month. Evaluate for compliance to diet, check for weight gain and activity potential.*

Sondra Ferguson, R.N.

Pamela Kay Owen

VII

Excerpts from Guidelines to Patient Teaching

Comfort in the role of patient educator can be facilitated by the development of guidelines that can be used to outline content to be taught. These guidelines should be utilized as *examples* of material which can be taught to a particular patient; they should *not* be seen as rigid standards or mandates to be taught. For instance, a patient may need to learn about an item in the middle of a guideline first, and then progress to the beginning of the outline.

Documentation of the teaching-learning process is facilitated with the use of flow sheets. Several examples of flow sheets are included in this appendix.

HEALTH TEACHING PROGRAM: PREOP PREPARATION

Principles

It is the goal of preoperative teaching to instruct all surgery patients before surgery; to decrease apprehension and promote recovery. Routine preop, prep, and recovery room procedures are explained to the patient; including coughing and deep breathing, postop exercises and relaxation skills, IVs, suction tubes, pain, medications, and other postop expectations; according to the type of surgery and the physician's requests and procedures.

Goals

1. Have group presentations available for preop general education, followed with individual instruction.
2. Give preop instruction to allay fears, apprehension, and anxiety, and to promote comfort postoperatively and hasten recovery.
3. Present the patient with information on what to expect.
4. Assist the patient to cooperate effectively in his own recovery.

5. Promote increase in patient turnover, for more efficient utilization of hospital facilities.

Objectives

1. To facilitate recovery after surgery.
2. To supply information to improve patient's understanding of his part in recovery.
3. To alleviate fears that hinder recovery.
4. To describe in general simplified terms what the patient can expect to see and do postoperatively.
5. To answer questions that develop, and to clarify misconceptions.
6. To demonstrate and practice any postop exercises and treatments for recovery.
7. To familiarize the patient with postop environment and equipment.
8. To allow time for and encourage verbalization of concerns.

PREOP TEACHING WORKSHEET

Diagnosis:
Surgery:
Discharge:
Background Data:
Home Call:
Address:
Phone:

Knowledge	1 P F	2 P F	3 P F	Comments
Preop Preparation				
Enema				
Skin prep				
Belongings				
Special tests				
Jewelry				
NPO				
Undergarments				
Gown				
Void				
Preop med (stay in bed)				
Surgery				
Define				
Time scheduled				
Family waiting room				
OR environment				
IV				
Anesthesia				
Suture line				
Dressing				
Drains/Tubes				
Foley				

Knowledge	1 P F	2 P F	3 P F	Comments
Recovery				
Recovery room environment	——	——	——	
ET tube	——	——	——	
Oxygen mask/mist	——	——	——	
Frequent V/S	——	——	——	
ICU	——	——	——	
TC & DB exercises	——	——	——	
Incision support	——	——	——	
ROM exercises	——	——	——	
Relaxation skills	——	——	——	
Pain & medications	——	——	——	
Activity/ambulation	——	——	——	
Sore throat	——	——	——	
Equipment & Treatments				
Wound care, stitches	——	——	——	
Peri care	——	——	——	
Sitz bath	——	——	——	
IPPB	——	——	——	
Other	——	——	——	

P=patient; F=family; 1=needs instruction on; 2=needs reinforcement on; 3=comprehends instruction/appropriate behavior; NA=not applicable (does not need instruction on)

HEALTH TEACHING PROGRAM: HYPERTENSION

Goals

1. Prevent progression and complications of disease.
2. Maintain balanced control.

Objectives

1. To provide information on basic anatomy and physiology of circulatory system.
2. To promote understanding signs and symptoms, and predisposing and risk factors.
3. To increase understanding of participation in and cooperation with prescribed medical management.

   I. Hypertension Teaching Worksheet
     A. Definitions
     B. Management/Control
  II. Anatomy Guide
 III. Physiology Guide
 IV. Definitions Guide
  V. Pulse Guide
 VI. Blood Pressure Guide
VII. Signs and Symptoms Guide
VIII. Hypertensive Record Guide

HYPERTENSION TEACHING WORKSHEET

Knowledge	1 P F	2 P F	3 P F	Comments
Definitions				
A&P	___	___	___	
Signs and symptoms	___	___	___	
Predisposing factors	___	___	___	
Risks	___	___	___	
Management/Control				
Medications (time, dose, storage, effects, administration)	___	___	___	
Diet	___	___	___	
Weight control/reduction	___	___	___	
Stress/fatigue	___	___	___	
Daily exercise/rest	___	___	___	
Smoking	___	___	___	
Constipation/straining	___	___	___	
Taking own B/P, pulse	___	___	___	
Follow-up importance	___	___	___	
Importance of balance	___	___	___	
Other Instructions				

P=patient; F=family; 1=needs instruction on; 2=needs reinforcement on; 3=comprehends instruction/appropriate behavior

HEALTH TEACHING PROGRAM: DIABETES

Goal:
Promote control and maintain control of diabetes.

Objectives:

1. To understand the importance of testing urine.
2. To gain knowledge about effective medication management.
3. To be able to maintain a therapeutic diet.
4. To know the signs of uncontrolled diabetes.
5. To maintain good health.

  I. Diabetes I Class
    A. Introduction Teaching Worksheet
        1. Definitions
        2. Complications
        3. Management balance
    B. Anatomy Guide
    C. Physiology and Definitions Guide
    D. Diabetic Complications Guide

    E.   Diabetic Hygiene Guide
II. Diabetes II Class
    A. Medication/Management Teaching Worksheet
        1. Activity
        2. Urine testing
        3. Medication
        4. Complications
    B. Urine Testing Guide
    C. Insulin Guide
    D. Insulin Syringe Guide
    E. Injection Site Record Guide
    F. Diabetic Record Guide
III. Diabetes III Class
    A. Diet/Management Teaching Worksheet
        1. Diet
        2. Exchange Lists
        3. Do's and Don't's
        4. Food Packaging
        5. Measurements
        6. Meal Planning

PATIENT EDUCATION LEARNING OBJECTIVES

The client will be able to:

1. Describe basic anatomy and physiology of diabetes (definitions) and signs and symptoms.
2. Define acidosis and hypoglycemia and their management.
3. Recognize controllability of diabetes.
4. Recognize importance of proper balance between exercise, diet, medication.
5. Recognize complications associated with disease process of diabetes.
6. Effectively follow medical management regimen prescribed by physician.
7. Understand and demonstrate skill in urine testing.
   a. Identify purpose of testing urine for sugar and acetone.
   b. Identify proper supplies for urine testing.
   c. Identify times to test urine.
   d. Use proper technique for urine testing and double voiding for collecting urine.
   e. Interpret results of urine test using proper color chart.
   f. Maintain testing supplies in tightly covered container to keep moisture out and without touching test tape ends and not using outdated tape or discolored tablets.
   g. Recognize the need for additional urine testing when ill, infection is present, or abnormal test.
8. Understand prescribed medication.
   a. Recognize need and use of glucagon.

    b. Identify use of insulin.
      (1) Identify type, dose, and times.
      (2) Select proper syringe and needle and handle properly.
      (3) Select proper site and identify rotation schedule and reason for rotation.
      (4) Properly prepare and inject insulin.
      (5) Identify proper storage of insulin and equipment.
      (6) Identify symptoms of insulin reaction and what to do.
9. Understand prescribed diet.
    a. Identify importance of selected diet.
    b. Recognize the function of CHO, fat, and protein.
    c. Identify food exchanges.
    d. Demonstrate skill in meal planning.
10. Understand available resources and supplies.
11. Identify influence of illness on control of diabetes.
12. Recognize need to contact physician.
13. Maintain a written record of urine test results, medications, and comments to show to physician.
14. Understand proper foot care, personal hygiene, and general health care.
15. Identify the influence of a change in exercise levels on medical management.
16. Recognize importance of informing others of diabetes and carrying proper identification.

DIABETES INTRODUCTION: TEACHING WORKSHEET

Knowledge	1 P F	2 P F	3 P F	Comments
Definitions				
A&P				
Signs & symptoms				
Complications				
Hypoglycemia				
Ketoacidosis				
Vascular complications				
Infections				
Pregnancy				
Management				
Balance of diet, weight, exercise, medication				
Hygiene: eye care				
Personal skin cleanliness				
Dental care				
Foot care				
ID bracelet or card				
Carry form of sugar				
Inform others				

Knowledge	1 P F	2 P F	3 P F	Comments
Regular Dr. appointments	___	___	___	

Note: Class Diabetes II instructs on urine testing, medication management
    Class Diabetes III instructs on diet management

Scheduled for class II _____
Scheduled for class III _____
Comments

P=patient; F=family; 1=needs instruction on; 2=needs reinforcement on; 3=comprehends instruction/appropriate behavior; NA=not applicable (does not need instruction on)

DIABETES MEDICATION/MANAGEMENT TEACHING WORKSHEET

Knowledge	1 P F	2 P F	3 P F	Comments
Activity	___	___	___	
Urine testing				
Times	___	___	___	
Technique	___	___	___	
Results	___	___	___	
Medication				
Oral Hypoglycemic	___	___	___	
Type	___	___	___	
Dosage	___	___	___	
Schedule	___	___	___	
Storage	___	___	___	
Insulin				
Type	___	___	___	
Dosage	___	___	___	
Schedule	___	___	___	
Storage	___	___	___	
Skin preparation	___	___	___	
Site rotation	___	___	___	
Syringe	___	___	___	
Vial preparation	___	___	___	
Drawing up	___	___	___	
Injection	___	___	___	
Sliding Scale	___	___	___	
Review complications & management of				
Hypoglycemia	___	___	___	
Ketoacidosis (Hyperglycemia)	___	___	___	

Return Demonstration: patient demonstrates skill at least twice
_____, 1. Urine testing
_____

_____ 2. Medication administration
_____

P=patient; F=family; 1=needs instruction on; 2=needs reinforcement on; 3=comprehends instruction/appropriate behavior; NA=not applicable (does not need instruction on)

DIABETES DIET/MANAGEMENT TEACHING WORKSHEET

Knowledge	1 P F	2 P F	3 P F	Comments
Diet	____	____	____	
Exchange lists				
Milk	____	____	____	
Vegetable	____	____	____	
Fruit	____	____	____	
Bread	____	____	____	
Meat	____	____	____	
Lean	____	____	____	
Medium fat	____	____	____	
High fat	____	____	____	
Fat	____	____	____	
Free foods	____	____	____	
Do's & Dont's	____	____	____	
Food				
Labels	____	____	____	
Packaging	____	____	____	
Purchasing	____	____	____	
Measurements				
Weight	____	____	____	
Volume	____	____	____	
Length	____	____	____	
Meal Planning	____	____	____	

Return Demonstration of Knowledge:
_____ 1. Identifies the 7 different exchange groups
_____ 2. Selects inhospital menu correctly
_____ 3. Correctly plans two-day home menu

P=patient; F=family; 1=needs instruction on; 2=needs reinforcement on; 3=comprehends instruction/appropriate behavior; NA=not applicable (does not need instruction on)

Guidelines for Patient Teaching

Guidelines for patient teaching may serve a dual purpose: first, as a guide for the educator to use with the patient (as in Appendix VII); and second, a well-developed guideline can also be used in quality assurance activities.

In the following guidelines, goals are stated for solving patient-care problems. These goals can then be used as criteria for quality assurance. The actions that follow the goals can then be used as definitions of the criteria, or patient's actions that demonstrate that the criteria have been met. The teaching plan becomes a permanent part of the patient's medical record.

DISCHARGE TEACHING PLAN FOR BURN PATIENT

Problem: Lack of knowledge concerning treatment and rehabilitation following thermal or chemical injury. Note: On discharge, the patient and/or responsible person will have achieved the following goals:

I. Goal: Performs routine skin care of healed burn and explains long-term care of healed burn

    Actions: 1. Cleanse involved area daily with Dreft or Ivory Snow

             2. Wash gently with wash cloth to remove dead skin

             3. Apply Nivea twice a day to provide lubrication

               a. Natural lubrication is lost after injury

               b. Purchase Nivea any local drugstore

               c. Cocoa butter is alternative

II. Goal: Demonstrate and explain the purpose of following procedures for burn wound care

    Actions: 1. Procedure

               a. Wash hands

               b. Removal of dressing and proper disposal; paper bag or newspaper

      c. Wash hands
      d. Cleanse open area gently with 4 x 4 pad using solution of Dreft or Ivory Snow
        (1). Basin (approximate size of bathroom sink) use 1 tbsp. Dreft
        (2). Bathtub, use 2 tbsp. Dreft
        (3). To remove dead skin and medicinal ointments
      e. Wash hands
      f. Apply prescribed dressing as directed
      g. Cleanse bathtub or basin with disinfectant such as Lysol or Listerine
      h. Wash hands

III. Goal: Explain purpose, complications, and care of pressure wraps; demonstrate application

    Actions: 1. Purpose
        a. Reduce scarring
        b. Increase circulation of affected area
        c. Decrease swelling of affected area
        d. Acewraps must be worn for extended length of time (6 to 12 months) to be effective
      2. Ace Wraps or Jobst garments
        a. Demonstrate proper application
      3. Complications
        a. Pressure wrap too tight will decrease circulation to area causing discomfort, numbness, and tingling. Rewrap properly
        b. Pressure wrap too loose will be ineffective. Rewrap properly
        c. If Jobst garment fits improperly, notify Burn Clinic
        d. Blistering of affected area under wrap is caused by rubbing
          (1). Do not break blisters: they provide protection and prevent infection
          (2). Apply Kerlex wrap to area under pressure wrap; this reduces friction and blister formation
          (3). Notify Burn Clinic if this is ineffective
          (4). Care of pressure wrap
            (a). Hand wash with Dreft or Ivory Snow in cold water
            (b). Towel dry
            (c). Lay flat or place over rod or clothesline
            (d). Do not use clothespins

IV. Goal: Explain method of caring for clothing that will be in contact with healed or unhealed area

    Actions: 1. Launder new clothing before use by machine or hand with Dreft or Ivory Snow

      2. Some dyes used in clothes will be irritating to skin and may cause itching (especially in socks). If so, wear white articles

      3. If you have open burns, wash all clothes separately from other family members with hot water and Dreft or Ivory Snow

      4. Rinse clothes twice

      5. Do not use fabric softeners or starch as they may be irritating to skin and cause itching

      6. Scarlet red will permanently stain clothing

V.   Goal: Explain following principles concerning medications ordered on discharge; name, dosage, frequency and pertinent side effects

     Actions: 1. Discuss name, dosage, frequency, and side effects for each medication (Specify medications for each individual patient)

VI.   Goal: Explain and demonstrate the exercise program designed by PT/OT

     Actions: 1. Discuss with PT/OT (Specify for patient)

VII. Goal: Explain following principles related to healed burn

     Actions: 1. Increased capillary permeability, which will begin to subside after 6 months

      2. Increased sensitivity to heat and cold

      3. Increased sensitivity to sun exposure
All healed areas must be protected by clothing to protect the skin and prevent sunburn

      4. Strong solutions or cleaning agents, e.g., Spic & Span, Lysol, Tide, will cause irritation, i.e., itching or burning
Wear rubber gloves for protection

VIII. Goal: Identify following symptoms, which should be reported to Burn Clinic

     Actions: 1. Healed area breaking open

      2. Decreased mobility of any joint due to tightness of healed skin

      3. Signs of infection
        a. Fever: general or localized
        b. Redness, pain, swelling or hardness in or around wound, or any other part of body
        c. Increased or foul-smelling drainage from wound

IX.   Goal: Have thorough understanding of and explain purpose of eating balanced diet

     Actions: 1. Instruct on basic 4 food groups

      2. Relationship of healing process or burn wound to dietary intake

      3. Consult dietitian if indicated

X.   Goal: Assist patient in identifying problems he may encounter on discharge and how he may cope with them

     Actions: (Specify for patient)

HANDOUTS GIVEN TO PATIENTS FOR HOME REFERENCE

Discharge Care

We on the Burn Team are happy to see that you are able to go home. To insure the speediest possible recovery, it is important that you are able to care for yourself and recognize problems that may interfere with your complete recovery.

If any of the following occur, please notify the Burn Clinic. Call the hospital and ask for the Burn Clinic. The nurse will be able to assist you.

1. Healed area breaking open. Cover with clean dressing.
2. Formation of blisters.
3. Signs of infection:
   a. Fever, temperature over 99°F.
   b. Redness, pain, swelling, hardness, or warmth in or around wound or any other part of body.
   c. Increased or foul-smelling drainage from wound.
4. Problems with your ace bandages and/or Jobst garment such as improper fit, formation of blisters, and/or opening of healed area underneath.

Please arrive at 11 A.M. for your first clinic appointment because you will need to register. If a family member can come with you, he or she can register for you and you may go to the Burn Clinic waiting room.

Skin Care for Healed Burn

These are your guidelines for your daily skin care of a healed burn. When you do your skin care this is the time to look at the involved areas and note if there are any changes that need to be reported.

1. Wash healed area every day with solution of 2 tbsp. Dreft (or Ivory Snow) and water.
2. Wash gently with washcloth to remove dead skin.
3. Rinse skin well after washing.
4. Dry thoroughly.
5. Apply Nivea lightly twice a day and more frequently if the skin is dry and flakey.
6. Do not put Nivea on open areas.
7. You can purchase Nivea at your local drugstore.

Ace Bandages

You have been taught to put on your own ace bandages while in the hospital but if you do have a problem with this at home, please notify the Burn Clinic. It is also important that you know how to care for them and understand problems that can occur.

1. If they are too loose they will be ineffective and must be rewrapped.
2. If they are too tight, they will cause discomfort, numbness, tingling, and puffiness and must be rewrapped.
3. They must be worn for a long period of time, probably 6 to 12 months to be effective, so please do not stop wearing them until your doctor tells you.
4. To care for your ace bandages:
   a. Hand wash with Dreft or Ivory Snow in cold water.
   b. Towel dry.
   c. Lay flat or place over rod or clothesline.
   d. Do not use clothespins.

Jobst Garment

You have been taught how to put on your Jobst garment while in the hospital but if you have a problem with this please notify the Burn Clinic. It also is important that you know how to care for them and understand problems that can occur.

1. If they are too loose, they will be ineffective, and you will require a new garment.
2. If they are too tight, they will cause discomfort, numbness, and tingling. Do not wear them if this occurs but notify the Burn Clinic as soon as possible.
3. To care for your Jobst garment:
   a. Hand wash with Dreft or Ivory Snow in cold water.
   b. Towel dry.
   c. Lay flat or place over rod or clothesline.
   d. Do not use clothespins.

Care For Burn Wound

These are your guidelines for the care of your burn wound. When you do your care this is the time to look at the involved areas and note if there are any changes that need to be reported.

Procedure for Burn Wound Care

1. Wash hands.
2. Remove dressing and dispose in paper bag or wrap in newspaper.
3. Wash hands.
4. Wash open area with gauze using solution of Dreft (or Ivory Snow) and water. Add 1 tbsp. Dreft to a basin of water of 2 tbsp. Dreft if you use the bathtub. Use a clean towel and wash cloth with each dressing change.
5. Rinse skin well.
6. Wash hands.
7. Apply dressing as described.

8. Wash basin or bathtub with disinfectant such as Lysol or Listerine. Wear gloves.
9. Wash hands.

Care of Clothing

When you are discharged you may find that healed burn areas are sensitive to harsh detergents, fabric softeners and clothing dyes. If you are sensitive, we suggest the following:

1. Launder new clothing before use by machine or hand with Dreft or Ivory Snow.
2. Rinse clothes twice.
3. Do not use fabric softeners.
4. If you have open burns or a healed area that opens, wash all clothes separately from other family members.
5. Scarlet red will permanently stain clothing.
6. If dyes used in clothing cause irritation, wear white articles.

DISCHARGE TEACHING PLAN FOR POSTPARTUM PATIENTS FOLLOWING VAGINAL DELIVERY*

Problem: Inadequate knowledge regarding postpartal period needs.
  I.   Goal: To explain physical body changes that will occur between delivery and her first postpartum visit.
    Actions: 1. Describe physical changes
        a. Uterus remains same size for 2 days then decreases in size so that by 10th day it cannot be felt.
        b. Uterus will return to its normal size in 6−8 weeks.
        c. Excessive passing of urine is normal.
        d. Sweating may be expected.
        e. Constipation may occur.
          (1). Increase liquid intake.
          (2). Include basic four in your diet.
          (3). Use a mild laxative if necessary.
        f. Hemorrhoids may be present. Take sitz baths for comfort.
        g. Vaginal discharge after delivery is termed lochia.
          (1). First few days discharge consists largely of blood (lochia rubra).
          (2). Color becomes pink from day 3 to day 10 (lochia serosa).
          (3). After 10 days discharge is whitish or yellowish (lochia alba).

*This plan becomes a permanent part of the medical record.

        (4). Discharge may continue for 4−6 weeks and menstrual period usually resumes 8 weeks after delivery.

      h. Fatigue is common and 2 or more rest periods must be included into daily routine.

II. Goal: Perform pericare and understand basic principles of feminine hygiene

   Actions: 1. Pericare instructions

      a. Remove peri pad from front to back; fold in paper bag; discard.

      b. After urinating or having a bowel movement:

        (1). Wipe with toilet tissue from front to back.

        (2). Separate legs as much as possible and pour warm water over perineal area.

        (3). Using a clean wipe for each stroke, wipe each side from front to back and once down the middle.

        (4). Apply clean pad from front to back touching only the outside of the pad.

     2. Take shower or tub bath daily.

     3. Douching and use of tampons are not recommended until after postpartum visit.

     4. Resume sexual intercourse when physically and emotionally comfortable.

III. Goal: To explain purpose of proper nutrition.

   Actions: 1. Instruct on basic 4 food groups

     2. Consult dietitian prn

     3. Increase protein and calorie needs for lactating mothers.

IV. Goal: Demonstrate ability to cope with emotional aspects of the postpartum period

   Actions: 1. Allow patient to ventilate feelings regarding infant and any physical or emotional changes she may be experiencing.

     2. Episodes of feeling blue are normal for 3−4 weeks.

     3. Crying spells sometimes occur.

     4. Call the OB Clinic Nurse if this does not improve.

     5. Consult Social Service if needed.

V. Goal: Describe signs and symptoms to be reported immediately to doctor or clinic nurse

   Actions: 1. Increased vaginal bleeding

     2. Foul-smelling discharge

     3. Pain in abdomen, back, or legs

     4. Redness or swelling of legs, stitches, or breast

     5. Sore, cracked, or bleeding nipples

     6. Fever or chills

       a. Instruct patient to take temperature.

       b. Report temperature 38°C or above to clinic nurse.

VI. Goal: Describe importance of keeping postpartum visit as indicated

   Actions: 1. Explain importance of postpartum follow-up.

a. Your physician will examine you to be sure your uterus has returned to its prepregnant size.

b. You may discuss any other concerns you have at this time.

2. Make appointment either with clinic or private doctor.

If Family Planning is desired:

VII.   Goal: Describe chosen methods of birth control and/or family planning.

Actions: 1. Have family planning counselor interview patient.

2. Reinforce information provided.

3. Assist patient to ventilate questions or concerns.

4. Give contraceptive of choice.

5. Give appropriate instruction sheets with contraceptive.

6. Explain that delivery and/or breast feeding does not reduce chances of pregnancy in next 4–6 weeks.

Index

Index

Guilt
  coping with, 291
  in psychosocial adaptation, 75

Handicapped patients
  health education resources, 249—250
  rights of, 45
Hand-trembler, in Navajo medicine, 89, 90
Health, defined, 99
Health care
  evaluation of institutional effectiveness, 153, 154—161, 162—164
  post-hospital provision of, 113, 114—127. *See also* Home care
Health-care team
  coordination of, 71—72, 73—74, 125, 219, 232, 233, 235, 267
  and discharge planning, 117—118, 125
  and family-centered teaching, 96, 97, 103, 265, 266
  liaison with home health agency, 123
  librarian as member of, 249, 250, 252
  patient education as function of, 225, 232, 309—310
  pharmacist as member of, 228, 229, 232
Health education. *See also* Patient education
  cost-effectiveness of, 181, 304—305
  distinguished from patient education, 310
  role of institutions in, 301—302
Health Library, Kaiser-Permanente Medical Center, patient education program, 250—251
Health maintenance organizations (HMOs), medication counseling in, 234
Hearing, in teaching-learning process, 63, 64
Heart disease
  arteriosclerotic, teaching method in, 30
  surgery, patient teaching materials for, 319—331
Hemophilia, and patient education, 305
HMOs. *See* Health maintenance organizations
Holistic approach, to care of critically ill
  and patient education, 256, 257—258, 267, 268—269
  stress in, 263
Home care
  and discharge planning
    nurse, 120, 121
    programs, 122—123
  and family's learning, 57
  health education, 233—234
    mobile library program, 251
    sources of, 249—250, 250—252
    videotape instruction, 190
  and medication counseling, 233—234
  quality of, 4
  selection of patients for, 118—119, 122
Home environment, as barrier to patient teaching, 113
Home health agencies. *See also* Community health agencies

feedback from, 125, 160
  as resource, 122—123
Home visit
  and discharge planning, 104, 122
  in evaluation of patient teaching, 140
Hospital administration
  cost-analysis in, 168—171
  and patient education, 147, 178, 205
Hospitalization
  of children, preparation for, 279—281
  effect of on self-concept, 7, 28, 29—30, 248—249, 262
  informational needs during, 3, 15. *See also* Learning needs, patient's
  and patient's rights, 299—300. *See also* Patient's rights
Hostility, in teaching-learning process, 75, 78
Humanistic view of man, and patient education, 95, 97
Hydrochlorothiazide (Oretic), sample notes for medication counseling, 241
Hypertension, 313
  patient teaching program for, 335—336

ICU. *See* Intensive care unit
Identity. *See* Self-concept
Identity change, in psychosocial adaptation, 77, 78
Illness
  as accidental crisis, 273
  effects of, 243, 248—249
    on family, 101
    on learning, 5, 28, 70, 74, 80, 82, 183, 255, 256—268
    on lifestyle, 2, 5, 7—8, 31, 100, 265
    on self-concept, 7, 28, 29—30, 76, 78, 248—249, 262
  orienting patient in, 292
  psychosocial adaptation in, 75—79, 265
Incompetent patients
  and disclosure, 43
  and informed (substituted) consent, 39—40
Industrial environment, and planning patient education, 17
Infants, and patient teaching, 274, 276
Infection control program, 160—161, 164
  and patient education, 161
Information. *See also* Informed consent; Patient education
  and compliance with prescriptions, 9. *See also* Prescriptions
  computer systems, 196—198
  in cost containment, 167—175
  documentation of, 41, 42, 46—47, 72. *See also* Documentation
  about family, 101—102
  fee for, advantages of, 179
  in guidelines for teaching cardiac surgery patients, 319, 319—329
  and law of disclosure, 42—44